Ju

Child Advocacy for the Clinician

An Approach to Child Abuse and Neglect

Child Advocacy for the Clinician

An Approach to Child Abuse and Neglect

Lawrence S. Wissow, M.D., M.P.H.
Assistant Professor of Pediatrics
The Johns Hopkins University School of Medicine
Director
Child Advocacy Program
The Johns Hopkins Hospital
Baltimore, Maryland

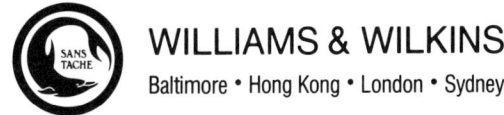

WILLIAMS & WILKINS
Baltimore • Hong Kong • London • Sydney

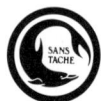

Editor: Laurel Craven
Associate Editor: Victoria M. Vaughn
Copy Editor: Bonnie Ashbaugh
Designer: Wilma Rosenberger
Illustration Planner: Lorraine Wrzosek
Production Coordinator: Barbara J. Felton

Copyright © 1990
Williams & Wilkins
428 East Preston Street
Baltimore, Maryland 21202, U.S.A.

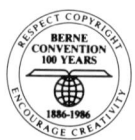

All rights reserved. This book is protected by copyright. No part of this book may be reproduced in any form or by any means, including photocopying, or utilized by any information storage and retrieval system without written permission from the copyright owner.

Accurate indications, adverse reactions, and dosage schedules for drugs are provided in this book, but it is possible that they may change. The reader is urged to review the package information data of the manufacturers of the medications mentioned.

Printed in the United States of America

Library of Congress Cataloging-in-Publication Data
Wissow, Lawrence S.
   Child advocacy for the clinician: an approach to child abuse and neglect / Lawrence S. Wissow.
     p.   cm.
   Includes index.
   ISBN 0-683-09204-9
   1. Child abuse. 2. Legal assistance to children. I. Title.
   [DNLM: 1. Child Abuse. 2. Child Advocacy. 3. Violence. WA 320 W816c]
   RC569.5.C55W57   1989
   616.85′822—dc20
   DNLM/DLC
   for Library of Congress   89-8967
                                                                                        CIP

90 91 92 93 94
1 2 3 4 5 6 7 8 9 10

For Stephen and Leah

Preface

Few cases can be as difficult for clinicians as those involving child maltreatment. Few cases are as likely to divide clinicians from their colleagues. Working with child maltreatment, or any form of family violence, places one apart, in a world of strong emotions and seemingly incompatible allegiances. Too often, the reward is to be regarded somewhat obliquely by one's peers. At best, one represents the seamy side of caring for children and families; at worst, one reminds people of the cruelty and conflict that lurk in and around them.

It is fair to say that as a medical specialty, the study and treatment of child abuse is in its infancy. Although medicine played a pivotal role in bringing abuse to public attention, clinicians still lack the diagnostic and therapeutic tools necessary to deal with the problem. The resultant feeling of uncertainty can add to the sense of isolation; one needs facts to face the withering emotional storm that results when the words "abuse" and "neglect" are mentioned. This book, then, has one major goal: to help frontline clinicians feel comfortable with the medical, social, and legal basis for intervention in cases of maltreatment or family violence. In outlining facts, this volume tries to distinguish clinical wisdom from research-based evidence. It provides data and references that will enable readers to draw their own conclusions and support them.

We have included a number of references to the legal literature, mostly to cases and to some law journal articles. Our hope is that these may be of interest to some clinicians and that they may provide guidance to attorneys who are willing to help with abuse cases but are not familiar with this area of the law. Readers will have to excuse one area of interdisciplinary schizophrenia: most references are given in the familiar "journal year;volume:pages" format, while legal references are in legal style (volume/title/first page, year). Clinicians and attorneys will also have difficulty figuring out the abbreviations for each other's journals or law reporters. Reference librarians can provide help with this task.

It goes without saying that we had to make some difficult decisions about what to include and how to organize the text. We have placed most of our emphasis on the process of diagnosis, and we have emphasized skills common to the evaluation of all types of maltreatment rather than writing separate sections on each type. To compensate for this organization, we have made the Index and Contents as detailed as possible so that readers can easily locate material on a specific subject. We hope these efforts have been successful; we look forward to hearing from readers with suggestions for improvements or corrections.

Contributors

Leon A. Rosenberg, Ph.D.
*Professor of Education
Associate Professor of Pediatrics and
Medical Psychology
The Johns Hopkins University
School of Medicine
Baltimore, Maryland*

Linda C. Anderson, J.D.
*Attorney-at-Law
Washington, D.C.
Former Chairperson
Child Abuse Committee
State Bar of Texas*

Acknowledgments

Portions of this book were orginally prepared for a child abuse training program commissioned by the Armed Services YMCA and the U.S. Navy Family Advocacy Program. Comments and guidance from professionals in both of those organizations, as well as from members of the U.S. Navy Medical Corps, were invaluable at that early stage. We also owe a great debt to our colleagues at the Johns Hopkins Medical Institutions, particularly those in the Division of General Pediatrics, and to the members of the Baltimore area medical, social services, and law enforcement communities who have helped us learn "on the job" and shared their experience with us.

Finally, no book on this subject could fail to include the trite-sounding but truly felt thanks to our families that is standard for texts written in one's "free" time away from other responsibilities. But the thanks is not for putting up with papers on the kitchen table or for watching the children while we wrote. Instead, it is for having taught us that if we cannot find enough time in the day to love and cherish our families, then the rest of what we are doing cannot be very important.

Contents

Preface vii
Contributors ix
Acknowledgments xi

1. Epidemiology and Definitions 1
    Problems in Defining Child Abuse and Neglect 1
    The Prevalence of Maltreatment 3
    Types of Maltreatment 4

2. Effects of Maltreatment on the Child 12
Leon A. Rosenberg and Lawrence S. Wissow
    Physical Injury 12
    The Psychological Impact of Maltreatment 12
    Responses to Maltreatment 14
    Adolescence and the Abused Child 17
    Specific Psychiatric Diagnoses in the Aftermath of Abuse 17
    Responses to Disclosure 19
    Responses to the Investigatory Process 20
    Abused Children as Adults 21

3. Interviewing Children: Psychological Considerations 23
Leon A. Rosenberg
    Investigation versus Assessment 23
    Interviewing the Child 23

4. Interviewing Children: Practical and Developmental Considerations 31
    Introduction 31
    Logistics 31
    An Approach to Interviewing Children about Maltreatment 33

5. Talking to Parents and Families 40
    Assessing the Family 40
    Basic Assumptions about Family Interactions 40
    The Process of Family Assessment 43
    Talking to Parents Suspected of Abuse 46
    Characteristics of People in Crisis 47
    Clinical Descriptions of Families in Abuse and Neglect 47

Contents

6. The Medical History and the Physical Examination ... 49
- The General Approach to Abuse and Neglect Cases ... 49
- Initial Medical History ... 49
- Physical Examination ... 52

7. Head and Internal Injuries ... 67
- Head Injuries ... 67
- Abdominal and Retroperitoneal Injuries ... 75

8. Injuries to the Genitals and Rectum ... 77
- Introduction to the Examination ... 77
- Female Genitalia ... 79
- Male Genitalia ... 85
- Perirectal Lesions ... 87

9. Skeletal Trauma ... 92
- The Skeletal Survey ... 92
- Bone Growth and Injury in Early Childhood ... 93
- Bone Lesions Highly Suggestive of Abuse ... 94
- Bone Lesions Seen in Intentional and Unintentional Injuries ... 96
- Differential Diagnosis ... 97

10. Sexually Transmitted Diseases and Forensic Procedures in Sexual Abuse ... 101
- Vulvitis and Vaginitis in Prepubertal Girls ... 101
- Infections with Specific Organisms ... 102
- Detection and Evaluation of Sexually Transmitted Diseases ... 114
- Forensic Procedures in Cases of Sexual Abuse or Assault ... 115

11. Neglect ... 121
- Parental Factors ... 121
- Medical Observations ... 122
- Making a Diagnosis ... 124
- Criteria for Social Service Involvement ... 125
- The Special Case of Educational Neglect ... 126
- Medical Neglect of Seriously Ill or Potentially Handicapped Newborns ... 128
- Legal Interpretations ... 130

12. Failure to Thrive and Psychosocial Dwarfism ... 133
- Introduction ... 133
- Etiologies of Failure to Thrive ... 133
- Diagnosis and Evaluation ... 140
- Treatment ... 147
- Long-Term Effects of Failure to Thrive ... 152
- Psychosocial Dwarfism ... 155

13. Emotional Abuse 158
    Reluctance to Recognize Emotional Maltreatment 158
    Goals of Emotional Development 158
    Forces Behind Emotional Development 159
    Obstacles to a Working Definition of Emotional Maltreatment . 160
    Diagnosing Emotional Maltreatment 160
    Consequences and Treatment 161
14. Corporal Punishment 163
15. Munchausen Syndrome by Proxy 167
    Characteristics 167
    Detection 169
    Treatment 170
16. Fatal Maltreatment 172
    Epidemiology of Homicide and Fatal Abuse in Childhood 172
    Fatal Abuse in Infancy 173
    Deaths of Older Children 175
    Physical Examination of Critically Injured Victims of Suspected Abuse 176
    Decision Making for Critically Injured Children 177
    The Autopsy 178
    SIDS and the Differential Diagnosis of Sudden, Unexplained Death of Children 179
    Prevention of Fatalities 182
17. Suspected Abuse or Neglect in the Prenatal and Perinatal Periods ..185
    Introduction 185
    Substance Abuse during Pregnancy 186
    Clinical Interventions 187
    Legal Considerations 190
18. Children as Abusers 195
    Child Perpetrators of Physical Abuse 195
    Children as Sex Offenders 196
    Implications for Clinicians 199
19. Reporting Suspected Child Maltreatment 201
    Reporting Requirements 201
    Liability and Reporting 204
    Confidentiality 205

20. Physician Expert Testimony 209
Linda C. Anderson
      Preparation for Court 209
      Courtroom Testimony 211
      The Purpose of Expert Testimony 214
      Sources on Which an Expert Opinion Is Based 215

21. Treatment Decisions 218
      Immediate Considerations 218
      Treatment Resources 221

22. Causes and Prevention of Maltreatment 225
      Causes of Abuse and Neglect 225
      Characteristics of Children at Risk for Abuse 227
      Prevention 229
      Summary 231

Index 233

1 Epidemiology and Definitions

PROBLEMS IN DEFINING CHILD ABUSE AND NEGLECT

On the surface, it would seem a simple task to write definitions for the various forms of child abuse.[1] Many forms of physical and sexual injury are now widely recognized as being abusive, and there is at least a growing willingness to discuss definitions of neglect and emotional maltreatment. The task turns out to be quite difficult, however. Neither professionals nor the public agree widely about what actions or omissions should be considered as abusive. The definitions that do exist are mostly in the form of laws, and those laws are frequently subject to differing interpretations. Not surprisingly, this lack of consensus plays a major role in the reluctance to uncover new cases of abuse and in the frequency of disagreements about what should then be done. An understanding of how people differ in their definitions of abuse can help clinicians anticipate the conflicts that arise when abuse is detected.

In the United States, specific legal definitions of child abuse are established at the state level. Most state definitions are based on federal law, the Child Abuse Prevention and Treatment Act of 1974 (PL 93-247). Section 3 of the act defines abuse and neglect as:

> . . .the physical and mental injury, sexual abuse, negligent treatment or maltreatment of a child under the age of 18 by a person who is responsible for the child's welfare under circumstances which indicate that the child's health and welfare is harmed or threatened thereby. . . .

Not only do actual state definitions differ on a number of points, but local social service agencies and individual practitioners vary in the way they interpret and implement the law. In addition, some state laws do not explicitly define certain kinds of abuse, such as emotional injury or medical neglect (Myers and Peters, 1987). Therefore, clinicians need to know details of the law where they practice and the specific policies or guidelines that are being used by local police or child protective service agencies. In the United States, laws that pertain to child abuse can usually be found as part of the state code, often under sections that pertain to family law, public health, or human resources. Parallel sections on criminal law may also offer definitions of specific types of abuse that are considered to be criminal acts. Individual agencies usually will have an operations or program manual that spells out definitions and procedures for their staff members.

In theory, laws and policies represent societal consensus. The individuals who shape the consensus, however, often continue to have divergent feelings. Although many factors enter into labeling a given act as child abuse, conflicts most often center on four issues: the nature of the act itself, whether the act caused harm, whether there was (or should have been) prior recognition that the act would cause harm, and whether the abuser was the child's caretaker.

The Nature of the Act

Societal judgments about whether a given act should in itself be considered abusive appear to depend on a combination of basic values, impressions regarding who is at fault, and innate feelings about harm to certain parts of the body. To cite some examples:

- There is widespread disagreement about whether corporal punishment is permissible discipline or reportable abuse. Some state abuse laws explicitly exclude it from their definitions, while others implicitly include it. Those who defend corporal punishment generally place a higher value on the autonomy

---

[1] There is little agreement about what global term should refer to all aspects of physical abuse, sexual abuse, emotional abuse, and the various possible forms of neglect. Some clinicians use "abuse" to refer to physical or psychologic acts, while "neglect" is reserved for omissions. "Maltreatment" is sometimes used as a global term for all kinds of harm to children and is sometimes restricted to acts alone. In this book, "abuse" will be used as a global shorthand for both acts and omissions, and specific definitions (e.g., physical abuse) will be used where appropriate.

of parents (and the need of adults to maintain order in their homes or schools) than they do on the risk that children could be harmed. Opponents, on the other hand, see it as an ineffective and unwarranted assault in violation of the rights of children.
- The belief that boys frequently solicit and enjoy sexual contact with adults contributes to underreporting of sexual abuse involving male victims (Finkelhor, 1984). The impression that a child has acted in a seductive or provoking manner is often used to blame the child for the abuse, despite recognition that it is adults, not children, who are supposed to be held accountable for their actions.
- Attempts to hurt certain parts of the body may be seen as abusive, while the same type of assault on another body part may be accepted. In one survey, professionals of different backgrounds generally found hitting a child on the head with a wooden stick to be worse than striking him or her elsewhere with the same object (Giovannoni and Becerra, 1979).

How Much Harm Is Required?

Must a child actually be injured to be considered abused, or are certain acts abusive even if they do not cause visible injury? A careful reading of the excerpt from PL 93-247 cited above reveals that either harm or the threat of harm is sufficient for an act or omission to be considered abusive. Although most states have adopted this language, a lack of consensus on what constitutes harm often means that children must already be injured in some demonstrable way before abuse or neglect will be judged to have taken place.

For example, the first National Study of the Incidence and Severity of Child Abuse and Neglect (National Incidence Study, or NIS) (Burgdorf, 1981) tried to follow professional opinion in defining the cases it would consider as involving maltreatment. Accordingly, acts such as tying up a child, expulsion from the home, or molestation with genital contact were considered abusive even if the child had no obvious sign of physical or mental harm. In contrast, acts that fell into the realm of neglect (failure to provide adequate food, shelter, or supervision) or emotional abuse, even though they could entail equally grave consequences, were considered maltreatment only if "serious" harm had already occurred.[2]

Who is a Caretaker?

Child maltreatment laws address injuries inflicted by caretakers, i.e., those persons, primarily parents, who have responsibility for a child's immediate or long-term welfare. Injuries inflicted on children by other individuals fall outside the jurisdiction of child protective service agencies and are matters for the police or juvenile justice authorities. The caretaker category usually includes any adult who lives or regularly spends time with the child or any person who has responsibility for the child for even brief periods of time (a babysitter or teacher, for example). Ambiguities frequently occur when the alleged abuser is a sibling of the victim or someone close to the victim's age. Overworked agencies may have an interest in using a narrow definition of caretaker as a way of controlling their case loads. Clinicians are often forced to negotiate with social service agencies or with police to have a case properly labeled. Cases of sibling abuse, for example, may have to be reported as parental neglect (failure to supervise the children) or as suspected abuse, but with recognition that the child perpetrator may also have been a victim.

Which Harms Can Reasonably Be Foreseen and Which Are Merely "Unfortunate"?

People frequently disagree when asked to classify a given act as abusive, neglectful, or merely unfortunate. If a parent "loses control" while punishing a child and causes serious harm, is that an intentional injury, is it unintentional but a risk that should have been recognized and avoided, or is it simply an unfortunate accident? If parents have no financial resources and have been evicted from their home, should the children be removed because the parents are not providing food and shelter? The traditional way of approaching these distinctions has been to place the critical emphasis on parental intent and to tolerate risk to the child in the interest of being fair to the parents. In contrast, Daro

---

[2]Serious harm meant "long-lasting impairment of bodily functioning or mental or psychological capacities" or the obvious need to provide immediate professional help to avoid future impairment.

(1988) and other students of treatment for abusing families suggest that it is the nature of the act or condition itself that matters, not the apparent motivation or extenuating circumstances. In other words, they maintain that certain situations in which children find themselves should by definition be grounds for public intervention, regardless of how the situation came to be.

THE PREVALENCE OF MALTREATMENT

As with many major public health problems, it is not easy to document the actual incidence or prevalence of child abuse. It is always difficult to obtain information on sensitive or highly stigmatized topics, and even more difficult when the problem takes place within the cloak of family privacy and the victims are children who cannot independently seek help. The single largest source of information about abuse is the annual compilation of official reports carried out by the American Humane Association (AHA). Reporting of suspected physical and sexual abuse was mandatory throughout the United States by 1967, although neglect was not uniformly reportable until 1979. The AHA attempts to collect reports from all of the states and territories, although only about two-thirds regularly participate. Consequently, even AHA figures are only estimates of the number of cases that annually come to the attention of child protection agencies.

In the last two decades, officially recognized cases of abuse have risen from a few thousand to over 1 million per year, or about two reports for every 100 children in the United States (Russell and Trainor, 1984). The sources of these reports have been relatively consistent over the years: about half come from the general public; schools, health professionals, the police, and social service agencies each contribute 11–12%.

When one attempts to relate the rate of reporting to the true extent of abuse, two questions quickly come to mind: Do all cases actually get reported, and do all reports ultimately turn out to be true? The seemingly paradoxical answer is that even though abuse appears to be hugely underreported, only about 60–70% of reports can be confirmed.

The best data available on the extent of underreporting come from the NIS, conducted first in 1979–80 and then again in 1986 (US Department of Health and Human Services [USDHHS], 1981, 1988). The NIS asked a national sample of professionals in schools, hospitals, police departments, and other social agencies to identify cases of suspected abuse or neglect and to note whether these cases, as required by law, had been reported to a child protective service agency. The NIS used very conservative definitions of abuse and neglect, including only relatively unambiguous cases in which a child had already suffered some demonstrable harm.

The most striking finding of the 1979–80 NIS was that, by their own admission, professionals reported only about 20% of all suspected abuse or neglect cases that they encountered. Schools were the least likely to report, calling in only 13% of their cases; hospitals had the highest response rate, although they reported only 56% of cases.

Race and income did not appear to be major determinants of which cases were reported, although in medical settings blacks and Hispanics were more likely to be reported than whites, and children from the highest-income families were less likely to be reported than those from lower-income groups (Hampton and Newberger, 1985). Age made a major difference. When reports from all types of professionals were combined, about 60% of suspected cases involving preschool children (ages 0–5) were reported, compared with less than a quarter of cases involving adolescents (ages 12–17). Among hospital-based physicians, about 80% of physical and sexual abuse cases (if they were diagnosed) were reported, compared with only 66% of physical neglect cases, 43% of emotional neglect cases, and 36% of emotional abuse cases. Physicians evidently did not consider neglect of education to be among their responsibilities, since they reported only 6% of the cases that they recognized.

If abuse and neglect are generally underreported, it would seem logical that most reports of suspected cases would be confirmed. Again, problems of definition make this difficult to ascertain. First, a great deal of evidence points to the fact that some cases reported by both professionals and the public are never included in official statistics. Most state laws require protective service workers to evaluate all reported cases, but many agencies have formal or informal systems of triage that give priority to more serious cases or those involving young children. Professionals seeking to make reports often find that they must bargain with intake workers or find ways to present the facts of a case so that the agency will be interested. Second, many states do not have explicit criteria for classifying a suspected case as confirmed maltreatment. Even those that do have explicit guidelines may not use their criteria in a uniform manner. Agency terminology may also vary among jurisdictions. In some states, for example, "confirmed" means that there is evidence that abuse actually took place; in other states it may simply mean that the family was found in need of some service that the agency could provide.

Given these problems, the AHA does not provide national estimates of confirmed or substantiated reports. Instead, it asks states to report whether a case was closed (in theory, because abuse or neglect was not found) or whether a family or child was offered services. In 1982, 49% of investigated cases were closed, 41% got services, and the rest either were still being investigated or had some other status at the time the AHA data were collected.

Where it has been possible to look at records more closely, a trend has emerged that evidence of abuse or neglect is being found in an increasingly smaller proportion of reported cases (Jason et al., 1982). Many authorities believe that this trend is is a function more of decreased investigatory resources than of an increased incidence of frivolous reports. The evidence for this conclusion is circumstantial, but it is built on observations that cases reported by professionals are consistently more likely to be offered services than are those reported by the public, just as cases of abandonment, sexual abuse, and serious physical abuse are more likely to result in services being offered compared to reports of minor physical abuse and physical neglect. The implication is that reports that are harder to ignore or involve more immediate crises (as opposed to long-term risks) are more likely to be officially recognized by an agency.

Given all of these considerations, what can be said about the actual incidence of abuse and neglect? The next section discusses evidence for each general type of maltreatment and some overall trends, discernible largely from the NIS and AHA data.

TYPES OF MALTREATMENT

NIS and AHA Data

Data from both the NIS (unreported cases) and the AHA (based on reports) underscore the fact that neglect, in its various forms, is the single most common form of maltreatment. The NIS found that about 50% of children identified by study participants were primarily victims of neglect, while the AHA found that about 65% of investigated cases, regardless of why they were reported, involved some form of material, educational, or supervisory deprivation. Abuse, both physical and sexual, was the primary form of maltreatment in about 37% of cases noted by NIS participants.

AGE

Although infants are most commonly thought of as victims of abuse or neglect, the NIS found that the rate of maltreatment among adolescents (ages 12–17) was twice that of children under 6. Infants were more likely than older children to be physically neglected, but other forms of maltreatment increased with age. Among boys, emotional and educational neglect rose sharply in adolescence, while for girls, physical and sexual abuse appeared to occur at a higher rate than among younger children. AHA figures tabulated from investigated cases confirm these trends (Table 1.1). Of note is that the proportion of cases involving physical abuse continues to rise during childhood, while neglect, although it decreases among older children, remains the single largest problem.

In addition to its relationship to type of abuse, age is also related to severity of injury. Nearly all of the fatal cases found by NIS participants occurred in the youngest and oldest age groups: 74% of the fatalities were among children under 6, and 23% were among those 15–17 years old. Several authors have noted that mechanisms of fatal injury vary with the age of the child (Christoffel et al., 1983; Paulson and Rushforth, 1986). Among cases investigated as homicide, infants and toddlers are more likely to die from either blunt trauma (beating or shaking) or neglect and abandonment (drowning, exposure, or burns), whereas older children are more likely to be killed with a deadly weapon such as a gun or knife (see Chapter 15).

Table 1.1. Cases Investigated by Child Protective Service Agencies, 1982: Percent of Children in a Given Age Group Found to Have Suffered Particular Types of Maltreatment[a]

Type of Violence	% of cases in given age group (yrs)			
	0–2	3–5	6–11	12–17
Physical injury	17	18	18	22
Sexual maltreatment	1	5	6	11
Deprivation of necessities	61	57	55	42
Emotional maltreatment	4	5	6	8

[a]Adapted from Table A-IV-3 of Russell AB, Trainor CM. Trends in child abuse and neglect: a national perspective. Denver: The American Humane Association, 1984. Figures may not add to 100% because miscellaneous categories are omitted and because a given child may have been found to have suffered more than one type of maltreatment.

SEX

Overall, males and females are equally represented among both incident and reported cases of maltreatment, although females are overrepresented among adolescents because of the increased prevalence of sexual abuse in this age group. Sex differences do seem to play a role in various kinds of abuse, however, as discussed below and in Chapter 20.

RACE

Although blacks are overrepresented in reported cases, analyses of reports and data from the NIS consistently find little if any racial differences in the estimated incidence of abuse or neglect. After adjustment for poverty, which appears to be a major causal factor for both neglect and physical abuse, white children generally have higher rates of abuse than do children from other racial groups (USDHHS, 1981).

Physical Abuse

Physical abuse was the first form of child maltreatment to be widely recognized by medical professionals. Caffey, in 1946, was among the first to suggest that the hitherto unexplained syndrome of subdural hematomas and long-bone fractures in infants might be caused by trauma (Caffey, 1946). Silverman (1953) later suggested that trauma was the most common cause of the occult bone abnormalities frequently found in infants, and 9 years later Kempe and co-workers published their landmark description of the battered child syndrome (Kempe et al., 1962). Although physicians originally viewed these reports with reactions ranging from skepticism to outrage, the concept of the battered child soon became not only an accepted medical diagnosis but also prima facie courtroom evidence that a child had been abused (Roberts, 1980).

Although the NIS found physical abuse the most likely to be reported of all types of maltreatment, other studies have found considerable disagreement among professionals as to which acts or injuries should be considered abusive. In a survey of professionals in the Los Angeles area (Giovannoni and Becerra, 1979), for example, physicians generally considered physical abuse to be much more serious than did attorneys. The two groups agreed more closely on the seriousness of burns and scalds, but attorneys were relatively less concerned about incidents of shaking and banging a child against a wall. As mentioned above, the widespread acceptance of corporal punishment makes it difficult for many observers to draw a line between acceptable and unacceptable intentional injuries to children.

Various definitions have been proposed as guides for determining when physical abuse has taken place. Gil (1971), considering the definition to depend on the act and not its consequences, called it the intentional, nonaccidental use of physical force, or an intentional, non-accidental act of omission aimed at hurting, injuring, or destroying a child. The NIS definition, which for research purposes insisted that harm had to have occurred, required either (1) the nonaccidental use of a "weapon, foreign object, or foreign substance," (2) injury resulting from slapping, spanking, punching, or biting, or (3) injury "foreseeably resulting from physical assault without use of an implement, e.g., child injured from fall caused by slap or shove, infant deliberately dropped or thrown" (Burgdorf, 1981). It is important to note that the NIS defined injury as being physical, emotional, or behavioral, even in cases of "pure" physical abuse.

The NIS, with its conservative requirement for harm, estimated that the annual United States incidence rate for physical abuse was 3.4/

1000 children, or about 208,000 cases per year. Other studies have estimated much higher rates. Among the best known is the National Family Violence Survey, originally performed in 1975 and repeated in 1985 (Gelles, 1987). The Family Violence Survey interviewed parents in households that had two adult caretakers and at least one child between the ages of 3 and 17. The families responded to Straus's Conflict Tactics Scale, which asked them to remember times when they disagreed with or were angry with another family member and what they had done about it. They were specifically asked whether they had engaged in one of several specific violent acts and, if so, how often (Table 1.2).

In 1975, 36 of every 1000 families (1146 were included in this part of the study) reported that on one or more occasions adults had engaged in what the researchers called "very severe" violence toward their children: they had kicked, bit, punched, or beat up a child, or they had used or threatened to use a gun or a knife to harm a child. The national estimate for the number of victims of this type of abuse was about 1.7 million children per year. Less severe assaults were much more common. About 10% of the parents said that they had hit their children with an object such as a stick or belt; over half reported they had slapped or spanked their children. Of the violent episodes, 94% were reported to have happened more than once.

The more severe forms of abuse did seem to have decreased in frequency from 1975 to 1985. On the surface, this finding seemed encouraging; the authors cautioned, however, that it might be an artifact of how the study was conducted. By 1985, the proportion of single-parent households in the United States had risen. These households had the lowest incomes and thus, epidemiologically, an increased risk of abuse. Excluding them from the study may have underestimated the true extent of violence toward children.

Physical abuse is definitely not a homogeneous phenomenon. Gil (1971), in one of the first large-scale studies of the problem, identified a number of what seemed to be discrete subtypes, many of which might warrant different treatments. These included:

- Uncontrolled anger as a response to real or perceived misconduct by the child (the single most common).
- General resentment or rejection of the child, sometimes based on the child's atypical or difficult behavior but often, for some other reason, associated more with the parent.
- Quarrels between caretakers, often associated with intoxication, in which the child was injured either as an innocent bystander or as an object against which the adults could vent their anger.
- Children whose parents left them with inappropriate or inexperienced caretakers who became abusive.

Heterogeneity is also seen in abusive families who enter treatment programs. Daro (1988), examining data from a national study of federally funded treatment efforts, found that among families in which physical abuse had been reported, it was the sole form of abuse in only 19% of the cases; 76% also involved emotional abuse, and 39% also involved neglect. In other words, physical abuse was usually just one part of a constellation of family problems that involved other forms of maltreatment. In both Daro's study and the National Family Violence Survey, spouse abuse was frequently found when physical child abuse was present.

Neglect

Neglect is the single most commonly recognized form of child maltreatment. It comprised about 50% of the cases found by the NIS and was found in over 60% of investigated cases

Table 1.2. Proportion of Parents in Two-Caretaker Families Reporting Violence toward Their Children: Results from the National Family Violence Surveys, 1975 and 1985[a]

Type of Violence	No./1000 Families	
	1975 ($n = 1146$)	1985 ($n = 1428$)
"Very severe" (kicked, bit, punched, beat up, threatened with or used deadly weapon)	36	19
Hit with object such as stick or belt	134	97
Slapped or spanked	582	549

[a] Adapted from Table 4 of Gelles RJ. Family violence. 2nd ed. Newbury Park: Sage Publications, 1987.

reported to the AHA. Although cultural values are widely perceived as influencing views on neglect, there is fairly wide agreement across socioeconomic groups about what constitutes basic, necessary care and nurturing of children and what material and emotional resources are required for maintaining a home (Polansky et al., 1981). There is evidence that poor and minority families, far from being less concerned, see neglect of basic child care as more serious than do those who have higher incomes or are white (Giovannoni and Becerra, 1979).

For all its prevalence, neglect appears to be underreported to a greater extent than are other forms of maltreatment. The reasons for this are unclear. If there is, in fact, relatively little variation in value judgments about parental perogatives and excusable limitations of parenting, the explanation may involve perceptions of the risk or severity of harm involved in neglect. There is some evidence suggesting that, relative to other forms of maltreatment, reporting of neglect may be discouraged by protective service agencies. Neglect cases may be given low priority because they seem to represent less urgent threats or because they appear to be more difficult to treat. Only 54% of reported neglect cases ultimately receive services from child protection agencies, compared with 67% of sexual abuse and major injury cases (Russell and Trainor, 1984). There may also be less agreement about what omissions, beyond failure to provide basic food, shelter, and emotional availability, constitute neglect. Society currently finds some forms of neglect acceptable, just as some forms of assault on children (corporal punishment) continue to be found acceptable. In particular, there is only a slow and grudging acceptance of the failure to maintain a safe environment for children (for example, one free of poisons and falling hazards) as a form of neglect (see Chapter 11).

Neglect is usually divided into several categories according to its manifestations. Clinicians and legal authorities may differ as to whether these acts or omissions alone constitute neglect or whether the child must, as a result, have suffered some harm. Many classifications have been offered; the following scheme is adapted from the NIS (Burgdorf, 1981).

Abandonment includes expulsion from the home (temporary or permanent) or the chronic shuttling of a child among caretakers.

Inattention to health care may include delay or failure to seek care for an obvious illness, failure to allow reasonable diagnostic maneuvers, or failure to follow through with reasonable, prescribed treatments. It may also include failure to obtain preventive care when the parents could reasonably be expected to know that preventive care was appropriate or when that care had been recommended at a previous encounter with the health care system.

Inadequate supervision involves leaving children (generally under school age) alone or with only a preteenage child as supervisor. Adult supervision may not be expected at every moment; however, leaving the premises, even if the child is in some presumedly safe place, is potentially neglectful. If the child is in a hazardous place, such as the bathtub, even a very brief absence may be catastrophic. Even older children whose parents are chronically unaware of their whereabouts may be considered inadequately supervised (for example, children who regularly take an inordinate amount of time to return home from school and whose parents have no knowledge of their activities).

Avoidable inattention to hazards includes the failure to protect children from poisons, exposed wiring, and dangerous structural aspects of homes, such as open windows and staircases. It also includes "reckless disregard" of potential hazards, such as driving with a child passenger while intoxicated.

Deprivation of necessities includes failure to provide adequate food, clothing, or shelter or failure to attend to a child's personal hygiene to the point where the child becomes ill (has irreparable dental disease, for example) or infested.

Educational neglect includes failure to enroll a child in school, failure to facilitate attendance or cooperate with needed educational plans (such as conferences designed to obtain special school services for the child), and failure to respond to chronic truancy.

Apparently permitting or condoning maladaptive behavior such as substance abuse, prostitution, or deliquency may be considered neglectful. Parents may not necessarily be able to control these behaviors, but they must make reasonable efforts to try to control them or to seek help.

Emotional neglect may be difficult to separate from emotional abuse. (There may be no real utility to making the distinction.) The NIS defines emotional neglect as either outright rejection or "conspicuous" absence of support or care about a child's emotional well-being.

Neglect is apparently more likely than other forms of maltreatment to occur alone, at least in cases that receive treatment. In the study by Daro (1988), of all families in which neglect was found, it was the only problem in 39%. In another 56% it was found in conjunction with emotional abuse, which in some cases may in fact be a form of neglect. When neglect did occur with another form of maltreatment, that other form was usually (in 19% of cases) physical abuse. Again, these figures are based on cases that received treatment; hence, these combinations may reflect professional perceptions of who needs treatment rather than the actual occurrence of maltreatment in the general population.

Sexual Abuse

As with other forms of maltreatment, it is widely believed that the true extent of sexual abuse is grossly underreported. Estimates of its prevalence depend very much on to whom and how questions are asked. In 1982, sex abuse was involved in about 7% of all reported cases of maltreatment compiled by the AHA. It also made up about 7% of the incident cases found in the 1979 NIS, involving an estimated 7/10,000 children per year in the United States.

Sexual abuse may be more likely than other forms of abuse to remain hidden (Daro, 1988). Visible scars are rare, victims often assume responsiblity for what has happened to them, and adults often act with disbelief when children make disclosures. It is therefore not surprising that prevalence estimates gathered from population surveys vary in relationship to how interviewers approach the question (Peters et al., 1986). In response to general questions such as "Were you ever sexually abused?," 5–20% of women report some sort of unwanted sexual experience during childhood. Surveys using more detailed probes have gotten positive answers from as many as 50–60% of women. Fewer studies have asked these questions of men, but from 3 to over 30% have reported an experience during childhood.

Definitions

Researchers, clinicians, and social service agencies have yet to arrive at a single, satisfactory definition of sexual abuse. There is perhaps most agreement on which *acts* are abusive. Most legal and clinical definitions include both contact and noncontact acts. Contact acts include those that are intrusive (any degree of penile penetration or contact by the abuser, or taking the victim's penis into one of the abuser's body orifices) and those that involve fondling of the breasts, genitalia, or rectum. Noncontact acts include exhibitionism, involvement in child pornography, attempts to involve a child in sexual activity, and deliberate exposure of children to sexually explicit materials or adult sexual activity.

While clinicians frequently find it sufficient to lump all of these acts under the single rubric of sexual abuse, law enforcement officials may be required to make fine distinctions among them. A child may not be able to tell the difference between vulvar coitus and actual penetration of the vagina, but in many jurisdictions the law views the latter act as a much more serious crime. Unfortunately, law enforcement personnel, who often are the first to investigate incidents of alleged sexual abuse, may interpret the law as downplaying the importance of acts that do not involve penetration. It is often the physician's job to educate prosecutors and police officers that "lesser" forms of sexual abuse can have just as devastating consequences.

Most clinical and legal definitions assume that a caretaker has sexually abused a child regardless of whether he or she was the actual perpetrator or simply allowed abuse to occur. Parents who encourage or fail to prevent their children from engaging in prostitution, for example, would be defined as abusers themselves. Less clear is the role of the parents when young children engage in potentially voluntary sexual activity. The NIS considered parents abusive if they allowed, or failed to try to prevent, a child under the age of 15 from engaging in sexual activity with a partner who was 2 or more years older.

Clinicians and law enforcement authorities also may not agree on the upper age limit for child sexual abuse or assault. As Peters and co-workers (1986) point out, even though laws may define a child as anyone under 18, society has taken an ambivalent approach to adolescent sexuality. The belief that teenagers frequently solicit sex with older individuals, or are at least capable of giving consent, contributes to a de facto lowering of the age limit, often to as low as 15.

This haziness concerning age makes it important for clinical definitions to include consideration of whether the sexual contact was coerced. Sexual contact with children younger than midteen or involving close family members is considered abusive regardless of whether the perpetrator found the victim willing. With older teenage victims, it may sometimes be reasonable to consider whether consent was obtained. This is obviously a difficult issue, however, since initially consenting individuals may subsequently be forced to partake in other acts against their wills.

Similar disagreements occur over whether sexual contact between children of similar ages constitutes abuse (see Chapter 18). A first step is to separate age-appropriate genital exploration from acts that are harmful or that mimic adult sexual activity. Perpetrators who are close in age to their victims (researchers usually define this as 5 years or less difference for victims under 13) are often found to be victims themselves. On the other hand, unwanted sexual contact can be traumatic regardless of the age of the perpetrator (Peters et al., 1986) and thus warrant intervention.

Sex of the Victim

Although the majority of sexual abuse victims are female, a sizable minority are male. Abuse of boys appears to be even more underreported than abuse of girls. Population surveys find about 30% of victims to be male, whereas males were involved in only 17% of sexual abuse cases found in the 1979 NIS.

Abuse of boys appears to differ from that of girls. The overwhelming majority of abusers are male for both groups, but boys are more likely than girls to be abused outside the home (Finkelhor and Baron, 1984). Abuse of boys is also more likely to involve multiple victims, physical abuse, low socioeconomic status, and young perpetrators.

Age

While reports of sexual abuse increase during the teenage years, community surveys find that there are two peak periods of onset: ages 6–7 and 10–12 (Finkelhor and Baron, 1986). This discrepancy between surveys and reports is explained by victim accounts: the average time from onset to disclosure is 3–4 years.

Socio-economic Status

Sexual abuse appears to be a much more middle-class phenomenon than are other forms of maltreatment. In 1982, for example, 43% of all abuse and neglect cases cumulated by the AHA involved families receiving public assistance. For sexual abuse reports, only 29% received assistance. As mentioned above, there is some suggestion that abuse of males may be more common in lower socioeconomic groups, but this could also be an artifact of reporting.

Race

Both compilations of reported cases and research studies have consistently found no differences in the prevalence of sexual abuse between blacks and whites. Some studies have suggested that the prevalence may be somewhat higher among Hispanic families.

The Special Case of Child Prostitution

Child prostitution is often considered separate from child abuse because it involves individuals who do not have a caretaker relationship with the child. As discussed above, however, parents may be considered abusers if they do not take steps to prevent their children from engaging in this sort of activity. There is evidence that parents play a role in many instances of child prostitution (Weisberg, 1985). The common conception of child prostitutes is of runaways[3] who turn to sex and drugs as a means of earning money. Male child prostitutes especially, however, are likely to have begun their activities while still living at home, when their parents could conceivably have been aware of unusual conduct or absences. Even when prostitution does not start while the child is at home, the majority of runaways who turn to sex for a living report being expelled from home, aban-

---

[3] Runaway children themselves, whether or not they turn to prostitution, constitute an enormous social problem. In the United States, an estimated 1 million children, mostly teenagers, run away from home every year. Many have been victims of abuse, and many have spent much of their lives in foster homes.

doned by their parents, or leaving to escape physical or sexual abuse.

Emotional Maltreatment

Emotional maltreatment has been the most difficult form of child abuse to define. Many states do not explicitly include it in their reporting or criminal statutes, and others refer to it only as damage to or impairment of a child's emotional condition. California law (Penal Code, Sect. 11165–11174.5), for example, specifically refers to "willful cruelty" that includes "unjustifiable" mental suffering.

Helfer (1987) argues that the term "emotional abuse" is a misnomer and that children who are victims of any kind of maltreatment suffer emotional harm. He prefers to make "verbal abuse" a specific category and to classify other forms of emotional injury according to the type of abuse or neglect that they accompany. One possible classification includes verbal abuse and two forms that may fall best under the rubric of neglect. "Verbal assault" includes belittling, scapegoating, inconsistent discipline, humiliation, and consistent unrealistic expectations that lead to loss of a child's sense of competence and self-worth. "Psychologic unavailabilty of the parent" involves failure to provide emotional nurturing either passively, because of preoccupation with the parent's own problems, or actively, through constant threats to sever the parent-child relationship. "Chronic role reversal" involves forcing the child to take on the emotional parenting role and is often linked closely with scapegoating when the child, expectedly, cannot satisfy the parent's own needs for nurturing.

The 1979–80 NIS added patterns of excessive nonphysical discipline and the verbal threat of other forms of abuse to the category of verbal assault. It also included close confinement, such as tying up a child or locking a child in a room, closet, or other chamber, especially if this was done repeatedly, for prolonged periods of time or under frightening conditions such as darkness.

Together, emotional abuse and neglect accounted for about 30% of the incident cases known to the NIS. Of the cases that were known to medical professionals in hospital settings, only about 40% were reported to protective service agencies (Hampton and Newberger, 1985). In general, emotional maltreatment seems more likely to be reported by professionals who have long-term contact with families than by those who encounter children in acute care situations. Physicians frequently see behavior that might be considered emotionally abusive, but they may not be able to say whether the incident observed is part of a more pervasive pattern of family functioning.

Interestingly, although emotional maltreatment is less consistently reported than physical abuse, there is more public consensus that it is harmful. In a poll conducted for the National Committee for the Prevention of Child Abuse, nearly 75% of those asked thought that repeated verbal abuse of a child was likely to lead to emotional problems, while only about 40% had that worry with respect to corporal punishment (Daro, 1988).

Although emotional maltreatment occurs at all ages, it is more common among adolescents than among younger children. This trend is found in both incident cases (from the NIS) and official reports (tallied by the AHA).

In the National Clinical Evaluation Study (Daro, 1988), more than 50% of all abuse and neglect cases were felt to involve emotional maltreatment, compared with about 17% of reported cases compiled by the AHA. Only about 5% of cases receiving therapy involved emotional maltreatment alone. One possible interpretation of this difference is that although emotional maltreatment contributes to the seriousness of other forms of abuse, agencies tend to give cases involving emotional maltreatment alone a lower priority.

References

Burgdorf K. Operational definition of child maltreatment. Technical report 2. DHHS publ. (OHDS) 81-30326). Washington, DC: US Government Printing Office, 1981.

Caffey J. Multiple fractures in the long bones of infants suffering from chronic subdural hematoma. AJR 1946;56:163–73.

Christoffel DD, Anzinger NK, Amari M. Homicide in childhood: distinguishable patterns of risk related to developmental levels of victims. Am J Forensic Med Pathol 1983;4:129–137.

Daro D. Confronting child abuse: research for effective program design. New York: The Free Press, 1988.

Finkelhor D. Child sexual abuse. New York: The Free Press, 1984.

Finkelhor D, Baron L. High-risk children. In: Finkelhor

D, ed. A sourcebook on child sexual abuse. Beverly Hills: Sage Publications, 1986:60–88.

Gelles RJ. Family violence. 2nd ed. Newbury Park: Sage Publications, 1987.

Gil D. Violence against children. J Marriage Fam 1971;33:637–657.

Giovannoni JM, Becerra RM. Defining child abuse. New York: The Free Press, 1979.

Hampton RL, Newberger EH. Child abuse incidence and reporting by hospitals: significance of severity, class, and race. Am J Public Health 1985;75:56–60.

Helfer RE. The developmental basis of child abuse and neglect: an epidemiological approach. In: Helfer RE, Kempe RS, eds. The battered child. 4th ed. Chicago: University of Chicago Press, 1987:60–80.

Jason J, Andereck ND, Marks J, Tyler CW Jr. Child abuse in Georgia: a method to evaluate risk factors and reporting bias. Am J Public Health 1982;72:1353–1358.

Kempe CH, Silverman FN, Steele BF, Droegmueller W, Silver HK. The battered child syndrome. J Am Med Assoc 1962;181:17–24.

Myers JEB, Peters WD. Child abuse reporting legislation in the 1980s. Denver: The American Humane Association, 1987.

Paulson JA, Rushforth NB. Violent death in a metropolitan county: changing patterns of homicide 1958 to 1982. Pediatrics 1986;78:1013–1020.

Peters SD, Wyatt GE, Finkelhor D. Prevalence. In: Finkelhor D, ed. A sourcebook on child sexual abuse. Beverly Hills: Sage Publications, 1986:15–59.

Polansky NA, Chalmers MA, Buttenwieser E, Williams DP. Damaged parents: an anatomy of child neglect. Chicago: University of Chicago Press, 1981.

Roberts M. Annotation: admissibility of expert medical testimony on battered child syndrome. 98 ALR 3d 306, 1980.

Russell AB, Trainor CM. Trends in child abuse and neglect: a national perspective. Denver: The American Humane Association, 1984.

Silverman FN. The roentgen manifestations of unrecognized skeletal trauma in infants. AJR 1953;69:413–426.

US Department of Health and Human Services, Office of Human Development Services. Executive summary: national study of the incidence and severity of child abuse and neglect. DHHS publ. (OHDS) 81-30329. Washington, DC: US Government Printing Office, 1981.

US Department of Health and Human Services, Office of Human Development Services. Study findings: study of national incidence and prevalence of child abuse and neglect: 1988. Washington, DC: US Government Printing Office, 1988.

Weisberg DK. Children at risk: a study of adolescent prostitution. Lexington, Massachusetts: DC Heath & Co, 1985.

2 Effects of Maltreatment on the Child
—Leon A. Rosenberg and Lawrence S. Wissow

Attempts to delineate the impact that maltreatment may have on a child inevitably run into two theoretical and methodological questions: would all kinds of maltreatment be expected to have the same effect, and would maltreatment at different times in a child's life be expected to have a greater or lesser effect. Only a few of the many studies that examine the effects of maltreatment have taken these questions into account. Although this means that much still remains to be learned about the effects of maltreatment, a good deal of research supports the clinical impression that abuse and neglect may have serious, long-term consequences for many, although not necessarily all, of their victims.

PHYSICAL INJURY

Physical injury is the most obvious result of maltreatment and often the reason that abuse comes to public attention. Injuries occur both from inflicted trauma and from neglect. The extent of inflicted injury can only be estimated, but it appears to be high. Homicide is one of the five leading causes of death in the United States for persons between ages 1 and 17 (Anonymous, 1982). Not all of these deaths result from child abuse—most of those among children over 3 years old are caused by acquaintances or others outside the family. Homicide rates among children ages 1–4, however, are rising faster than are rates among older children, and rates of infant homicide (about 4.8/100,000 children) continue to be nearly as high as the much more publicized homicide rate among teens (see Chapter 16).

It is harder to estimate the extent of nonfatal injuries that are attributable to maltreatment. In the 1970s, when fewer children were reported as being victims of abuse, about 30 children were felt to suffer significant inflicted injury for every child that was killed. About 10% of children who were injured but survived were felt to have permanent brain injury (Kempe, 1976).

Child neglect may also result in injuries and death. Children may be left in the hands of inexperienced or inappropriate caretakers or in unsafe environments that put them at risk of ingestions, falls, burns, drownings, or shootings. These sorts of events, which are frequently labeled "accidents," are the leading cause of death among persons less than 15. Each year in the United States they result in about 12,000 deaths and 6 million injuries (Baker et al., 1984). The proportion directly attributable to parental negligence is not known.

THE PSYCHOLOGICAL IMPACT OF THE MALTREATMENT

By far the greatest impact of maltreatment is on social, emotional, and cognitive development. In some cases, abuse probably has a direct impact: a child's brain is damaged by a blow, he or she runs away to escape an abusive situation at home, or the child fails to get an education because the parents will not help with homework or attend conferences with a teacher. In most cases, however, maltreatment probably works indirectly. It can change the way children feel about themselves and the way they see the world. That altered perception then leads children to fail socially, emotionally, and educationally.

The impact of maltreatment is influenced by several factors that act alone and in combination: the child's level of psychological development (closely correlated with chronologic age), the duration of maltreatment, the psychological meaningfulness of the perpetrator to the child, and the specific nature of the abuse.

Duration plays a major role in determining whether the child will be responding to a fairly isolated psychological trauma or to a continuous experience. Although the former may be traumatic, the latter much more powerfully teaches the child expectations about relationships with those on whom he or she depends. The longer the duration of abuse, the more likely that successive stages in development will be disrupted and the greater the observed negative impact on psychological functioning.

The psychological meaningfulness of the perpetrator to the child is not something that is easily defined by such terms as "mother" or "babysitter." The issue is not the adult's title but the role that he or she plays in meeting the child's basic dependency needs. The more important the adult is to the total care of the child, the greater will be the impact of maltreatment by that adult.

The nature of maltreatment also influences impact. The extent of neglect, or the degree of pain and fear involved in physical or sexual abuse, alters the extent of depression or anxiety generated in the child. As discussed below, the various forms of maltreatment have many influences in common, most likely because individual forms of maltreatment usually do not occur in isolation. There also appear to be some unique effects.

The interaction of these factors is best perceived within a developmental framework. Several major theories of child development have been proposed; much of the discussion that follows is drawn from the work of Piaget and Erikson. More extensive discussions have been written, both from particular theoretical positions (Goldstein et al., 1979) and on the basis of empirical work (Wolfe, 1987).

Infancy

The predominant force in the life of the newborn is the infant's total state of dependence, and the primary psychosocial task of the period is to establish trust in those on whom the infant is dependent. An important corollary of this trust, it is thought, is that the infant comes in some way to realize that he or she is worthy of being cared for. Serious challenge to these basic dependency needs can produce catastrophic results: extreme withdrawal or apathy that may be associated with growth delay (see Chapter 12) or extreme irritability that disrupts normal patterns of sleep and rest. Infants may also become hypervigilant, a condition that on the surface mimics generalized irritability but is in fact a more selective response to potential danger. Such infants have periods of normal responsiveness but show a much lower threshold for a generalized startle response when in the presence of a particular person. Of course, it is hard to trust third-party reports of the phenomenon because they can be self-serving; for example, the grandmother may report that the infant is comfortable with her but cannot relax in the presence of the child's mother, who happens to be the observer's daughter-in-law. Even in early infancy, however, a selective reactivity can be observed that suggests an exaggerated vigilance directed toward certain cues and not others. Those cues are usually people. The child's selective negative response appears to be most often associated with a deviant or threatening relationship between the infant and an individual of psychological importance.

One of the major reflections of infant development is the phenomenon of attachment. The importance of this phenomenon to the impact of maltreatment lies in the fact that patterns of attachment (or the underlying psychodynamics that they reflect) appear to influence the ways that older children handle stressful events and relate to helpful or powerful figures in their lives (Minde, 1986). These types of abilities are critical to normal psychosocial development.

Attachment is manifested by the infant's need for the presence of a particular person and by an increase in anxiety when that person is absent. Perhaps most important is the child's ability to use the person as a secure "home base" from which to explore. Distinct patterns of attachment—secure and "anxious" or "avoidant"—are felt to evolve from fairly specific types of parenting. Secure attachment results from responsive and consistent care, whereas anxious attachment comes from either active rejection or inconsistent and ambivalent responses to the child's needs (Egeland and Farber, 1984).

Toddlerhood

Toddlerhood is a time when children's cognitive and physical abilities start to grow enormously. As toddlers learn to navigate the world around them, they begin to test their independence. This is part of the process of individuation, the psychological separation of the child from the parent. Children at this age, however, do not necessarily have a great deal of understanding about their own actions or why things happen around them. One of the ways that they learn about themselves is from how they are treated by important caretakers. This gives a great deal of emotional power and meaning to the actions of the caretaker toward the children. For example, toddlers or even older children cannot classify a parent's hostility toward them as being the parent's personal problem. Instead, they introject parental attitudes, meaning that they take them on as their own. The child who perceives hostility toward self from the parent introjects a derogatory attitude toward self and becomes hostile toward self. Individuals must reach a much later level of development (well into adulthood for many) before they can differentiate between myself-as-I-know-myself and a parent's negative view, with the concomitant ability to declare that the parent's view is wrong because I know myself better. Positive or negative feelings toward self can influence the child's mastery of important skills, determining whether he or she will approach new developmental tasks confidently or withdraw expressing an expectation of failure.

Toddler behavior can be extremely taxing for parents, especially those whose own views of self and ability to draw interpersonal boundaries are impaired. One of the major developmental issues of toddlerhood is "compliance" (Erickson and Egeland, 1987). Toddlers have to learn how to strike a compromise between their new skills and parental rules. At the same time, parents must learn how to give their children room to grow while maintaining safety and order. This struggle is made even harder because toddlers frequently express their wishes by being negative—a strong affirmation of their own desires and importance—and their main response to new situations may be ambivalence—a manifestation of their desire to do more, coexisting with their fear of separation from the parents.

Preschool

Preschool children begin to develop more sophisticated language and play. The main developmental tasks of this period are to amplify the self-reliance and initiative that began to appear in toddlerhood and to develop relationships with other children. Like toddlers, however, preschoolers have a very self-centered view of why things happen. When things go wrong, toddlers tend to blame themselves. They see their parents, not justice or fairness, as the arbiters of what is right and wrong. Thus, when parents say that the child is "bad," there is a risk that the child will incorporate this label into his or her view of self.

Elementary Age

Elementary age children have as their main tasks to develop a sense of competence with both cognitive and social skills. Children of this age are having their first extended contacts outside the family and learning how to play and work in groups. The success of these early peer relationships appears to have great meaning for later, adult relationships (Shirk, 1988). Elementary-age children come to have a better understanding about what causes events. They are less likely to blame themselves but more likely to blame others and to have little insight into their own actions.

RESPONSES TO MALTREATMENT

Threats to the child's basic sense of security engender an emotional response that can range from anxiety-based behavioral inhibition to angry acting out. To a large extent, these responses are attempts by children to adapt to the environment created by their caretakers. A child's withdrawal and social isolation may be cultivated by parents who prefer a quiet, unobtrusive child. In contrast, other parents may be stimulated to great anger by a child who is relatively unresponsive or who does not demonstrate need or appreciation to a sufficient extent. Children of this latter type of parent may respond by becoming aggressive.

Apparent Delays in Development

The child whose adjustment pattern emphasizes withdrawal may demonstrate delays in language development and in acquisition of self-care skills, problems that then lead to late development of social skills. The child functions as if total development is below age expectancy and gives the impression of cognitive impairment. Such children function in the IQ range of 65–80, an indication that special educational services may be required. On first examination, they may seem identical to children who have organic bases for developmental delay, but many will demonstrate gains in ability once their emotional environment improves.

Depression

An overall picture of limited cognitive development may mask a depressive component of the adjustment-through-withdrawal response to abuse. Classic symptoms of depression are not often seen or easily identified in very young children. The usual symptoms found among older children and adults can be masked in a variety of ways (Pfeffer, 1986; Harris, 1987). Manifestations include severe apathy in infants and a lack of responsiveness or appearance of chronic sadness in toddlers and early-school-age children. In somewhat older children, one may observe sleep disturbance, periods of agitation, excessive over- or undereating, and strong feelings of negative self-worth. Attention-seeking behavior, although outwardly aggressive, is often a response to the negative self-concept and strong expectation of rejection that is integral to childhood depression.

Aggressive Behavior

Aggressive or acting-out behavior is the most visible response to maltreatment. It is not simply a matter of behavior modeling, although children obviously are influenced by the negative behaviors of their adult models. Of greater importance are two other factors: (1) the rage stimulated by the frustration of basic dependency needs and (2) the child's need to obtain mastery over anxiety. Rage is often expressed as hostile and aggressive behavior. Aggression may be become self-directed, resulting in self-disparaging attitudes and self-destructive behavior. It may also be aimed at objects in the environment such as household pets or inanimate objects. When aggression is aimed at other people, it is more likely to be directed toward safer targets, such as teachers and smaller children rather than toward the abusive caretaker. Not only might this latter course present an increased risk that the child will be physically harmed in return, but in the child's eyes it also risks loss of the child's only source of emotional support, no matter how deficient that source might seem to outside observers.

Anxiety

The maltreated child is never simply angry but is always dealing with a significant degree of anxiety. The child can achieve some reduction of immediate anxiety by experiencing a sense of control over his or her environment. When the victim of sadistic behavior acts in a sadistic manner toward a younger victim, the child is not becoming an abuser as a result of having been abused. Rather, the child is most likely reenacting experiences that were terrifying for him so as to achieve a sense of control. The abject panic that a child experiences when being unexplainably hurt by a parent is mitigated, to some degree, when that child inflicts the same torture. It is not at all uncommon to see 3- and 4-year-old victims of serious maltreatment act as the aggressors in sadistic play with dolls to a degree that adult observers find quite disturbing. A child at this age may also direct such activity against an infant sibling. Anxiety will also be expressed at this age as sleep and eating disturbances, deterioration in peer relationships, and regressive behavior.

Management of these issues is complex and demanding because we are not simply dealing with the modeling of deviant behavior but with the child's emotions as well. The child needs better models of adult behavior, but proper clinical care also requires appropriate attention to the youngster's anxiety by addressing basic issues of security and self-worth.

Special Responses to Sexual Abuse

Sexual abuse produces symptoms of anxiety in the same manner as other forms of maltreatment, but some symptoms may be more directly related to the sexual experience (Browne and Finkelhor, 1986). Play acting of sexual activities with dolls, being sexually provocative with other children and adults, and very frequent masturbation are frequently noted among young sexual abuse victims. In the Minnesota longitudinal study described below, young girls who had been sexually abused were more likely to become quiet and dependent than were victims of physical or emotional abuse, who were often overly hostile or aggressive (Erickson and Egeland, 1987). Male victims seem especially prone to reenacting their victimization, often with younger children (Rogers and Terry, 1984). Children who have been physically hurt sexually may become bowel retentive and express extreme fears of going to the bathroom. Such children may become fearful of being touched or examined by a doctor or develop unusual fears of activities that happened in association with abuse.

Finkelhor and Browne (1985) have summarized the repercussions of sexual abuse into four "traumagenic dynamics." Although, as they note, there are fewer studies to support the model than one would like, it offers a framework for seeing how the impact of sexual abuse is both similar to and different from the effects of other forms of maltreatment.

One of the four dynamics is traumatic sexualization, a term that refers to the child's premature and deviant introduction to his or her own sexual feelings and the role of sexuality in human relations. Sexually abused children may develop unusual fears or beliefs about their genitals or about their sexual identity. They may come to see sex as a primary or only means of meeting basic security needs and carry this orientation into later life. The risk of sexual and social dysfunction in later years is also related to two other dynamics, powerlessness and stigmatization. Both operate in other forms of maltreatment but may have special meaning in a sexual context. Violation of the child's body, especially in the emotionally sensitive genital or anal areas, may engender even greater feelings of vulnerability than sporadic physical abuse or inability to predict the whims of an unstable parent. Stigmatization is also often more extreme in sexual abuse. In some cases, the abuser himself will induce shame by telling the victim that he or she has somehow been the provocateur. The prolonged secrecy required of victims and the fact that normal social contacts are often limited may lead to a sense of being different and bad. After disclosure, revulsion expressed by friends or family members may further reenforce feelings of shame and guilt. Betrayal, the fourth dynamic, may act during the time that abuse is taking place but, unfortunately, often continues after disclosure. The fact that trusted individuals have used or misled the child or have refused to believe a disclosure seriously undermines the child's future abilities to trust and form close relationships.

Empirical Data

Studies of abused children have generally confirmed the clinical observation that maltreatment leads to alterations in normal psychosocial development. One of the richest sources of information about the effects of maltreatment has been the Minnesota Mother-Child Project, an effort that has followed about 250 "high-risk" mothers and their children from before birth through early school age (Erickson and Egeland, 1987; Egeland et al., 1983). About 60 of these mothers were felt to have abused or neglected their children in some way during the first years of life, offering a chance to compare those families with families whose children were not mistreated. The most striking early finding was a difference in attachment patterns. By 18 months, children who had been abused or neglected were much more likely to be anxiously than securely attached. These attachment behaviors seemed linked to serious social problems. When these children were 4–5 years old, they were observed while playing with other children (Troy and Sroufe, 1987). Children who had been anxiously attached in infancy, when paired with each other, almost always fell into victim-bully roles, becoming physically aggressive with each other, displaying verbal hostility, and sometimes appearing to seek out punishment from another child. Increased anger among the children who had been abused was also seen in school and social settings. Other researchers have also found that children with a history of both abuse and neglect are more likely to threaten or hit others and are more likely to respond negatively to authority figures (Reidy, 1977). This increase in aggression seems to be an ominous sign for future social development: children who are aggressive tend to be less well liked and are more likely to get into trouble with adults. Aggression has a tendency to become a general way of interacting with others, and it is a style that tends to maintain itself as an individual gets older.

Aggressive tendencies may not be the only reason why some abused or neglected children do poorly in social situations. In psychological testing, children who have been abused display less ability to detect changes in other people's feelings and less ability to respond to social cues (Barahal et al., 1981). In the Minnesota study, kindergarten teachers consistently found abused children to be unpopular with their peers and to have difficulty understanding their roles in the classroom.

Another possible reason for poor social performance is the abused child's distorted sense of "locus of control," or the feeling that what one does can influence what happens, as opposed to a feeling of powerlessness and the perception that the actions of others control one's life. Individuals who have a healthy, internal sense of locus of control can take some credit for things that go well and shoulder some of the blame when things go poorly. Those with a poor, external sense of control are unable to derive self-esteem from success, and they are likely to become angry and blame others for failures. In psychological testing (Barahal et al., 1981), abused children tended to take little credit for good things and to strongly blame others for bad ones. This tendency, the researchers postulated, may be of critical importance, since having an adequate sense of locus of control was considered necessary to the development of empathy for other people and for the ability to see matters from other people's perspective. It is important to be able to take pleasure in one's own achievements and to appreciate that others might want to as well, and it is hard to consider another person's point of view if one blames them for everything bad that has happened. Empathy appears to be a critical factor in controlling social behavior. One of the consistent findings in studies of violent adolescent sex offenders, for example, is a lack of empathy and understanding of the victims (see Chapter 18).

Lack of social skills and self-esteem also plays a role in the poor intellectual achievements of many abused children. In the Minnesota study, abused children were inattentive and impatient in kindergarten classes. They had difficulty understanding what was expected of them in class, and more than half of those who had been neglected or physically abused were referred for special education. Many of these children, however, had shown intellectual problems much earlier in life. Children whose parents were emotionally abusive or neglectful started out normally on developmental testing during the first year of life, but by 24 months their scores had declined significantly. As toddlers they had great difficulty approaching new tasks. When faced with a challenge, they became anxious and were easily frustrated. Some came to show little interest in new situations, whereas others became overly distractable. Importantly, when their mothers tried to help them, the children became more negative and noncompliant rather than being comforted. Other long-term studies of children who were neglected or abused in childhood have also shown a pattern of decreased intellectual performance (see Chapter 12).

ADOLESCENCE AND THE ABUSED CHILD

Preteens and teenagers have progressed through many life experiences and may have responded to maltreatment in a variety of ways. Because adolescents carry with them these results of earlier emotional learning, patterns of behavior seen in adolescence often are related to behaviors observed during earlier stages of development. However, as children grow older, they have more opportunities to interact with people outside the family. Some of these interactions may counteract earlier experiences, while others may reinforce them.

Adolescents are dealing with the stress of moving toward complete independence as well as adjusting to the reality of sexual identification and interaction. The child whose response to stress includes aggressive acting out becomes a more serious problem because such behavior can now reach a significant level of danger both to self and to society. By adolescence, feelings toward self have become extremely well crystallized. There has also been a complete generalization of the child's expectations regarding the behavior of adults. Patterns of adjustment, no matter how maladaptive, are well ingrained and extremely difficult to change regardless of the degree of social and behavioral difficulties they produce. This fact points out the importance of identifying and treating school-age children who may be abused.

The range of symptoms seen in preteens and teenagers runs the gamut of behavioral and emotional disturbances and cannot be presented as specific to maltreatment. Among adolescent boys, acting out or aggressive behavior is more common than isolated or withdrawn behavior. Girls show a tendency toward depression. A component of depression, however, is often identified in angry boys as they become older, thus the risk of self-destructive behavior and the potential for suicide increases. Sexual fears and confusion regarding sexual identity may be also be expressed, but they may be related to many causes other than maltreatment.

SPECIFIC PSYCHIATRIC DIAGNOSES IN THE AFTERMATH OF ABUSE

The psychological examination of an abused or neglected child does not always result in diagnosis of a specific mental illness. Many such children function well enough despite maltreatment, and as a result their behaviors do not meet the criteria for any particular diagnostic syndromes. When they do, the diagnoses fall in several categories, none of which is uniquely associated with maltreatment. Quite common are the disruptive behavior disorders of attention-deficit hyperactivity disorder (ADHD), the conduct disorders, and oppositional defiant disorder. ADHD is usually seen as having an organic cause, but the stress of maltreatment may serve as a catalyst to its behavioral expression. The appearance of chronic depression in some children leads to a dysthymic diagnosis. More prevalent are the anxiety disorders: separation anxiety disorder and overanxious disorder being seen more frequently than avoidant disorder of childhood or adolescence. Less severe or persistent reactions to maltreatment may meet the criteria for one of the adjustment disorders, which emphasize anxiety, depression, conduct, emotions, or a specific symptom such as inhibition in school functioning.

Post-Traumatic Disorders

The post-traumatic stress syndrome described in victims of catastrophic events includes a reexperiencing of the trauma in dreams or thoughts, suffering from guilt, hyperalertness and sleep disturbances, and possibly the compulsion to renact the trauma (Green and Berlin, 1987; Foy et al., 1984). Victims may also come to avoid recalling the trauma by avoiding specific activities and discussion or by blunting their general emotional responsiveness. A parallel rape trauma syndrome that is more specific to sexually related stresses has also been described (Burgess and Holmstrom, 1974). These syndromes have gained fairly widespread acceptance as clinical entities that may often be helpful in identifying victims of abuse and orienting their treatment. On the other hand, their acceptance as medical-legal diagnoses whose presence serves to prove that abuse has taken place has been much more limited (Cohen, 1985–86). This is a prime illustration of how medical and legal standards of proof may differ.

The symptoms of post-traumatic stress in children may differ from those of adults. Children's dreams, for example, may be more general nightmares of attack and threatened loss than specific visions of the stressful event itself. Their reliving of the stress is more likely to occur through repetitive play. The following case illustrates some manifestations of post-traumatic stress in a young child:

> A three-year-old female had been physically and sexually abused over a period of time. Abuse included being tied up tightly and having objects placed in her anus and vagina, producing significant pain. For some time after the maltreatment terminated and the child was in a safe environment, she became panicky when dressed in clothing that fit snugly around her waist or neck, and she vigorously avoided wearing anything that was not loose fitting. She became extremely bowel retentive and indicated that she greatly feared having anything come out of her rectum. The discomfort she felt when having to pass large and hard feces produced a panic response. In her play activity, she repeatedly tied up her dolls and stuffed animals and then pushed pencils and other pointed objects into what would be their vaginal or anal areas. She complained of frequent nightmares in which monsters attacked her and/or her parents. She would insist that she and her mother cross the street if she saw a man approach who had a mustache. She declared that all such men were her assailant. The unexpected approach by any male produced a near-panic response. She also became very uncomfortable whenever she heard a child cry.

The Accommodation Syndrome

Child maltreatment is associated with an adjustment process that is unique to the child's experience and often causes difficulties in diagnosis. In the area of sexual abuse, this process has been called the accommodation syndrome (Summit, 1983), but the concept is applicable to the entire range of maltreatment experiences. For the child, maltreatment is typically a life-long process, and the youngster's survival requires adaptation to such a life. Children are taught to be submissive and obedient to authority figures and to believe in the omniscience of adults. They have no choice but to perceive the family environment as representing the set of rules by which they must live, and the nature of the parent-child relationship guarantees that they will not perceive the rest of the world as being any different from the world presented to them by their caretakers. A child's efforts to adapt will center on an attempt to maintain the parent-child relationship according to these standards.

Accommodation to abuse also includes self-blame. Much of this behavior comes from the psychodynamics discussed above, but some also derives directly from the actions of the abuser, who frequently succeeds in shifting responsibility for the abuse to the victim. The victim is told that disclosure will destroy the family, hurt one of the parents, or cause the abuser harm. The victim is caught between his or her own needs and the fear of either hurting others or losing loved ones. As a result of accommodation, children who have been physically abused do not run away from home or seek assistance. They may actually stay close to their parents and concentrate on attempting to appease them. Sexually abused children may act as if the sexual relationship with the parent is simply a part of their lives that they must accept in order to survive.

Separation Problems

One would think that maltreated children, at least by the time they reach the age of 7 or 8, would concentrate on putting distance between themselves and a potentially threatening parent. Avoidance may be an adaptation demonstrated by some children, but paradoxically the maltreatment process can easily produce a pathological need for closeness. The child may cling to the parent and have difficulties separating. Separation fears represent fears of being rejected. The child acts as if the parent will disappear, manifesting a final, total rejection, if the child allows the parent out of sight.

RESPONSES TO DISCLOSURE

Ambivalence and Recanting

As a direct result of the conflicts described above, the child who actually reports abuse or in anyway cooperates with those who have come to offer assistance is placed in a situation that is extremely stressful. It can be best described as an intense approach-avoidance conflict. Asking for help offers the immediate expectation of diminished pain and the hope of receiving emotional support. Unfortunately, asking for help also puts the child in the position of attacking a significant adult, often a parent. As if this were not difficult for an individual of any age, one should recall that children have no choice but to introject the experience of abuse as evidence of their own unworthiness. Even when the child appears angry with the abusive parent, he or she may not feel worthy of being helped or believe that outsiders will perceive the parent as being wrong. Instead, the fact that the child feels motivated to say something threatening about the parent is incorporated into the child's sense of being a bad person, often at a level below conscious awareness. As a result, children who disclose abuse, often in a moment of crisis or anger, often later retract their statements.

The possibility of recanting becomes even greater when children are exposed to suggestions that they are not believed. Children may get this impression during the usual course of investigation following a disclosure, when they may be interviewed by a series of medical, social service, and legal professionals. Even if each interviewer tries carefully to be supportive and empathetic, these children frequently perceive being made to repeat their stories over and over again as a sign of distrust (Avery, 1983; Berliner and Barbieri, 1984; Landwirth, 1987). Many children will be unable to tolerate this perceived lack of support and will recant to escape the situation. These same children may have also received the message, both from the accused parent and from other adults who are significant in their lives, that recanting is strongly desired. We now recognize that recanting reflects both within-the-child emotional conflicts and within-the-family emotional pressures (Summit, 1983; Avery, 1983).

Timing of Disclosure

The pattern of disclosure reflects the conflicts experienced by abused children. It is rare for a child to simply say "I have had enough" and to disclose the situation to an appropriate party. It is more common for the disclosure to be stimulated by other experiences. For example, injuries may become apparent to someone in authority, such as a teacher or physician. The child will be questioned regarding the possibility of abuse, perhaps for the first time. Some children will reach for help at this point and disclose, but many will be unable to respond to the treating physician. Their unusual pattern of avoidance and denial, however, may result in further investigation. Voluntary disclosure sometimes happens when the child is older and has apparently coped with the situation for many years, but the situation in the family suddenly changes. For example, teenage girls reveal years of incest when they see the father indoctrinating a younger sister into the activity. Disclosure may also come when the child is furious about some type of restriction and impulsively attacks in the process of expressing anger toward the parent. This is such a common phenomenon that specific warning must be given not to discredit the child's statements because they are made within the framework of adolescent anger toward a restrictive parent (Summit, 1983).

RESPONSES TO THE INVESTIGATORY PROCESS

One of the reasons most frequently given by clinicians for not reporting maltreatment is that the formal social service and legal process does more harm than good (Schoeman, 1983; Saulsbury and Hayden, 1986). Both professionals and families alike may feel that outside involvement in a case is likely to stigmatize the family, punish rather than treat the abuser, and subject the victim to further public trauma. Although one might argue that all of these risks are potentially justified by the chronic nature of abuse and the high rate of recidivism among some types of offenders, certainly the risk of further trauma to the child is a very real consideration. As discussed above, disclosure itself creates conflicts and stresses for the child. Participation in legal proceedings raises the possibility of further stress: the child mistakenly believing that he or she is the one being arrested; anxiety associated with seeing or having to confront the abuser; and the likelihood of repetitive questioning, sometimes from skeptical investigators or aggressive attorneys.

Legislators and courts have responded to these concerns by establishing procedures designed to make some accommodation for children within the legal environment. The laws and precedent outlining these procedures vary greatly from jurisdiction to jurisdiction, and most are sufficiently new that their ability to withstand legal challenge remains to be tested. Not all are available in any one location. Having a general idea of what may be available, however, can help clinicians better coordinate their efforts with those of the social service and legal system. The various courtroom and procedural reforms that may be invoked in abuse cases fall into the following categories (Whitcomb et al., 1985):

- Exclusion of general spectators (and sometimes the press) from the courtroom; laws barring disclosure of the victim's identity.
- Provisions for avoiding direct courtroom confrontation of the victim by the abuser. The Sixth Amendment to the United States Constitution guarantees the accused the right to confront his or her accuser. Many jurisdictions now have laws allowing children to testify via closed-circuit television so that they can be seen by an alleged abuser but not vice versa. Limits apply to when this procedure can be used, and questions remain as to how well it will withstand constitutional challenges at the state or federal level.
- Videotaping statements by victims. Videotapes have proved useful to avoid multiple interviews during investigation, to aid in pretrial maneuvering, and as some protection from recanting, but they have generally not been seen as useful substitutes for testimony in actual court proceedings. At least one reason is that the interview, performed for clinical purposes, generally uses techniques that would not be acceptable in court.
- Exceptions to rules barring hearsay testimony. Again, these may serve to avoid having a child appear in court or, more frequently, to avoid having the child speak in court about painful or embarrassing details of abuse. Some jurisdictions have enacted laws creating special hearsay exceptions for cases of sexual abuse, while others have expanded exceptions used in other types of cases (see also Chapters 6 and 20).
- Provision of victim advocates or friends of the court, who help the child and family understand the judicial system and become familiar with the courtroom and its procedures. Some advocates may accompany the child to depositions or to court or help negotiate alternative mechanisms (such as closed-circuit testimony) for the child's participation. The advocate's purpose is not to further the prosecution but to further justice by helping child participate in the most atraumatic and effective way possible.
- Streamlined investigatory procedures to avoid multiple interviews. Some jurisdictions have designated teams or centers in which abuse cases can be efficiently evaluated, while others have interagency agreements that allow sharing of information or coordination of interviews.
- Court procedures that give priority to abuse

cases so that pretrial delays are kept to a minimum.

Although few objective data are available, one study by Runyan and colleagues (1988) suggests that at least some courtroom proceedings can be therapeutic. Children who had experienced juvenile or family court proceedings had a decrease in anxiety compared with children who were still awaiting criminal trials or other interventions.

One major hope from any legal proceeding is that the verdict of the court will serve to vindicate the child's claims and thus serve as a powerful signal to child and family regarding the abuser's responsibility for what has happened. In theory, the child, when properly prepared, has the opportunity to state what has happened in an open and accepting forum. Even a confrontation with the alleged abuser, in a controlled setting, may help to improve the child's self-esteem. Taking a case to court, however, especially a criminal charge against the abuser, has many risks. Even if the abuser is found guilty, after sentencing some of the child's initial feeling of vindication or even revenge may be replaced by guilt. Alternatively, if the sentence is seen as too light or if the abuser is acquitted, the child may lose faith in the judicial system or again become a scapegoat for other members of the family. For these reasons, the decision to prosecute an abuser or to have the child testify in a family or juvenile court proceeding must be made very carefully. Before the decision is made, the child and supportive family members must have some understanding of how courts work. Perhaps most important, they must understand the different standards of proof required in clinical work, family and juvenile courts, and criminal proceedings. They must come to grips with the fact that it may be perfectly clear to them that abuse has taken place, but that proving the identity of the perpetrator "beyond a reasonable doubt" may be difficult.

Attorneys and family members must discuss their goals for legal action. In any given situation, a range of charges, associated with a range of possible outcomes, may be filed. Most sexual abuse cases, for example, are settled by a plea bargain in which the alleged abuser waives his or her right to a trial and agrees to plead guilty to what is usually less than the maximal charge that might have been filed (Whitcomb et al., 1985). Sometimes this tactic seems to deny the child his or her day in court or give the abuser what seems to be an inappropriately light sentence; undoubtedly some plea bargains represent part of society's general unwillingness to face the problem of abuse. Most, however, probably result from careful decisions that weigh the uncertainties and possible trauma of a trial against specific goals for the family's short- and long-term benefit. Many families, however, and even some professionals, judge the outcome of a proceeding in terms of its immediate impact on the abuser. The stiffer the sentence, the greater the feeling of vindication and retribution. In the long run, however, the certain knowledge that an abuser will have a criminal record, or the leverage of a provisionally suspended sentence to mandate the abuser's separation from the victim and participation in a bona fide treatment program, may be more important and ultimately less guilt provoking.

ABUSED CHILDREN AS ADULTS

Empirical Data

There is evidence that the social, psychological, and intellectual deficits originally triggered by maltreatment may last into adult life. For example, a study on post-traumatic effects found that individuals who had had behavioral problems as children (many of which may have been related to abuse) were more likely to suffer from post-traumatic stress syndrome if they suffered trauma as adults (Helzer et al., 1987). More striking, however, was the finding that those who had had problems as children were also more likely to encounter trauma as adults. Those who were soldiers in Vietnam were more likely to see combat, and those were were civilians were more likely to have been beaten or mugged in the 18 months prior to being interviewed. Although the link between childhood problems and adult trauma is not known, it again suggests that maltreatment in childhood may lead, through a chain of other developmental problems, to difficulties in functioning later on.

In parallel to the Minnesota longitudinal study's findings among young children (Egeland et al., 1983), adults who report having been sexually abused as children appear more likely to develop depression, suicidal ideation, and somatic disturbances such as eating disorders or excessive anxiety than others do in the general population (Browne and Finkelhor, 1986). These individuals may also suffer from serious problems with self-esteem, often combined with ongoing sexual dysfunction.

Is There a Cycle of Abuse?

Perhaps the most widely publicized long-term outcome of maltreatment is the observation that many adults who are found to abuse their children report that they were themselves abused in childhood (see Chapter 22). Evidence does suggest that abused children are more likely to become abusers but that the majority will not. Perhaps the most important finding is that children can to some extent be protected from abnormal or abusing home environments by finding an adult who can relate to them in a normal, warm, consistent fashion. Teachers, relatives, or official "big brothers" can all play a role in helping modify maladaptive ways of seeing the world. This help probably has to arrive very early, however. Once the child is set in a pattern of poor social interactions and decreasing school achievement, intervention may be too late.

References

Anonymous. Child homicide—United States. MMWR 1982;31:292–294.

Avery M. The child abuse witness: potential for secondary victimization. Crim Just J 1983;7:1–48.

Baker SP, O'Neill B, Karpf RS. The injury fact book. Lexington, Massachusetts: Lexington Books, 1984.

Barahal RM, Waterman J, Martin HP. The social cognitive development of abused children. J Consult Clin Psychol 1981;49:508–516.

Berliner L, Barbieri MK. The testimony of the child victim of sexual assault. J Soc Issues 1984;40:125–137.

Browne A, Finkelhor D. Initial and long term effects: A review of the research. In: Finkelhor D, ed. A sourcebook on child sexual abuse. Beverly Hills: Sage Publications, 1986:143–179.

Burgess AW, Holmstrom LL. Rape trauma syndrome. Am J Psychiatry 1974;131:981–986.

Cohen A. The unreliability of expert testimony in the typical characteristics of sexual abuse victims. 74 Georgetown Univ Law Rev 429, 1985–86.

Egeland B, Farber EA. Infant-mother attachment: factors related to its development and changes over time. Child Dev 1984;55:753–771.

Egeland B, Sroufe A, Erickson M. The developmental consequences of different patterns of maltreatment. Child Abuse Negl 1983;7:459–469.

Erickson MR, Egeland B. A developmental view of the psychological consequences of maltreatment. School Psychol Rev 1987;16:156–168.

Finkelhor D, Browne A. The traumatic impact of child sexual abuse: a conceptualization. Am J Orthopsychiatry 1985;55:530–541.

Foy DW, Sipprelle RC, Rueger DB, Carroll EM. Etiology of post-traumatic stress disorder in Vietnam veterans: analysis of premilitary, military and combat exposure influences. J Consult Clin Psychol 1984;52:79–87.

Goldstein J, Freud A, Solnit AJ. Beyond the best interests of the child. New York: The Free Press, 1979.

Green MA, Berlin MA. Five psychosocial variables related to the existence of post-traumatic stress disorder symptoms. J Clin Psychol 1987;43:643–649.

Harris JC. Don't overlook depression in children and adolescents. Contemp Pediatr 1987 ♂ rch:70–90.

Helzer JE, Robins LN, McEvoy L. Post-traumatic stress disorder in the general population. N Engl J Med 1987;317:1630–1634.

Kempe CH. Approaches to preventing child abuse. Am J Dis Child 1976;130:941–47.

Landwirth J. Children as witnesses in child sexual abuse trials. Pediatrics 1987;80:585–589.

Minde K. Bonding and attachment: its relevance for the present day clinician. Dev Med Child Neurol 1986;28:803–806.

Pfeffer CR. The suicidal child. New York: Guilford Press, 1986.

Reidy TJ. The aggressive characteristics of abused and neglected children. J Clin Psychol 1977;33:1140–1145.

Rogers CM, Terry T. Clinical intervention with boy victims of sexual abuse. In: Stuart IR, Greer JG, eds. Victims of sexual agression. New York: Van Nostrand Reinhold, 1984.

Runyan DK, Everson MD, Edelsohn GA, Hunter WM, Coulter ML. Impact of legal intervention on sexually abused children. J Pediatr 1988;113:647–653.

Saulsbury FT, Hayden GF. Child abuse reporting by physicians. South Med J 1986;79:585–587.

Schoeman F. Should child abuse always be reported? Hastings Center Rep 1983;Aug:19–20.

Shirk SR. The interpersonal legacy of physical abuse of children. In: Straus MB, ed. Abuse and victimization across the life span. Baltimore: The Johns Hopkins University Press, 1988:57–81.

Summit RC. The child sexual abuse accommodation syndrome. Child Abuse Negl 1983;7:177–193.

Troy M, Sroufe LA. Victimization among preschoolers: role of attachment relationship history. J Am Acad Child Adol Psychiatry 1987;2:166–172.

Whitcomb D, Shapiro ER, Stellwagen LD. When the victim is a child: issues for judges and prosecutors. National Institute of Justice, Office of Development, Testing, and Dissemination. Washington, DC: US Government Printing Office, 1985.

Wolfe DA. Child abuse: implications for child development and psychopathology. Beverly Hills: Sage Publications, 1987.

3 Interviewing Children: Psychological Considerations
—Leon A. Rosenberg

This and the following chapter are designed as guides to the primary care clinician who interacts with children who may have been abused, or who must interpret the findings of other professionals who interview these children. The chapters are not meant to be "cookbooks" for conducting psychiatric or forensic interviews. The skills involved in those tasks must be developed with experience and expert supervision. On the other hand, many of the considerations and maneuvers involved in formal interviewing are applicable to general interactions with abused children and can help both to gather information and to promote therapeutic relationships.

INVESTIGATION VERSUS ASSESSMENT

Assessment and investigation should be perceived as different processes following different rules. Investigation is carried out to meet legal requirements, while diagnostic assessment seeks to meet clinical requirements. The investigating process has as its goal determining whether a court should be asked to place a child under its protection or whether a criminal charge should be made against an individual. The diagnostic assessment is concerned with determining the basis of a child's behavior and developing a therapeutic plan. The techniques of investigation and assessment overlap, however, because both must be carried out in a manner that can, if necessary, withstand scrutiny in a court of law. The assessment of a child who may have been abused must anticipate that a report to legal authorities may have to be made and justified. Even if the child is known to be abused and the authorities are already involved, establishment of an effective treatment plan may require legal support and thus an assessment that can be defended in court. This chapter provides background for techniques that serve both assessment and investigation: methods of probing that do not lead, and tools for assessing the child's competency as an observer. Chapter 4 discusses practical aspects of carrying out an interview.

INTERVIEWING THE CHILD

The assessment process relies heavily on direct interviewing skills, although supportive materials can be obtained from indirect sources such as storytelling, artwork (drawings of people or of family activities), and diagnostic doll play. The interview technique is generic to clinical assessment and is not designed specifically for dealing with issues of maltreatment. It seeks to examine children's views of themselves, relationships with caretakers and siblings, management of feelings, and perceptions of caretakers.

Guilt and Shame

The abused or neglected child is always struggling with a variety of emotional issues, including guilt and shame, no matter how irrational that may seem to the observer. Regardless of the child's age, it is often helpful for the interviewer to indicate his or her awareness of these feelings and to show support and acceptance despite these "bad things." Indicating that the interviewer is aware that something significant has occurred, without specifying exactly what, and that the interviewer is concerned for how upsetting this must be can often allow the child to share sensitive material. For example, simply indicating to a young girl that one understands that her father is no longer in the home and that she may have some feelings about that situation is a powerful statement of acceptance that counters her sense of guilt for having "caused" the father's departure. Dealing with the child's shame (guilt) is necessary even when there is a spontaneous disclosure, as during a physical examination when interviewing is going on but is not the primary process at that moment. A concerned look on the physician's face, for example, will not be automatically perceived by the child as concern but will more likely be interpreted as doubt or rejection. The youngster needs to hear clear statements of concern and acceptance of his or her immediate feelings of fear and embarrassment. Doubt expressed by the examiner ("Tell me again what happened?," accompanied by a puzzled expression) will immediately increase the child's already significant struggle about the wisdom of disclosure.

Progressive Confrontation

The most helpful interview is one that gives an overall picture of the child's relationship with parenting figures and does not restrict itself to a specific experience of alleged maltreatment. This not only gives valuable information, but it enables the child to speak about the parent-child relationship in terms of less challenging issues before approaching topics that would stimulate a more serious guilt component. Dealing with typical areas of the parent-child relationship also allows use of a process of progressive confrontation to apply some reasonable pressure on the child to reveal uncomfortable material.

Discussion of punishment can serve as a basic example of progressive confrontation. Initially, the child can be told that all children, even the best, get into difficulty at home and have to be punished by their parents. After obtaining agreement to that statement, the interviewer can ask about the different ways in which parents in general might punish children in general. That response can lead directly to questions about how this child's parents punish him or her and for what reasons. A sudden refusal on the child's part to cooperate with the examiner or a statement that the child absolutely never gets into trouble and never gets punished should be dealt with by increased confrontation. This means firm but pleasantly presented statements indicating a great deal of surprise that this particular child absolutely never gets punished since the child and interviewer have already agreed that all children get punished at some time by all parents. This must not be done with the appearance of trapping the child but rather with a tone emphasizing the examiner's surprise as well as positive regard for children who sometimes get punished.

Sometimes the approach has to originate even further away from the child's current life experience by utilizing family doll play. For example, a 5 year old would not talk about punishment interaction within the family, so the interviewer engaged the child in play with a set of family dolls. The interviewer insisted that it was time for the boy doll to be punished by a parent doll because "all boy dolls do something wrong sometimes." This resulted in the child having each parent doll severely beat the boy doll. The interviewer's knowledge of the child's history then led to the statement, "I think that this little boy [doll] got burned. Is he crying?" The youngster then immediately started talking about being burned by a cigarette by his stepfather and being extremely angry. With a good deal of emotion, he talked about being injured in a variety of ways by the stepfather. Although the youngster was now able to more openly discuss punishment issues within the family, his sense of guilt was still present and the feelings he expressed toward his stepfather remained ambivalent rather than consistently angry. Basically, at some emotional level the youngster perceived himself as being a bad person who deserved the punishment he had been receiving.

Fantasy versus Reality, Truth versus Lies

When the allegedly maltreated child discloses abuse during an interview, it is appropriate for the examiner to be concerned about the child's ability to differentiate between reality and fantasy. When the child is clearly reality oriented, it is appropriate to wonder whether the child can differentiate between the truth and a lie and recognize the value of telling the truth. This is not just a concern for the clinical assessment process; the credibility of the clinician's court testimony depends in part on his or her ability to demonstrate that these issues have been appropriately investigated.

When summoned to court, the clinician's testimony includes much of what would be categorized as hearsay: the child told me this, the child told me that. This material is often admitted into family or equity court because it constitutes a basic part of the clinician's examination of a child. For example, it is often argued that one cannot plan treatment for the youngster unless the identity of the maltreating person is discussed with the child and, hence, that identification actually becomes part of the diagnostic statement. However, the clinician's faith in the validity of the child's statements regarding who hurt him and how the incident occurred will be directly challenged by a defense attorney. A common challenge is to suggest that the younger the child, the more he or she lives in a world of fantasy. Other challenges include the assertion that children lie all of the time and that therefore their statements generally cannot be trusted.

In response to these challenges, clinicians are often tempted to take a developmental perspective and examine at what age children can typically deal with the abstract concepts of reality, fantasy, truth, and lies. This determination may be useful as supporting information, but as a specific rebuttal it is a waste of time. First, regardless of general developmental principles, each child is unique and how any one child deals with truth and reality must be determined by clinical interview; it cannot be reliably estimated from chronologic age. Second, how well the very young child can deal with these concepts is strongly related to the skill of the interviewer. Poor interviews may obtain little useful information, even from competent children.

Children as young as 2½–3 can demonstrate a consistent reality orientation. They may believe in Santa Claus, but they also clearly know when they have been hurt and who has hurt them. A child in this age range may have a great deal of difficulty answering the question "What is the difference between real and make believe?" However, the same child shown a toy car and asked whether it is real will answer no. A series of objects can be presented, ranging from those that are real to those that are make-believe or toys. The questions can move from "Is this a real airplane or a make-believe airplane?" to the next level, "Can this airplane really fly?"

The same can be done for the concept of truth versus lies. One has to listen to what the child says and use some ingenuity. For example, one 2½ year old was unable to understand the introduction of these two concepts no matter how they were presented. However, when he was asked "You are a girl. Is that true, yes or no?," he quickly answered no, establishing his ability to identify a statement as being true or not. The child was then presented with two same-sex child dolls and engaged in a game in which one doll told things to the other doll that sometimes were not and sometimes were true. The youngster's role in this game was to tell how the second doll felt. It was easy for the youngster, without any prompting, to talk about how bad the doll felt when it was being told nontruths and how good it felt when it was being told the truth. The statements used related to activities within the life experience of the child and were always kept simple: sex of the doll, presence or absence of easily identified clothing on the dolls, announcement of actions by the other doll that clearly did not happen ("You hit me!"). At the conclusion of play, the interviewer could convincingly state that the child understood the difference between truth and lies and understood the value of telling the truth.

The younger children are, the more limited their experience with the real world. Hence, they will accept certain false statements that are made by respected figures or that deal with concepts that they cannot test for themselves. One 3-year-old child, for example, agreed with the claim that the interviewer could fly. However, throughout the interview the youngster had consistently and accurately differentiated between truth and lying. When asked why he thought that the interviewer could fly, he said, "Because you are the doctor." He indicated that he did not know anyone else who could fly but that he had seen it done on television. He was not sure that people could really fly, but he suspected that there might be an occasional person who was able to do so. Hence, when the nice and powerful doctor said that he was able to fly, the child agreed. Such moments of confusion are easily understandable and do not indicate that children cannot validly report specific personal experiences such as being hurt by someone.

Anxious Elaboration

Maltreated children do occasionally present the interviewer with unusual statements that cannot possibly be factual. Sometimes these will be deliberately silly responses aimed at testing the clinician's willingness to set limits. If the child's statements are playful, they will not be accompanied by negative feelings, and the child will clearly be having fun. Most of the time, however, these statements will be manifestations of anxious elaboration, or the tendency to confuse one's fears with reality. For example, a 3-year-old child was able to describe in ever increasing detail the sadistic sexual abuse to which she had been exposed. As she shared this during therapy sessions, she obviously experienced an increase in anxiety. She began to talk about other things that were done to her, including "and he made all of my hair fall off." It was known that the abuser had not removed all of her hair. Did her fanciful statement negate everything that she said earlier? The answer is clearly no. As her anxiety became more severe, the child began to confuse actual experiences with threats made by the abuser. The clinical examination clearly indicated that we were dealing with a child who was highly anxious but not psychotic. She was demonstrating an anxiety-based elaboration based on experiences that were emotionally devastating.

When such elaborations occur, it is best to recognize the increase in the child's anxiety by uncritically accepting the statement, indicating sympathy and awareness of the frightening nature of what the child is relating, and then moving on to another topic. Until anxiety has decreased, the child may be unable to differentiate between actual memories and what are "scary ideas" that perhaps did not really occur.

Differentiating between Truth and Coaching

There are many situations in which people attempt to make children lie. A parent may drill a youngster on what to say to the interviewer in an attempt to block an investigation or influence a custody decision. Critics of children's competence go farther and suggest that the issue is not just one of trying to get the child to lie, but that there is a possibility of "programming" or "brainwashing" a child to the point where he or she actually believes that certain things have or have not happened. This goes well beyond telling a child to say something because "Mommy wants you to" or "Daddy will punish you if you don't." The claim is that the child actually can come to believe that Daddy put his fingers in her vagina and hurt her, even though it never happened and the entire belief system is based on Mommy's verbal training of the child.

The notion of brainwashing is well loved by defense attorneys but lacks scientific or clinical support of any significance. Laboratory studies on programming language have indicated that subtle reinforcement techniques can do such things as increase the frequency with which a subject may use personal pronouns or words denoting feelings (Krasner, 1958; O'Brien and Holbern, 1979; Primac, 1980). Those changes in frequency, however, are very hard to maintain without consistent reinforcement, and the procedure followed in one successful experiment often fails in another. The most these studies show is change in the frequency of occurrence of a category of words, a far cry from a child learning to believe that "Daddy put his fingers in my vagina and hurt me." The clinical literature contains fears that such a process could occur, either with no data presented or with speculations made on the basis of materials that could be interpreted in a variety of ways (Schuman, 1986, 1987). In contrast are reports of case surveys indicating false accusations by children to be rare but false recanting (recanting in spite of independent verification of the abuse) to be a more significant problem (Goodwin et al., 1978; Summit, 1983; Benedek and Schetky, 1984; Berliner and Barbieri, 1984; Paradise et al., 1988). This is not to say that external factors cannot influence the type of allegations made by or on behalf of children, but that these effects are relatively small compared with the tendency of children to tell the truth when they disclose abuse. Rates of substantiation of allegations of sexual abuse, for example, *are* related to whether or not they occur within the context of a child custody conflict. In the study by Paradise et al. (1988), substantiation was defined as a positive determination by (1) medical evidence, (2) investigation by child protective services, or (3) the perpetrator's admission. Within a custody conflict, substantiation was obtained for 73% of cases; for cases in which custody was not an issue, the substantiation rate was 95%. The inability to substantiate an allegation does not guarantee that the statement is untrue, and the substantiation process itself may lead to false-positive conclusions. However, by these commonly accepted standards, three-quarters of allegations made in the context of custody disputes and brought to the attention of the social service system were felt to be valid.

The quality of the relationship between the child and the alleged abuser can also play a role when another individual wishes to influence the child's perception of the alleged abuser. It is commonly believed that given several months, one parent can "poison the mind" of the child against the other parent. In reality, attacking a positive relationship between a child and a parent will usually cause backlash, with the child becoming angered and threatened by the manipulating parent rather than learning to hate the parent that is loved. If, on the other hand, the relationship between the child and one of the parents is negative, then it is more possible for the other parent to manipulate the attendant fears. For example, a 2-year-old child who had been physically hurt by her father, but never in the genital area, could possibly be maneuvered by the mother to refer to the vaginal area as yet another area where father hurt her. Basically, a harmful relationship already exists, and a parent attempts to take advantage of it to make the other parent look worse. This is very different from a child being "programmed" to believe that harmful experiences actually occurred when the actual relationship was a normal one. Hence, it is of value to obtain a history from each parent independently. This technique allows the examiner to more fully explore the quality of each parent's relationship with the child.

The Child's Memory

Beyond the extreme of "brainwashing," there is the concern that young children are significantly more suggestible than adults. Research in this area with children as young as age 4 has made use of many different types of tasks: recall of real-life events, recall of filmed events portrayed realistically, recall of filmed events such as cartoons, and recall of material shown in film strips. The manner of testing recall has varied as well. In general, results have indicated that, depending on situational factors, both adults and children can be susceptible to suggestion and that it is not the case that children are always more susceptible than adults (Loftus and Davies, 1984). In one study, children as young as 6 were as successful as older subjects in discriminating what they had been told or had imagined from what they had seen or heard. Six year olds, however, did have more difficulty distinguishing what they had imagined from what they had themselves said or done. The authors concluded that "children do not have a general deficit in discriminating the origin of information in memory" (Johnson and Foley, 1984). Much more research is needed, but it is clearly inaccurate to categorize children's memory as either dominated by fantasy or easily distorted through suggestion.[1]

Attempts have been made to specifically categorize the information that would lead to a decision that a child has or has not been coached. Although there are conflicting views on this point, there is strong support for reliance on awareness of the emotions demonstrated by the child during the interview and the independence and spontaneity of the child's language. These qualities can be confirmed as the interviewer approaches the topic of abuse at different points in the conversation, from different directions, and with different questions about various aspects of the experience. In an appropriate way, children must be asked how the experience felt, where it happened, when it happened, who was dressed or undressed, and other details. If these questions are presented in the form of an interrogation, one greatly increases the possibility of defensive recanting. However, if the questions are presented within a supportive atmosphere, with the interviewer seeing the child two or three times over several days, they can be presented without the child feeling threatened.

Inconsistency with regard to specific detail, in contrast, is not an important factor in the evaluation. The memory research noted earlier suggests that while there are conditions under which a child's memory for the basic event may be accurate, there will be some limitation on the amount of detail that can be recalled. The process of anxious elaboration can also influence the recall of detail. The interviewer is looking for consistency not in descriptive facts but in the feelings demonstrated by the child as memories are elicited. Children can be trained to make a specific statement, but they cannot be coached on how to respond to a variety of approaches to the same experience or to express appropriate emotion with each approach to the

---

[1] Clinical surveys do note appropriate concerns for the occasional psychotic child. Psychosis involves severe impairment in reality-testing function, and thus memory for all events will be suspect. Psychosis in children is relatively rare, but it does take clinical skill both to identify it when present and to differentiate between such a severe process and the transitory confusion seen in highly anxious children.

topic (Benedek and Schetky, 1984; Faller, 1984; Bresee et al., 1986; deYoung, 1986).[2]

In the following clinical examples, the expression of emotion plays a significant role in differentiating between truthful statements and those that are the result of coaching.

> A 6½ year old child announced that he wanted to live with his grandparents because it would be "better" than living with his mother. That statement was immediately accepted by the interviewer, and no challenge was made. However, the interviewer went on to ask the different ways in which things were good and bad in the grandparents' home and in the home of the mother. The child consistently related many positive experiences in the mother's home as well as some appropriate discomfort associated with things mother would not give the child or with punishment she would administer. In contrast, the child had a great deal of difficulty elaborating on positive experiences in the grandparents' home. The original question about where the child would rather live was then rephrased in terms of the positive and negative characteristics expressed by the child. The child began to look tense, stared at the floor, and repeated his original one-sentence preference for living with his grandparents in the manner of a child who has memorized a line for a play.
>
> A 2½-year-old child had consistently talked about being afraid and angry at her father, whom she described as having hurt her in the vaginal area. Each time she discussed it, there was firm and consistent expression of angry feeling. Whenever possible, she would avoid the topic of her father and happily engage in other activities with the examiner. After staying away from the topic of the father for a while, we were engaged in a dollhouse game. The child was manipulating a female doll inside the dollhouse and repeatedly asked the interviewer to come to the door of the dollhouse and say "Knock, knock." In response, the child would ask "Who is there?" The interviewer started by giving a neutral response, and a positive interaction would occur at the door of the dollhouse. After this was repeated several times, the interviewer responded to the question "Who is there?" by saying "Daddy." The child was quite startled and demonstrated a great deal of fear. She immediately screamed "No, he'll hurt me, he'll hurt me."
>
> An 8-year-old girl consistently reported sexual fondling by her father during court-ordered visitation. Through therapy and separation from the father, the youngster had become comfortable discussing these issues. Although she was more interested in fun activities than in dealing with the issues any further, she expressed a willingness to receive a letter or a taped message from her father, since she had not seen him for several months. She appeared mildly anxious when agreeing to this but was reassured when told that the therapist would be with her when she saw the material. Her exposure to a letter, which was a supportive and well-written statement containing nothing of direct threat, led to a significant increase in anxiety. Nearly reaching a panic state, she reexperienced the fear stimulated by the threats her father had made to ensure her silence.

Characteristics of a History of Sexual Abuse

Sgroi (1982) points out several characteristics of an account of sexual abuse that, when present, lend credence to a child's story. (1) Sexual abuse usually involves multiple incidents over time; single episodes are less common. (2) Sexually abusive activity usually progresses from less invasive to more invasive; adult pedophiles and incest offenders (as opposed to rapists) usually start with fondling or exposure and, as they gain confidence, move to digital and finally genital penetration. Stories that allege first-time penetration are less likely to be true in these settings. (3) Secrecy and coercion are fairly constant elements of intrafamilial or pedophile abuse. When asked, children may be able to supply details of how these were invoked by the abuser. (4) Older children can usually give explicit details of the abuse that took place. Inability to do

---

[2] The effects of simply bad interviewing cannot be predicted. It is assumed that children can be confused by interviewers who are threatening or who give purposely misleading information. Just how far that confusion can take the child is not known, but it should be obvious that an interviewer is expected to be nonthreatening and to not make statements that suggest specific answers (as in "I know your father touched you down there; now show me on the doll how he did it"). There are no data to indicate that a child will simply agree with whatever a bad interviewer suggests or demands, although defense attorneys always argue that this occurs. However, the entire discussion of lie versus truth and the effects of coaching assumes that the interviewer is a professional who has experience in interviewing children, who understands the effects of bias, and has the degree of self-awareness necessary for recognizing and controlling his or her own feelings during the interview.

so in an otherwise verbal child may be a reason to doubt a story.

Behavior in the Clinical Setting

The observable behavior of the abused child can be quite variable and confusing. As a result of the accommodation syndrome (see Chapter 2), a maltreated child may act happy and comfortable in the presence of the maltreating adult. This behavior can be seen even when the youngster expresses a great deal of hostility toward the maltreating parent during separate interviews. For example, a 7 year old consistently played happily with her father in the waiting room before each diagnostic interview. However, during each interview the youngster expressed continued fear of the father and an underlying rage toward him. Her intellectual explanation of the contradiction, as presented to her by the examiner, was that the easiest way to deal with her father was to smile and make believe that all was well. She explained the process primarily in terms of a conscious manipulation of her father in order to protect herself. Further clinical examination found a great deal of ambivalence in the child's feelings toward her father. In her case, this ambivalence expressed itself in terms of overt happiness with the father, while her anger was expressed in settings that both were separate from him and seemed safe.

Are There Tests That Can Help?

Research continues to investigate the possibility that specific procedures can identify an adult highly likely to act in a maltreating manner (Caldwell et al., 1988) or to take the range of factors accepted as being related to the issue of truthfulness and put it into a test form. Thus far, there are no instruments of accepted reliability and validity that can substitute for clinical judgment. The use of general personality measures to examine the effects of maltreatment on children has a longer history, with some areas of success and some areas of limitation. Of particular interest are the projective tests, such as human figure drawings (Burns and Kaufman, 1970; DiLeo, 1970; Schildkraut et al., 1972), the Thematic Apperception Test (Bellak, 1975), and the Rorschach (Halpern, 1953). For a great many years, the clinical diagnostic process has taken advantage of the individual's ability to express underlying emotional conflicts through indirect means, with the indirection enabling these conflicts to be expressed without being so severely defended. Fantasy itself is a defense mechanism allowing the individual to find a means of expressing emotional conflict that does not require direct conscious acceptance of the presence of the conflict. Fantasy expressions can be sampled through human figure drawings, family drawings, word associations, sentence completion, storytelling in response to ambiguous pictures, and imagining what might be seen in very ambiguous inkblots. These techniques are referred to as projective tests, and there has been a great deal of experience in their use with children.

Projective testing deals with the child's perception of his or her world as influenced by the emotional distortions caused by underlying conflicts. Projective data do not give one a clear picture of the child's actual experiences, but rather reveal the child's emotional response to those experiences. For example, a child who perceives a hostile and threatening interaction when the projective material would be expected to stimulate maternal or nurturing responses is giving a clear picture of a deviant parent-child relationship. Details of that relationship may or may not be forthcoming. A child whose fantasy productions emphasize aggression and conflict, with maternal figures who are punitive toward children in storytelling fantasies, who are pictured as threatening and aggressive in human figure drawings, and who are consistently associated with violence on other projective techniques, is describing an extremely threatening maternal figure. Such an emotional description may have been caused by actual experience of physical maltreatment at the hands of the mother or by exposure to psychological abuse not involving any physical harm. Such measures can greatly aid in the clinical assessment of the maltreated child, but they do not serve as independent indicators of the presence or absence of maltreatment.

References

Bellak L. The T.A.T., C.A.T. and S.A.T. in clinical use. New York: Grune and Stratton, 1975.

Benedek ET, Schetky DH. Allegations of sex abuse in child custody. Paper presented at the Annual Meeting of the American Academy of Child Psychiatry, 1984.

Berliner L, Barbieri MK. The testimony of the child victim of sexual assault. J Soc Issues 1984;40:125–137.

Bresee P, Stearns GB, Bess BH, Packer LS. Allegations of child sexual abuse in child custody disputes: a therapeutic assessment model. Am J Orthopsychiatry 1986;56:560–569.

Burns RC, Kaufman SH. Kinetic family drawings (K-F-D). New York: Bruner/Mazel, 1970.

Caldwell RA, Bogat GA, Davidson WS. The assessment of child abuse potential and the prevention of child abuse and neglect: a policy analysis. Am J Comm Psychol 1988;16:609–624.

deYoung M. A conceptual model for judging the truthfulness of a young child's allegation of sexual abuse. Am J Orthopsychiatry 1986;56:550–559.

DiLeo JH. Young children and their drawings. New York: Bruner/Mazel, 1970.

Faller KC. Is the child victim of sexual abuse telling the truth? Child Abuse Negl 1984;8:473–481.

Goodwin J, Sahd D, Rada R. Incest hoax: false accusations, false denials. Bull Am Acad Psychiatry Law 1978;5:276–296.

Halpern F. A clinical approach to children's Rorschachs. New York: Grune and Stratton, 1953.

Johnson MK, Foley MA. Differentiating fact from fantasy: the reliability of children's memory. J Soc Issues 1984;40:33–50.

Krasner L. Studies of the conditioning of verbal behavior. Psychol Bull 1958;55:148–170.

Loftus EF, Davies GM. Distortions in the memory of children. J Soc Issues 1984;40:51–67.

O'Brien JS, Holbern SW. Verbal and non-verbal expressions as reinforcers in verbal conditioning of adult conversation. J Behav Ther Exp Psychiatry 1979;10:267–268.

Paradise JE, Rostain AL, Nathanson M. Substantiation of sexual abuse charges when parents dispute custody or visitation. Pediatrics 1988;81:835–839.

Primac DW. Reducing racial prejudice by verbal operant conditioning. Psychol Rep 1980;46:655–669.

Schildkraut MS, Shenker IR, Sonnenblick M. Human figure drawings in adolescence. New York: Bruner/Mazel, 1972.

Schuman DC. False accusations of physical and sexual abuse. Bull Am Acad Psychiatry Law 1986;14:5–21.

Schuman DC. Psychodynamics of exaggerated accusations: positive feedback in family systems. Psychiatr Ann 1987;17:242–247.

Sgroi S. Handbook of clinical intervention in child sexual abuse. Lexington, Massachusetts: Lexington Books, 1982.

Summit RC. The child sexual abuse accommodation syndrome. Child Abuse Negl 1983;7:177–193.

4 Interviewing Children: Practical and Developmental Considerations

INTRODUCTION

Types of Interviews

History taking has a major role in the diagnosis and care of any medical condition, but it assumes a critical role in cases of suspected abuse and neglect. Often there is little or no physical evidence that abuse has taken place. The victim of abuse is often the only person who can give an account of what has happened. There are at least three main types of interviews with children suspected of being victims of maltreatment. (1) The general medical "history of the present illness" (discussed in Chapter 6) is usually obtained by a physician or other clinician at the time of a comprehensive medical evaluation. It is usually part of a series of conversations about the child's past and present illnesses and is often followed by a physical examination. Its goal is to make an initial diagnosis and to develop a plan for further diagnosis and treatment. Information about abuse often surfaces here, although it is usually not probed for specifically. (2) A psychological interview (discussed in Chapter 3) is also a general diagnostic and therapeutic procedure aimed at determining the cause of a child's behavioral or emotional problems. The interviewer may probe for evidence of maltreatment, but only as part of a broader evaluation of the child's functioning. (3) A forensic interview, in contrast, is a procedure aimed specifically at eliciting legally admissible evidence of maltreatment. It is usually carried out by a specially trained social worker, psychologist, or child psychiatrist and sometimes by a police officer or prosecutor. It may involve special techniques such as the use of anatomically detailed dolls if sexual abuse is suspected.

Although each type of interview has its own goals, the medical-legal aspects of child maltreatment and the psychosocial nature of its manifestations force the general medical interviewer to adopt techniques developed for psychological and forensic procedures. The purpose of this chapter is to help front-line medical clinicians develop better skills for general history taking in cases of suspected abuse and to help them arrange for and interpret the findings of appropriate psychological and forensic evaluations.

The Initial Interview

Essential to the success of any interview (and important therapeutically) is that children and their parents feel that they are working with competent professionals who care and want the best for them. The initial interview sets up their expectations for further interaction with the medical, social service, and legal systems. The first interview may also have special importance for gathering information. In a crisis state, victims may reveal more than they are likely to reveal later. Many of these revelations may be directly admissible in court, although under normal circumstances they would be regarded as hearsay (see Chapter 6). Subsequently, remorse, guilt, and conflicting interests may make the victim more reserved. On the other hand, the first interview often reveals little. It is rare that all details of a case are divulged initially. It is important for the clinician to accept this as a matter of course and not reveal any sense of frustration or haste to the interviewee. The interview will be judged successful if it has allowed the child or parent to become acquainted with the clinician and to feel that he or she has a protected and understanding place in which to talk about problems.

LOGISTICS

Who Interviews and How Many Times

It is important to minimize the number of interviews a child undergoes and the number of individuals conducting them. Usually, however, at least two interviews are required, one medical and the other forensic. The medical interview is often carried out by whichever clinician happens to be seeing the patient for emergency or general medical care. If this individual feels inexperienced or uncomfortable with abuse cases, he or she should try to arrange for someone else to talk with the child. As early as possible, all parties to the case (police, social service representatives, and medical staff) should agree to share information and appoint the most comfortable and skilled among them to conduct the forensic interview. This is often facilitated if the interview can be video- or audiotaped or conducted in a room with a one-way observation window.

Setting

The atmosphere should be as stress-free and quiet as possible. If the interview must be carried out in an urgent care area, an examination room that is out of the main stream of traffic is preferable to one that is vulnerable to disturbances or noise. It is also important that the setting convey a feeling of privacy. A room with closed doors and windows is preferable to an area enclosed only by curtains. Interviewers should avoid sitting behind desks or otherwise dominating child patients. If the clinician cannot sit with the child at an appropriately sized table, the interview may be conducted on a carpeted floor.

One should always try to conduct the interview in a setting separate from that in which the abuse is suspected to have taken place. When family members are suspected as perpetrators, interviews in the home should be avoided because the setting may have a strong emotional meaning for the child. It may also be more difficult to ensure privacy. A child may feel less willing to speak if there is the possibility that a parent may "accidentally" come into the room at any moment.

Accompanying Persons

Ideally, children should be interviewed individually. If the child cannot separate, one can propose that another professional accompany the child. This has the advantage of providing an independent observer and witness to what is said in the course of the interview. If the presence of an unknown person is not acceptable to the child, a parent or other trusted adult may attend. Any observer should sit behind or alongside the child and be warned to make no audible reaction to anything that the child says or does. In no case should the alleged perpetrator (if already identified) be allowed to accompany the child.

Ideally, each parent, child, and relative involved in a case should be interviewed separately, without a chance to hear each other's statements. This is often not possible in the rushed setting of the initial medical examination but can sometimes be done by asking a social worker or another member of the medical team to interview a parent or sibling while the primary clinician is interviewing the child. If the parent and child must be seen together, it should simply be remembered that this situation is less likely to result in a disclosure of abuse. If abuse is strongly suspected, separate interviews must be scheduled as a part of immediate follow-up.

Equipment

Even for short medical history interviews, it can be important to have some age-appropriate toys or play materials available. Children can often overcome a hesitancy to speak if they converse while playing. Toys also help decrease anxiety and thus improve behavior in the examining room, which facilitates conversation with parents and helps reduce the general level of stress for both parents and clinician. Available items might include small blocks, pots and pans, toy cars, dolls, puppets, crayons and paper, and child-size furniture. Depending on the techniques used, formal forensic interviews may require toy telephones, a dollhouse with dolls and furniture, and anatomic drawings or anatomically detailed dolls.

Anatomically detailed dolls are widely used in the evaluation of children suspected of sexual abuse, and several protocols for their used have been developed (Boat and Everson, 1986). Although many clinicians do not use this type of doll, careful use may help some children better express what has happened to them (Freeman and Estrada-Mullaney, 1988). Anatomically detailed dolls appear to be best used with preschool and school-age children (about ages 3–10) and, within that age group, those who prefer to demonstrate with the dolls rather than talk or draw. The dolls, like other toys, help to decrease anxiety by providing the child with a familiar object and giving the child and clinician something to talk about. Many types of dolls are available, some more pleasant and less strikingly detailed than others. By following the suggestions discussed below, as well as more detailed published guidelines, the dolls can be used in ways that facilitate conversation but do not lead the child. Given the present state of knowledge about interviews that make use of dolls, what the child does with the dolls (sexual positioning, exploration of body orifices) is clinically less interpretable (and thus legally less useful) than what the child says while manipulating them. Although some authors feel that certain specific actions with dolls are indicative of abuse (White et al., 1986), surveys of professionals who use doll interviews find varying degrees of consensus about the weight that should be placed on particular observations. Boat and Everson (1988), for example, in a survey of social service, law enforcement, and medical professionals, found wide agreement that penetrating any of a doll's orifices or simulating genital-genital or oral-genital contact was abnormal and suggestive of abuse. Likewise, there was general agreement that touching a doll's genitalia or breasts or simulating kissing was normal behavior and not suggestive of abuse. In contrast, the survey respondents were divided on whether being anxious about the dolls or placing them on top of each other was abnormal. Thus, the goal of the interview, even one using dolls, remains verbalization by the child, with the dolls serving primarily as facilitators of verbalization.

Recording the Interview

Video- or audiotape recording (with consent) can be useful in an interview as long as the equipment is unobtrusive, since taping allows other professionals to see or hear the interview and review its interpretation. Depending on local law and practice, such recordings may or may not be admissible as courtroom evidence. Any plans to use recordings as evidence should be discussed with a lawyer who is familiar with local child protection laws. In most cases, the interview will not be directly useful in court (Whitcomb et al., 1985). Even trained forensic interviewers may use clinically acceptable encouragement and reenforcement that help children disclose but that are fodder for challenges by opposing attorneys. Children may also reveal facts or make statements that, taken in isolation, appear to discredit their competency as witnesses. Recordings may be useful, however, in pretrial discussions, for their mere existence can confirm to the alleged abuser or skeptical family members the fact of the child's disclosure. Whether electronic recording is used or only the interviewer's notes, it is critical that some record be made of exactly what questions were asked and what the child responded. If dolls or other equipment are used, witnesses or recordings should be able to document that acceptable techniques were employed.

A good witness or tape can be used to avert or rebut charges that a child was coached. The interview witness usually cannot testify in court about the child's statements, since that would mean allowing introduction of hearsay evidence. If defense attorneys allege that the child was coached or that the interview technique was improper, however, the witness's testimony can be admissible because it is necessary to rebut the challenge. Thus, if a credible witness or interview tape is available, the defense must choose between using the "coaching" challenge, which risks the introduction of potentially damaging testimony, or trying to find another way to discredit the interview (Freeman and Estrada-Mullaney, 1988).

AN APPROACH TO INTERVIEWING CHILDREN ABOUT MALTREATMENT

The following discussion draws heavily on two sources, Boat and Everson (1986) and Berliner et al. (1985), and represents only one of many possible ways to structure an interview. The developmental considerations and interview steps apply to all kinds of conversations with children. Special aspects relating to forensic interviews, especially in cases of sexual abuse, are also noted.

Of foremost importance is that the interviewer be as comfortable and calm as possible. It is his or her job to convince the child that talking about an otherwise taboo subject not only is reasonable but will be therapeutic. Having a plan for how to conduct the interview, being familiar with the child's vocabulary, and using a developmentally appropriate approach will all help build this comfort. It is also vital that the interviewer not lead, prompt, coach, or coerce the child into making any sort of statement. Maintaining this restraint can be very difficult if time is limited or the interviewer has strong convictions about what has happened. A corollary principle is that each interview session not last too long; most young children cannot sustain attention or separate from their parents for more than a half hour, and after this time discomfort is likely to increase.

Developmental Considerations

The style and content of an interview must be geared to the child's developmental level. The following paragraphs give some background and guidelines for approaching children of various ages. Communication skills, common fears (Wittmer and Crouthamel, 1986; Morris and Kralochwill, 1983), and normal psychosexual development (Rothchild, 1969; Rutter, 1971) are noted. Sexual development and its relationship to maltreatment is also discussed in Chapter 18.

INFANCY AND TODDLERHOOD (UNDER 3 YEARS)

Infants and toddlers may understand a great deal of what is said to them, but their ability to respond is very limited. The oldest may be able to point to objects or answer simple questions. Interviews with children of this age are usually centered on play. The sessions are usually short (15 minutes or so), and the child often requires the accompaniment of a parent or trusted adult. Observations of how the child behaves toward adults or plays with toys or dolls may be more important than what the child says. These observations must be interpreted cautiously, however, and alone are usually not sufficient to document that abuse has taken place.

Infants and toddlers are very interested in all parts of their bodies. Self-stimulation of the genitals may normally occur as early as the first few days of life, although it is not certain whether the associated arousal conveys a specific sort of pleasure, as it does in older children and adults. Boys are capable of having erections from the first days to weeks of life. Young children have many other sources of stimulation and pleasure, such as sucking and learning control over elimination. Older toddlers are curious about adult genitalia and take opportunities to touch and view their parents'.

Children at this age are often fearful of loud noises, large moving objects, and changes in their environments. As they get older, they come to be afraid of strangers (onset usually at about 7 months, with less after 18 months) and of separation from close caretakers (from 5 months on). They also become aware of the possibility of harm to their bodies, especially the genitalia.

PRESCHOOL (AGE 3–5)

Children of preschool age think concretely and are apt to make literal interpretations of what is said to them. They tend to not understand metaphors or analogies. Their sense of elapsed time or formal time of day may be poor, but they can often sequence events, especially those related to major activities such as waking up, going to preschool, or going to bed. They are socially and emotionally dependent on older family members and may have few contacts outside their immediate family. Under normal circumstances, however, they will experiment with independence and desire a certain amount of autonomy once they feel that they are in a safe environment.

Preschoolers are very aware of anatomic differences between boys and girls, and they may be very curious about body parts and where babies come from, especially if there are infant siblings in the home. They will take advantage of opportunities to explore their own genitalia and those of peers, although they are increasingly wary of touching adult genitalia. Preschoolers may act out adult sexual activity if they have witnessed it, but normally this behavior will not involve force or occur repeatedly. A sizable minority of preschoolers will engage in some homosexual play that has no apparent bearing on future sexual orientation. Many children will express a desire to be like the opposite sex. Exhibitionism is also common, with the buttocks vying for the genitals as the preferred portion of the anatomy to display.

Behavior in the home may be marked by oedipal dynamics: competition with the same-sex parent for the attention of the opposite-sex parent. A boy may talk about marrying his mother and a girl her father, although desires to marry the same-sex parent may also be expressed. Hugging and intimacy between the parents may evoke protests or even oppositional behavior from the child. Both boys and girls may express a desire to have babies, especially if there is a newborn in the home. The origins of these behaviors are not fully understood, but their appearance and resolution probably play an important part in development of the child's idea of male and female social roles.

Major fears involve bodily harm and integrity. Preschoolers have vivid imaginations and easily conjure up visions of monsters or ghosts, especially in the dark. Nightmares and night terrors are relatively common, although they are unlikely to have a sexual content under normal circumstances. Specific fears may develop; fear of high places and deep water are common, while other fears, such as being shot or kidnapped, may depend on exposure to discussions of these situations. Preschoolers may be either frightened or simply curious about death. The use of euphemisms such as "went to sleep" may provoke problems at bedtime.

Children in this age range may manifest abuse in many ways. Physically abused or neglected children may seem fearful of or overly attached to adult caretakers. Sexually abused children may change their behaviors, act out sexual activity, or ask developmentally inappropriate questions. It is important not to assume that sexual contact itself has been unpleasant for them, although such contact is at best likely to be confusing. Much of a child's reaction stems from the coercion or secrecy imposed by the abuser rather than from the sexual nature of the contact.

Interviews with preschoolers are usually short and often require the presence of a familiar adult. Toys or drawing materials are particularly useful to decrease anxiety. After a short introductory period, the interview must be brief and to the point. The interviewer should back off at the first sign of resistance. The child will often need extra reassurance that no harm will come to the perpetrator.

SCHOOL AGE (6–PREPUBERTY)

School-age children have better communications skills than do preschoolers but they still have only limited use of symbolism and analogies. They are better at sequencing events and being aware of formal time. Although preschoolers know about secrets, school-age children are better at keeping them. An important part of their thinking is the perception that they are somehow responsible for everything that happens around them. Pseudo-maturity can be a problem for clinicians interviewing older school-age children and adolescents. Children, especially those who have lived with role reversal or have been forced to be very independent, can seem to be stronger, less in need of support, and more capable of understanding nuances of adult behavior and speech than they truly are. Although school-age children begin to have relationships with friends and adults outside the home, they continue to have a strong feeling that adults, especially their parents, are all-powerful and all-knowing, and they fear being cut off from the support of loved ones.

Children in this age range have a heightened interest in sexuality but have usually been taught that this is an embarrassing or guilt-laden area. Their interest is therefore usually discreet and involves urges to touch or look at peers of either sex. Self-stimulation continues to be common but is frequently associated with anxiety if adults have labeled it as bad. In settings where adult sexual relations take place in communal living quarters, children often mimic these adult roles and activities.

Up to age 7 or 8, day-to-day social play usually involves friends of both sexes. Beyond that age, children begin to play more with children of the same sex, and relationships with opposite-sex children begin to take on dynamics foreshadowing adult social roles. Many children have a "sweetheart" by age 10–12, although the sexual nature of this relationship varies a great deal with environmental influences. Peer pressures or parental reenforcement may encourage sexual exploration. Depending on the social setting, a significant proportion of children have attempted intercourse by the early years of puberty.

Fears in this age group continue to involve bodily harm, but they expand to involve social issues as well. Anxieties may involve the possibility of war or other catastrophes as well as peer or achievement problems in school. Fear of death and fear of harm to loved ones become more explicit than among younger children.

School-age children usually know that abuse, especially sexual abuse, is wrong. They may not reveal it, however, because they feel powerless to control adults or because they have been offered rewards such as toys or money. Abuse may be manifested by behavior changes (regression, aggression, stylized adult behaviors, or changes in relationships with peers) or by excessive fearfulness, especially of situations in which the child once felt comfortable.

Interviews with school-age children require time at the outset to build trust and rapport. Since sexual topics are difficult for them, it may help to allow discussion to take place while the child is playing with some unrelated toy or is drawing. Children of this age usually will be able to separate from a caretaker. It may be necessary to reassure the child that he or she will not go to jail or get in trouble for what has happened or what may be said.

PUBERTY (ABOUT 9–12) AND OLDER

Adolescents have strong desires to be accepted by their peers, and for the first time they develop emotional attachments outside the home that rival family ties. Common fears involve social and sexual development as well as mortality. Self-consciousness may have a major impact on their behavior and relationships.

With the onset of puberty, children begin experiencing more overt sexual feelings toward others, although many find both these feelings and spontaneous bodily reactions such as erections to be disturbing. Internal conflicts over sexual arousal and masturbation may be very troubling to teenagers. Homosexual activities (group masturbation among boys and crushes on other females among girls) are relatively common among young teenagers and are not predictive of adult sexual orientation.

Pubertal children often have good communication skills and are able to relate events in time sequence. Like adults, they may be helped by prompts that involve major events or parts of their daily schedules. Memory for specific events may be elicited by asking the teenager to first think of details of the scene (such as smells, clothing worn, and the time of day) before talking about what actually happened. Once the account begins, the interviewer should not interrupt and risk losing other details. Follow-up questions are saved until the end of the story and then asked in reverse order (details mentioned at the end of the story are questioned first). This technique is reportedly more successful than conventional questioning in eliciting facts (Leary, 1988).

Interviews of adolescents differ from sessions with younger children. The interviewer may need to maintain some professional distance and formality to help the child overcome embarrassment. It may be necessary to match the sex of the interviewer to that of the victim and to reassure the child that he or she is normal and not guilty of having provoked the abuse. Older children may do best if they can write out their stories or communicate them in some other indirect way.

Teenagers' pseudo-maturity and their need to feel in control can make it difficult for clinicians to speak with them. Much conversation may take place at an adult level, but the clinician should be aware of the teenager's strong need to feel accepted and secure and of a tendency to overgeneralize and adopt strong beliefs. As described in Chapter 3, barriers and denial can be gently confronted in the context of support and appreciation of the teenager's personal qualities. Other tactics include exploring problems that are likely to occur in families in which teenage behavior problems or abuse are taking place. Approaches range from asking simple questions, such as "Has the drinking of either of your parents ever created a problem for you?," to presenting more elaborate questionnaires that probe for family social problems (Biek, 1981).

Steps in the Interview

1. Greeting and Introduction

If the interview has been scheduled in advance, the interviewer will often have had a chance to explain to the parents what the procedure will be and how long it will take. Care should be taken to reveal as little as possible about the content of the interview or how it will be conducted so that parents—with good or bad intentions—will not attempt to coach the child.

A first chance for assessment comes when the clinician approaches the parents and child in a waiting area. The clinician has a brief chance to assess the child's mood and level of development and adjust the introductory remarks accordingly. The interviewer should take a few minutes to greet the child and the adults in the waiting area. This courtesy gives the child a chance to observe the interviewer in a safe setting.

The greeting should be appropriate to the child's developmental level and mood. Older children can be extended a longer, more formal greeting during which the clinician says a few things about him- or herself and what is going to happen. Younger children need only a brief introduction and a statement such as "I'd like to talk with you for a while."

At this point, the child can be asked to accompany the clinician to the interview room. If the child insists, an adult may be allowed to come along, provided that person agrees to the ground rules discussed above.

2. First Contact with the Child

While making some opening remarks, the interviewer assesses the child's developmental level, emotional needs, and desire to talk. With younger children, the interviewer usually takes the lead and proceeds; older children may need more explanation, which should include additional information about the clinician's background and how his or her work helps children.

Older school-age and pubertal children may need initial conversation about why they are being interviewed. It is wrong to assume that they know or have the correct explanation; they may think that they are the ones suspected of doing something wrong. The clinician can be reassuring and acknowledge that talking about sensitive issues can be difficult. It is important, however, that the interviewer not make assumptions about the child's feelings toward the suspected perpetrator; the child may not be angry and may in fact be fearful that the perpetrator will be harmed. With younger children, a casual and reassuring patter may help diffuse anxiety. The clinician's objective is to project the feeling that hearing about abuse is not upsetting or startling.

3. Assessing the Child's Abilities

At many points in the assessment of abuse cases it becomes important to establish a victim's credibility as a witness. Interviewers need to provide evidence for their belief that a victim's account is true. For child victims, credibility includes general knowledge and awareness of day-to-day activities. Boat and Everson (1986) suggest asking the following questions and documenting the responses. These questions also serve to break the ice and start off conversation on a neutral topic. Alternatively, if the child is playing with a toy, general questions about the toy can be raised and then generalized to other toys and day-to-day activities.

Older children can be asked a few general identifying questions that establish their mental status: where they go to school, favorite activities, family structure, and some generally known facts such as what city they are in or the name of the President. Younger children (preschoolers) require a more detailed assessment of cognitive abilities:

- Can the child name and distinguish people? Ask the child to give his or her name and to name other family members.
- Can the child name and distinguish locations? Ask the child "Where do you live?," "Where are we now?," "Where do you go to school?"
- Can the child name objects and semiabstract concepts? Ask the child to name some toys in the room and demonstrate what they do. Ask the child for his or her preference between two objects or colors.
- Can the child sequence events? Ask the child "When do you get up?," "When do you go to bed?," and "When does it get dark outside?" and then ask the child to state which of these comes first in the day.
- Does the child know the meaning of the word "touch"? Ask the child (without demonstrating) to touch his or her nose or your hand.
- The concepts of real and imaginary can also be explored (see Chapter 3).
- Observe the child exploring toys. Be neutral and encourage activity. Avoid use of the words "special," "play," or "let's pretend" when talking about the toys; these words may have meaning for the child in the context of abuse, and they may make it appear to observers that the interviewer is encouraging fantasy or imaginary accounts rather than factual statements. Avoid touching the toys yourself; you want to observe the child's spontaneous activity. If anatomically detailed dolls are being used, they should be visible and available at this time so that the child can begin to explore them. It is best to have a set of four dolls, two adults and two children of each sex.

4. Establishing a Common Vocabulary

Children and even many adults may not use or understand "proper" words for genitalia or other body parts. Students of the subject have documented over 600 English-language synonyms or euphemisms for vagina and over 300 for penis (Rawson, 1981). Clinicians must not only learn a child's vocabulary but use it without being embarrassed themselves.

A variety of techniques are available with younger children. One approach is to draw the outline of a "gingerbread" person, including the navel (which demonstrates that the person is undressed). Starting with nonsexual parts, the clinician and the child can draw in various portions of the anatomy, and the child can be asked to name them. A similar procedure can be followed with dolls (Boat and Everson, 1986):

- Direct the child's attention to the dolls (if not there already) and show one to the child. Ask the child to say whether it is a girl or boy doll and to give the doll's name. While pointing, ask the child to name some general body parts (eyes, nose, ears, etc.). Ask "What do we do with _____ (use child's word)?"
- Take off the doll's clothing (starting at the top) and ask child to name and describe the use of nipples, breasts, navel, genitalia (use dolls of both sexes). One can follow up names given to genitalia with "Ever hear it called anything else?," "Who calls it that?," and "Have you ever seen a grownup's _____?" (Freeman and Estrada-Mullaney, 1988). Allow the child to play with the dolls for a few minutes and observe for interest in any particular site. Interest in the genitalia is probably normal, while many (but not all) observers feel that avoidance or anxiety associated with a naked doll is unusual among normal children.
- If the child acts out anything sexual with the dolls, ask "What are they doing?" and ask the child to name each doll involved. Go beyond "daddy" or "uncle." Ask for their names or where they live. Ask "Who showed them how to do that?"

5. Asking Questions

Sometimes the vocabulary session elicits a story from the child. If not, or if the interviewee is an older child, more direct questions may be necessary. One needs to do this without leading or zeroing in on sensitive topics that will cause the child to be silent. Ideally, one never directly asks "Did anyone abuse you?" The goal is to direct the conversation in such a way that the child spontaneously reveals the abuse.

If there is some knowledge of the setting in which the abuse may have occurred, a good way to begin is to ask some general questions about that setting: "Who do you ever go visit?"; "What do you do there?" Avoid questions that are likely to elicit only monosyllabic responses. The child's facial expressions and body language may indicate that a sensitive or important issue has been approached. If so, it is prudent to back off and ask a few similar questions about less threatening topics and then work back to the abuse setting. Alternatively, children can be asked if they would rather show something with the dolls or tell the interviewer indirectly on a toy telephone. Older children may prefer to write answers.

One way to encourage responses in a certain area without leading is to reflect statements and emotions back to the child, offering an opportunity for elaboration. The interviewer should try not to show sudden interest in any particular statement or to reveal any judgment about things the child says.

6. Specific Questions about Abuse

The risk of leading or of getting rote answers is greatly increased if direct questions about abuse are asked, but such questions are sometimes required as a final step in an investigation. If the child is upset or lacks rapport with the interviewer, it may be better to break off and try another session rather than press on with specifics.

Initial direct questions can involve yes-no answers about touching and other activities. These are general questions not involving the identity of any particular person ("Has anyone touched your _____?" or "Has anyone ever hit you?"). If any question is answered yes, ask "Who?" and "Show me where?" If dolls are being used, the child can be asked to demonstrate.

Failure to get positive answers to these questions usually indicates the end of the interview, especially for a first session. Specific questions about specific individuals should be avoided ("Did Uncle Bill ever put his ding-dong in you?"). There is a great risk of leading the child, getting a false answer, or jeopardizing further testimony. Further questions should be deferred and other members of the treatment team consulted.

7. Wrap-up

The child should be given reassurance regardless of what has or has not been disclosed. Praise can be given for helping, along with reenforcement that disclosure of any fact or feeling was the right thing to do. The child should be asked about any particular worries or fears; older children can be told what will happen next in the evaluation. If it is believed that the child is still at risk of injury or wishes to speak at greater length, he or she may be given a way to contact the interviewer or another provider. Any dolls that have been used should be dressed and carefully put away to show respect for the individuals they represent. Younger children who do not seem anxious to leave can be given a chance to draw or engage in some other relaxing activity to decrease tension built up during the interview. They may want to take a picture they have made as a reward.

Documenting Findings

An important part of the interview is the record made of it. Even if there is an audio- or videotape record, the interviewer will usually make a written record of what was said. The record of a forensic interview may be more detailed than that of a medical history; however, the rules are the same for both:

- The record should give only facts and not opinions or secondhand information unless these are clearly marked as such.
- The writer should limit the contents of the record to findings directly related to the problem at hand. The record may become public in court and will certainly be seen by many health care and social service providers. Any family matters that are not directly related to the case should be excluded.
- The time and place of the interview should be given, as well as the names of all persons present.
- The child's statements should be recorded word for word whenever possible, along with a notation as to whether the statement was spontaneous or in response to a question (in the latter case, the question should be given as well).
- The child's affect (excited, upset) at the time the statement was made and afterward should also be noted.

References

Berliner L, et al. Initial approach to the sexually abused child. In: Evaluation of the child sexual assault patient in the health care setting. Supplement 1. A manual for trainers. Seattle: University of Washington School of Social Work, 1985.

Biek JE. Screening test for identifying adolescents adversely affected by a parental drinking problem. J Adol Health Care 1981;2:107–113.

Boat BW, Everson MD. Using anatomical dolls: guidelines for interviewing young children in sexual abuse/assault investigations. Chapel Hill: University of North Carolina, 1986.

Boat BW, Everson MD. The use of anatomical dolls among professionals in sexual abuse evaluations. Child Abuse Negl 1988;12:171–179.

Freeman KR, Estrada-Mullaney T. Using dolls to interview child victims: legal concerns and interview procedures. NIJ Rep 1988;207:2–6.

Leary WE. Novel methods unlock witnesses' memories. New York Times 15 Nov 1988:C1, C15.

Morris R, Kralochwill T. Treating children's phobias: a behavioral approach. New York: Pergamon Press, 1983.

Rawson H. A dictionary of euphemisms & other doubletalk. New York: Crown Publishers, 1981.

Rothchild E. Emotional aspects of sexual development. Pediatr Clin North Am 1969;16:415–428.

Rutter M. Normal psychosexual development. J Child Psychol Psychiatry 1971;11:259–283.

Whitcomb D, Shapiro ER, Stellwagen LD. When the victim is a child: issues for judges and prosecutors. Washington, DC: US Government Printing Office, 1985.

White S, Strom GA, Santilli G, Halpin BM. Interviewing young sexual abuse victims with anatomically correct dolls. Child Abuse Negl 1986;10:519–529.

Wittmer D, Crouthamel CS. Overcoming the common fears of childhood. Contemp Pediatr 1986; September:76–90.

5   Talking to Parents and Families

ASSESSING THE FAMILY

Families can be frightening to clinicians who usually see children for isolated episodes of medical illness. At best, getting involved with a family means taking time to hear a story from multiple perspectives; at worst, it means resisting efforts to embroil the clinician in family conflicts. Considering the family as a whole, however, is vital when evaluating issues of potential abuse and neglect. Most important, it may offer an opportunity for actually preventing maltreatment. Much of what is known about the etiology of abuse and neglect suggests that the origins lie in dysfunctional family relations such as parents' conflicts with their own parents or inappropriate casting of a child as scapegoat for the family's problems. Interactions surrounding routine medical problems often create opportunities to explore these relationships.

The ability to explore family relationships may also be useful at the point at which maltreatment is suspected. With the opportunity to indirectly approach issues associated with maltreatment, the clinician can gain insight into the causes of abuse in this particular family and determine the approaches to which the family may be most receptive. Family interviewing techniques can also help the clinician guide conversations when concerns for maltreatment are discussed. Clinicians are often caught in a cross fire of angry accusations and finger pointing. Disputes frequently erupt that shift the focus of discussion away from the child's problems or sabotage efforts to obtain needed information. Trained observation of these maneuvers can yield valuable information about the family, and an awareness of the dynamics may help to modulate the interaction and guide it back on course.

BASIC ASSUMPTIONS ABOUT FAMILY INTERACTIONS

Family functioning can be viewed within any one of several theoretical frameworks. The orientation presented here is based largely on the work of two pioneers in the field of family therapy, Salvador Minuchin and Jay Haley. More faithful renderings of their work, and synopses of other work about and with families, are available in several of the texts included in References.

Influences on Behavior

A common theme among those who work with families, and one that has traditionally set these clinicians apart from more psychoanalytically oriented mental health workers, is that an individual's behavior is influenced not only by internal (unconscious, or intrapsychic) thought processes but also by moment-to-moment interactions with other individuals (extrapsychic influences). Psychoanalytically oriented clinicians accept the influences of other individuals, but mostly as forces in the past that now shape a person's perceptions and thought processes. Family-oriented theorists accept the importance of these past influences, but they see them as acting in conjunction with the demands and roles that the person is now subject to. This multigenerational orientation fits closely with the type of assessment required in maltreatment cases. An important corollary of the family-oriented view is that influences on behavior are seen as circular rather than linear. In other words, less emphasis is placed on what person A does or did that makes person B act in a particular manner; more is given to identifying what A and B do together that perpetuates the unpleasant aspects of their relationship.

Family Structure

A family's structure is defined by the sometimes unspoken, sometimes explicit demands and rules established by its members (Minuchin, 1974). These regulations determine who leads and who follows, who communicates with whom, and, to some extent, what each family member sees as possible in his or her life. The structure is often reinforced by family myths or assumptions, such as "X is lazy" and "people generally don't like us," or by implicit contracts, such as "your father needs to be in charge" or "as long as I tolerate his drinking he won't leave me." Positive versions of such myths and contracts can help hold a family together and organize its functioning; problems occur when myths depart from reality, when contracts perpetuate inequities, and when the assumptions that underlie family life cannot be altered to suit new circumstances.

The ties between family members give many characteristics of a single organism to what otherwise appears to be a group of separate individuals. For example, families have developmental stages through which they must progress (Scharff and Scharff, 1987). The roles of various family members change as children are born and grow up and as grandparents age and die. Long-standing conflicts can arise when the family structure is unable to take on increasingly mature configurations.

Perhaps the most powerful property of families is homeostasis, the tendency to resist change in the family structure and in individual roles (Jackson, 1957). Clinically, the most important aspect of homeostasis is that attempts to help a family member who has psychiatric or behavioral symptoms are often resisted by the family. The individual's illness or problem has taken on a crucial role in how the family functions, and rather than restructure itself, the family tries to maintain its old configuration. For this and other reasons, family-oriented clinicians see symptoms in one family member as actually belonging to the entire family. The symptomatic individual may or may not be the member whose problems truly need to be addressed. Only an assessment of the entire family can determine where the symptomatic individual fits within the family structure and thus what the etiology of the symptoms might be.

Family Subsystems

Several subsystems of individuals make up the larger family system (Minuchin, 1974). A given individual may belong to more than one subsystem, but in a well-functioning family, individuals will have a clear idea of which subsystem's rules they are following at any particular time. The well-adjusted family with children usually has three distinct subsystems: the spouse or caretaker system; the parent-child system; and the sibling system. Each has an important purpose (Allmond et al., 1979). The spouse or caretaker system provides the adults with mutual support and thus encourages and distributes their authority. The children are not included among this group of individuals who take a leadership role in the household. The parent-child system, on the other hand, provides a setting in which the children are assured of having access to their parents and the benefit of operating under the protective authority of adults. The sibling system provides the children some degree of independence, giving them a limited but ever-increasing realm within which to function without the direct intervention of adults.

Boundaries

The formation and function of subsystems can be seen largely as a matter of the boundaries or walls that individuals or groups of individuals place around themselves. At one extreme, individuals in a subsystem or in an entire family can be enmeshed; that is, they cannot separate from each other emotionally and sometimes physically. One person's feelings are quickly and intensely experienced by others, with the result that there is no flexibility or buffering in times of crisis. One person may feel that he or she knows another so well that there is no longer a need to solicit the other person's opinions or ask how that person is feeling. Such individuals may come to confuse their own feelings with those of the other. An enmeshed individual's sense of loyalty and dependence can be so great that he or she passes up opportunities for growth and development in exchange for maintaining the feeling of belonging.

At the other extreme, disengaged individuals do not relate to each other at all. Stresses and supports are not shared, and others in the family may be left to handle crises alone. There may be little awareness of how others are feeling and little response to even blatant calls for help. An entire subsystem can become disengaged from the rest of the family, with the result that other family members are effectively excluded from family life. The ideal boundary is somewhere between these extremes: enough relating takes place for support and security of the group, and enough distance is present to allow for growth and protection of the individuals.

The relative strength of boundaries gives family subsystems a rough priority in family functioning. The caretaker subsystem potentially has the strongest boundary. It has to contain and buffer the many life stresses experienced by the family's adults, and it must create a united, consistent pattern of family leadership. Difficulties can arise when other subsystems develop stronger boundaries, when new, strong subsystems evolve (especially those that cross generational lines), and when the subsystem arrangement becomes unclear (Haley, 1976).

Children as Bearers of the Family's Symptoms

Children frequently become the individuals consciously or unconsciously delegated by the family to display symptoms of its dysfunction. In some cases, the adults in the family may be aware of their difficulties and simply feel more comfortable using a child as a means of making first contact with the helping professionals. Probably more common, however, are various uses of children to fulfill individual or group psychological needs within the family system (Wachtel and Wachtel, 1986). Children may be designated as scapegoats to account for individual or family failings, or they may be used to act out roles that a parent either would like to play or would prefer to deny in himself or herself. For example, parents who have difficulty expressing anger or dealing with authority figures may encourage rebellious or even antisocial behaviors by their children. Children can also be cast in roles that fill a void in the parents' lives. The role reversal often seen in abusive households may result from this phenomenon. In many abusive families, children are used by adults to provide nurturing and support that are not available from a spouse or from the adult's own parents. Not only does this make difficult demands on the child, it also makes him or her the object of the anger and ambivalence the parent feels toward those who actually should be providing support.

Children can also play a role in what some family-oriented clinicians call triangles, that is, relationships between two people into which a third has been recruited to alleviate stress or mediate communication. Concentrating attention on a "bad" child may help a couple avoid having to speak with each other and address their own difficulties. A couple can also fight with each other by using the child as a battlefield. They can compete for the child's loyalty or criticize aspects of the child's behavior that they identify with the opposing spouse. Perhaps most devastating to the child are attempts to involve him or her in an alliance with one parent that excludes the other. These relationships subordinate the child's normal development to the emotional needs of the parent and may, in part, be responsible for problems such as school phobia and incest.

One of the difficulties faced by medically oriented clinicians when they confront children with behavioral problems is that the behaviors do in fact often seem irritating and even obnoxious. No matter how troubled the family, it is tempting to assign at least some blame to the child and to focus treatment on the child and empathy on the parents. Family-oriented clinicians, however, emphasize not only that this is exactly what the family wants to happen but also that families can induce children to adopt behaviors that suit the family's needs. Family myths that consistently characterize a child as bad or lazy can ultimately cause the child to behave in that manner. Mixed messages and other maladaptive communication techniques can subtly encourage behaviors that are formally not sanctioned. Some clinicians also believe that children can play an active part in maintaining their dysfunctional role in the family. They may not flee the situation, seeing loyalty to the family as more important than their own mental health, or they may on some level come to realize their importance to the stability of the family structure and, out of mistaken benevolence, refuse to change (Haley, 1976). Money and Werlas (1976) have proposed that at times the parents and child together enter into a delusional world whose basic assumptions necessitate the problem behaviors. A similar premise, incorporated by Summit in his sexual abuse accommodation syndrome (discussed in Chapter 2), is that children's problem behaviors cannot be taken at face value; The motivations for them and the roles they serve in the family must be considered.

Cycles of Dysfunctional Behavior

Haley (1976) and others point out that both individuals and families often find themselves repeating patterns of behavior that seem to be solutions to problems but in fact serve only to engender further difficulties. These behaviors require several "actors" to learn their parts and then recreate them in an alarmingly consistent fashion. In one example developed by Haley (1976) and Allmond et al. (1979), the stage is set by the parents' decision that the oldest child must help in the care of her younger siblings. The child does this, but predictably things go poorly because the younger children refuse to recognize the eldest as an authority figure. The parents return and berate the oldest child for being incompetent. She then withdraws from contact with her siblings, causing a loss to which they react by developing behavior problems that strain the parents' caretaking resources. The oldest is again recruited to help care for the siblings, which starts the cycle again. Ultimately the oldest child starts to develop behavior problems herself, which prompts either punishment or a request for medical consultation. Identifying such cycles, and the role that each individual plays, may cast light on why a given child has developed symptoms.

THE PROCESS OF FAMILY ASSESSMENT

Clinicians in acute care settings may not carry out the in-depth assessments conducted by family therapists or even by some social service workers. A great deal of information can be obtained in a relatively short period, however, even if only one member of the family is present.

Setting the Stage

Whether the family has been invited to come as a group for an interview or whether one or more family members simply happen to be in a hospital room or at an acute care visit, specific recognition of each individual conveys the message that the clinician finds each person's viewpoint important. Allmond et al. (1979) suggest greeting each person by name and, if possible, making physical contact, such as shaking hands.

Observing the Process of Communication

Traditional medical interviews depend heavily on the content of communication. The goal is to elicit specific statements that reveal important points of medical history or symptoms. Unfortunately, content is not always useful in evaluating behavioral or emotional problems. Individuals may not be able or willing to discuss their concerns openly. Watching how the family communicates, however, may give clues both to the ways family members manipulate each other and to the roles and systems that make up the family structure.

One of the first clues to how the family is structured may be how they enter the interview or examination room and how they seat themselves in relationship to one another. One can observe whether the parents sit together, whether the children stay close to or apart from the parents, and whether one particular child (for example, the one with the "problem") is seated closer to one parent than the other.

Asking for a Statement of the Problem

The discussion can be opened by asking the family members to talk about why they have come for help, avoiding use of the word "problem" (Allmond et al., 1979). When the family has not gathered specifically for a therapy session (because a child has been injured, for example), the clinician's opening remark might be to ask to get to know the family better. In both cases, however, first statements should demonstrate that the clinician is interested in hearing from everyone and that blaming and finger pointing are not intended parts of the assessment process. The clinician may systematically ask each person for a statement; if the "problem" child is present and is old enough to fear that the session is meant to be a form of punishment, that child may be asked to begin.

Dysfunctional Communication

As the discussion begins, the clinician can observe who does most of the talking, who seems to be consulted for permission to talk, and who seeks to control the conversation. Several specific types of dysfunctional communication techniques may be observed (Table 5.1). Speakers may consciously or unconsciously use these techniques to maintain power in the family or to avoid meaningful discussion of troublesome issues. Nearly everyone uses such strategies to some extent, but some individuals persist in using them even when asked to speak more clearly. The fact that they are used can give the clinician clues to how problems develop within the family and offer opportunities for restructuring family relationships by asking individuals to change the manner in which they speak. For example, when

Table 5.1 Patterns of Dysfunctional Communication: Types of Statements That Can Be Used to Subvert or Avoid Meaningful Discussion[a]

1. Overgeneralization.
    He never does that.
    She always is that way.
    Nothing ever works for me.

2. My views reflect universal feelings.
    I just can't image. . .
    Doesn't everyone feel that way?

3. My understanding of things is complete; no other information exists that could enlighten the situation.
    So what's that have to do with it.

4. I'm really not willing to change the way I see things.
    That's just the way things are.
    That's the way things have always been.

5. Everything is black or white.
    If he loved me, he would (wouldn't) do that.

6. Isolated aspects of a person's behavior are indicative of the person's worth and character.
    He doesn't like to clean up his room (and thus is lazy/bad/unloving).
    He yells or gets angry when I try to discuss things (and thus is hostile/uncooperative/selfish).

7. I am so smart and perceptive that I know what other people are thinking (especially my spouse or children).
    What she really means is. . .
    I know what you really want.

8. Other people should be able to ready my mind.
    You know how I feel about that.
    Why do I always have to tell you how I feel?
    You know what I mean!

[a]Adapted from Allmond, BW; Buckman, W; Gofman HF. The family is the patient: an approach to behavioral pediatrics for the clinician. St. Louis: CV Mosby, 1979; Satir V. Conjoint family therapy: a guide to theory and technique. Rev. ed. Palo Alto: Science and Behavior Books, 1967:65–67.

addressed to an individual should be addressed to that person, not made via the clinician or another person; there will be no blaming of other people; and there will be no dredging up of past sins (these may or may not be relevant to the problem at hand, but discussing them often serves as a strategy to avoid talking about more pressing concerns).

Asking Questions

With more than one family member present, launching the discussion of the problem and pointing out some difficulties with communication style may be sufficient to get the family to reveal details of relationships. The clinician can have a greater opportunity to observe, and push the family members to reveal more about themselves, by insisting that he or she not be the conduit through which group communication flows. If the conversation stalls or if only one family member is present, some specific questions can be asked to stimulate thoughts about how the family operates. Wachtel and Wachtel (1986) suggest use of some of the following questions:

- If X has a problem with Y, who would X tell?
- Who does X confide in?
- How would X get word of Y's feelings about something?
- When the parents fight, do the children get involved? What do they do?
- What acute and chronic stresses are being placed on family members or on significant persons such as grandparents, who mistakenly may be considered to be outside the immediate family? Stresses can include financial, health, and job problems, behaviors of certain individuals, or life cycle events such as marriage, the birth of a new child, or the death of a parent's parent.
- Who worries most about problems, and how do they react? Who tries to offer solutions, who supports whom, and who sides with whom in laying blame?
- Beyond what individuals say they feel, what do they actually do?

Another technique for learning how the family functions is asking for an account of a typical day in the home, starting in the morning and finishing with the last person asleep. The clinician can get a picture, for example, of

a speaker is implying that he or she already knows what X would say if asked a particular question, the clinician can say "Maybe you could let X tell us how she feels herself." At times, the clinician may have to make explicit rules about discussion during the evaluation (Allmond et al., 1979): one person speaks at a time; there will be no speaking for other people; statements whether the father actually takes part in any home activities and whether a child's reluctance to attend school is exacerbated by a chaotic or nonexistent morning routine.

The Genogram

The goal of each technique mentioned above is to give the clinician a mental image of how a family is organized and which persons actively influence its activities. Sometimes, if a family seems particularly complicated, if its members seem blocked in their efforts to observe their surroundings, or if there is time for a truly in-depth assessment, working with them to complete an actual drawing of the family tree may be helpful. Family genograms look very similar to a geneticist's pedigree, but they are used to prompt the family to systematically explore its history for myths, cycles of behavior, and unspoken but powerful alliances. One of the genogram's major uses is elicitation of important details that the family knows but has not considered relevant to the problem at hand. Genograms also reinforce the fact that the clinician regards the entire extended family and its history as important to the assessment.

Genograms may be simple or detailed. Systems of notation and lists of pertinent questions are available (McGoldrick and Gerson, 1985). An easy way to start is to sketch the family tree, filling in names, ages, dates of birth and death, dates of marriages and divorces, major health problems, and occupations. Families can be asked whether they remember any stories about particular individuals or if they remember who was close to whom or who admired whom. Histories of maltreatment, unusual death, or removal of children are of special importance. When the family claims that they know very little about a particular individual or branch of the family, the clinician can "wonder out loud" about why that might be the case (Wachtel and Wachtel, 1986). Contrasts with the parallel family trees of cousins, aunts, or uncles may also yield insights into the family's expectations or fears.

Beyond Assessment

This chapter is not intended to be a guide to actually carrying out family therapy; this process is described in the texts referenced above and can be learned in a variety of formal and informal settings. On the other hand, even the assessment process can be helpful to a family if it empathetically helps them become aware of feelings, relationships, and communication styles that may have presented problems. The clinician maximizes this benefit by being aware of a few potential pitfalls.

First, the picture of family relationships drawn at the end of an assessment represents the clinician's hypotheses about the family's functioning, not necessarily the truth. Individuals may have withheld or not yet remembered key information. Alternatively, the clinician's initial interpretations may simply be wrong. Longer contact is usually required before a picture of the family can be clearly established. Second, it follows that the clinician must exercise restraint so as not to dispense a formulation or advice too quickly. Even if the clinician's formulation is correct, direct advice is likely to be resisted or to serve only as another focus for conflict among family members. Ending sessions with a review of the problem as the clinician sees it so far, with some suggested plans for further exploration and with an expression of appreciation for the family's efforts, can at least leave the family feeling hopeful and somewhat relieved. Allmond and co-workers (1979) stress the importance of trying to "touch" each family member with the feeling that he or she has at least been heard. They suggest that the clinician consider the feelings that each family member expressed during the session and to try to acknowledge those feelings by saying something to each person, such as "That does seem very hard" or "I can see why that makes you so happy."

Talking to families, especially about potentially abusive or neglectful situations, can be difficult emotionally for the clinician. Because family assessments focus on the process as well as the content of communication, they do not allow the clinician to hide behind objective questions and rigid control of the clinician-patient discussion. Family therapy techniques essentially require that the clinician become part of the family system, temporarily sharing many of its members' emotions and conflicts. Scharff and Scharff (1987) note several maladaptive responses that clinicians may find themselves using as a means of self-protection. A clinician may become angry with the family, either because of the nature of the maltreatment suspected or because the family's problems evoke frustration and anxiety. Once angry, the clinician may strike back at the family by unsympathetically assaulting its members with a harsh interpretation of their problems. It is important to demonstrate understanding of the family's dilemma, but discussion must be empathetic and tactfully timed.

Sometimes, as an attempt to appear accepting or as a way of denying anger, clinicians will not respond at all to what the family is saying. While it is important for clinicians to show that they are not shocked or scared by a family's story, it is necessary to make a response that acknowledges the seriousness of the problem and validates the family's expression of concern. Otherwise, the family may interpret a lack of response as evidence that the clinician has been "killed off" by its horrible story, and they may be fearful of making further disclosures.

Clinicians may also find themselves taking sides with one or more family members or consistently being reluctant to talk to certain others. This can happen for a variety of reasons. Perhaps foremost is a desire to rescue a child who is suspected of having been maltreated or to punish an individual who is seen as having been particularly cruel or controlling. More subtly, the family may succeed in making the clinician feel unwanted and ineffective, and the clinician's unconscious response may be to form an alliance with more accepting family members or shun those who are seen as rejecting.

TALKING TO PARENTS SUSPECTED OF ABUSE

Facing parents who are suspected of being abusers can be especially stressful. It requires a delicate balance of quiet assertiveness and genuine empathy for the pain of the situation. These encounters are never easy, although some guidelines may help one prepare.

Clinicians should clearly state that they are familiar with methods by which child maltreatment cases are evaluated. The clinician's role can be stated in a few simple words that convey credibility and confidence. Intervention should be presented as a positive step for the entire family, not as an exercise in establishing guilt. If one has reservations about the social service system, one should at least try to be neutral and not convey these reservations as a way of apologizing to the parents for having to intervene. Being negative undermines the clinician's credibility and effectiveness.

If the interview will touch on any topics beyond those required for the abuse victim's immediate treatment, the parents should be informed of the reasons for the interview and the legal procedures (such as reporting) that may be involved. Clinicians taking a medical history should avoid questions directed at establishing responsibility for a particular act of abuse. Such questioning is best left for police or protective service workers. Even when an interview session relates only to the victim's treatment, however, if the parents raise the issue, the clinician should be open about the fact that intentional injury is being considered as a cause of the child's condition.

Managing the clinician's own emotions may be the most difficult part of talking to suspected abusers. The clinician may be angry for having to handle a difficult and time-consuming case. As mentioned above, some abusers or injuries can evoke the interviewer's anger or disgust. One approach to mastering anger is remembering that professional conduct enhances the likelihood that the perpetrator will be properly identified and brought to justice. Inappropriate treatment by professionals advocating for the victim often becomes a courtroom defense for the perpetrator. Another response to one's own anger is to bear in mind that having an empathetic discussion with the abuser does not require condoning what that person has done. Clinicians sometimes prefer to express anger rather than risk appearing to show any support at all for a perpetrator. Saying "I can see how you feel" or "I can see how things must look from your point of view" can convey concern while maintaining the clinician's distance from the abuser's position.

Clinicians sometimes compensate for anger by becoming overly sympathetic or empathetic toward the suspected abuser. These tendencies are often exacerbated by the clinician's feelings of guilt when the abuser becomes uncomfortable during the interview. Challenging a parent's authority makes many clinicians uncomfortable. At some level, nearly everyone has conflicting feelings about the authority of their own parents. These feeling sometimes keep the clinician from asking difficult or personal questions. Questions asked in a tactful and sensitive manner should have the long-term effect of helping rather than hurting the interviewee. It may even be the case that an abuser is looking to the clinician to gently draw out an admission that is difficult to state openly.

One can best cope with anger and guilt by being candid about these feelings and sharing them with colleagues. Abuse cases often leave professionals feeling bad, sad, or incompetent. The problems involved evoke many taboo subjects and emotions, and rarely is there any clear-cut correct therapeutic course or rapid improvement of the situation. One of the key functions of a multidisciplinary approach to abuse cases is to provide support and feedback for each member of the team.

CHARACTERISTICS OF PEOPLE IN CRISIS

The disclosure or suspicion of abuse is often a time of crisis for all members of a family—the victim, the perpetrator, and others who are just becoming aware of the problem. Crises alter the way in which individuals function, and medical personnel must be careful about interpretating crisis behavior (Borgman et al., 1979).

Individuals in crisis may have difficulty focusing and organizing their thoughts. They may omit or dwell on details and seem confused. They may be unable to respond to what staff members consider logical suggestions and thus evoke the anger and frustration of those who seek to help them. Alternatively, individuals in crisis may be able to focus their energies but will concentrate on matters that to others seem unimportant given the current state of affairs. Sometimes energies may be focused impulsively and without apparent regard for whether an action is helpful or harmful. In any case, individuals in crisis need understanding so that they can be gently redirected or given time to regain control.

Hostility exhibited by an individual in crisis may come from a variety of stimuli, one of which is simply a feeling of lost control. Hostility of this type does not automatically represent an admission of guilt or a dislike for the staff. Staff members must temper their reactions accordingly and avoid precipitating a second crisis that diverts attention from the issue at hand. Hostility may be manifested by aggressive behavior or by extreme withdrawal and detachment. It may be that conversations or decisions must simply be deferred until the crisis has partially resolved.

All of the preceding characteristics of crisis mean that those involved are unable to function as well as they might under normal circumstances. Staff members may have to do things for patients that they would otherwise be expected to do for themselves. It is important that this dependence not be automatically interpreted as unwillingness to cooperate, and it is equally important that providers not count on patients in crisis to take critical steps in their own care such as arranging a follow-up appointment or finding adequate emergency shelter. A crisis is not a time to insist on patient "motivation" or to feel that one is being taken advantage of as a provider. Staff members must be careful not to usurp what control or competency the patient retains, but they must be willing to step in and provide direction until the crisis wanes.

CLINICAL DESCRIPTIONS OF FAMILIES IN ABUSE AND NEGLECT

Although the following descriptions may not be entirely supported by research evidence, they form a useful basis for organizing a clinical evaluation and formulating initial treatment plans.

Physical Abuse

Families in which physical abuse occurs may display a number of qualities, many of which stem from the parents' own lack of social and emotional development (Anonymous, 1979). The parents may themselves have been physically or emotionally abused as children. They feel that their needs for nurturing and dependence have never been met, and they react with anger to those who seek nurturing from them. They have poor social skills and cannot cultivate the supports they need. They may in fact seem to encourage rejection because that is less threatening to them than the challenge of forming a relationship.

Physically abusive parents thus are often socially isolated. They may seek to satisfy their emotional needs by placing unrealistic developmental or emotional demands on their children. When the children fail to meet these demands, the parents become angry and abuse may result. The demands may escalate if a parent has suffered a recent stress or crisis.

Intrafamilial Sexual Abuse

Sexual abuse often occurs in families that outwardly seem highly organized and functional (MacFarlane, 1979). In fact, these families are often isolated and have poor extra- and intrafamilial relationships that are worsened by alcohol abuse. The parents may have a strained and hostile relationship, with little or no sexual intimacy.

The abusing father is often outwardly well functioning. The same rigid interpersonal conservatism that makes him do well on the job may make his family relationships very difficult. He typically has low self-esteem and functions poorly on a social basis with other adults. These characteristics may not apply to stepfathers, who seem much more likely than biologic fathers to sexually abuse their daughters.

The role of the mother in intrafamilial sexual abuse, especially the assertion that she often is aware that the abuse is taking place, has been subject to much debate. It does seem likely, however, that mothers to some extent adopt a passive or powerless role that at least facilitates abuse. This may progress to a full abdication of the mother's role as the woman of the house, a role that, along with its sexual component, is turned over to the daughter. The mother herself may have been a victim of sexual abuse as a child or she may have been abused by a previous or present spouse. These scars on her development may have left feelings of helplessness and immobility; fearing the total dissolution of her family, the mother may consciously or unconsciously aid in perpetuating abuse. If there is a component of physical violence in the family, the mother may fear that any attempt to intervene will endanger her own or the child's safety.

Child Neglect

Neglectful mothers (fathers have been less well studied) may fall into one of several categories: those who are victims of the apathy-futility syndrome, those who are overly impulsive, the mentally retarded, the extremely depressed, and those few who are actively psychotic (Polansky et al., 1981). Apathetic mothers probably make up the single largest identifiable group. These mothers are passive, withdrawn, and verbally inaccessible. They see much of life as a futile endeavor; therefore, although they may be quite capable, they fail to carry out day-to-day tasks that others routinely perform. They may be intensely lonely and clinging but react to helpful suggestions with passive-aggressive behavior and resistance. A major weapon in their resistance to change is the ability to evoke feelings of futility in those who try to help them.

Overly impulsive parents may also come to neglect their children. Unable to formulate plans or think out difficulties, when faced with stress they develop maladaptive responses that often exacerbate their problems. They may be fully aware of their children's needs but unable to organize their own lives to meet them.

References

Allmond BW, Buckman W, Gofman HF. The family is the patient: an approach to behavioral pediatrics for the clinician. St. Louis: CV Mosby, 1979.

Anonymous. Characteristics of abusive families. In: Leader's manual, we can help, a curriculum on child abuse and neglect. National Center for Child Abuse and Neglect. DHEW publ. (OHDS) 79-30220. Washinton, DC: US Government Printing Office, 1979.

Borgman R, Edmunds M, MacDicken RA. Crisis intervention: a manual for child protective workers. DHEW publ. (OHDS) 79-30196. Washington, DC: US Government Printing Office, 1979.

Haley J. Problem-solving therapy: new strategies for effective family therapy. San Francisco: Jossey-Bass, 1976.

Jackson DD. The question of family homeostasis. Psychiatr Q Suppl 1957;31:79–90.

MacFarlane K. Sexual abuse of children. In: Leader's manual, we can help, a curriculum on child abuse and neglect. National Center for Child Abuse and Neglect. DHEW publ. (OHDS) 79-30220, Washington, DC: US Government Printing Office, 1979.

McGoldrick M, Gerson R. Genograms in family assessment. New York: WW Norton & Co, 1985.

Minuchin S. Families and family therapy. Cambridge, Massachusetts: Harvard University Press, 1974.

Money J, Werlas J. *Folie à deux* in the parents of psychosocial dwarfs: two cases. Bull Am Acad Psychiatry Law 1976;4:351–362.

Polansky NA, Chalmers MA, Buttenwieser E, Williams DP. Damaged parents: an anatomy of child neglect. Chicago: University of Chicago Press, 1981.

Satir V. Conjoint family therapy: a guide to theory and technique. Rev. ed. Palo Alto: Science and Behavior Books, 1967.

Scharff DE, Scharff JS. Object relations family therapy. Northvale, New Jersey: Jason Aronson, 1987.

Wachtel EF, Wachtel PL. Family dynamics in individual psychotherapy. New York: Guilford Press, 1986.

6 The Medical History and the Physical Examination

THE GENERAL APPROACH TO ABUSE AND NEGLECT CASES

It is impossible to give one all purpose approach to evaluating cases of suspected child maltreatment. Sometimes the clinician is asked to evaluate a case of known or highly suspected abuse, sometimes skeptical caretakers want abuse ruled out, and other (perhaps most) times, suspicions grow while a child is being examined for a totally unrelated complaint. In all of these situations, a few general guidelines remain constant.

First, as in any clinical encounter, the most important task is to assess the patient's need for immediate medical and psychological care. Other medical-legal considerations are important, but they are secondary to a consideration of the patient's immediate needs.

During the evaluation, the clinician must attempt to maintain both an appropriate level of suspicion and a neutral, objective attitude. One can be either too concerned about abuse or not concerned enough. It is easy to get angry and jump to a conclusion or to take an opposite course and rationalize an incomplete examination so as to avoid confrontation (see Chapter 5).

It is important to keep in mind that the physical exam and medical history are only part of the data that will ultimately be used to determine whether a child has been maltreated. Evaluations by other medical professionals, by social service agencies, and possibly by law enforcement officials may all enter into the final determination of whether abuse or neglect has taken place. In the primary or urgent care medical setting, the clinician's task is generally to establish, from the medical perspective, whether there is a reasonable basis for suspecting maltreatment. Proof is not required.

It is helpful to remember, and to remind parents and other professionals, that in only a minority of cases can medical findings stand alone as evidence of abuse. Indeed, in most cases there may be no medical findings at all. Consequently, one should never write "no evidence of abuse" as the conclusion of an initial examination. It is preferable to note that the examination found no abnormalities and to mention in the final assessment that this does not eliminate the possibility that some form of maltreatment has taken place.

Finally, it is important to fulfill one's medical-legal obligations. Findings must be carefully documented so that their meaning can later be evaluated in court or by other authorities. If abuse is suspected, the appropriate authorities must be notified. (These tasks are discussed later in this chapter and in Chapter 19.)

There are three main steps in the evaluation of a child suspected of having been abused: (1) the initial medical history and social assessment, (2) the physical exam and diagnostic testing, and (3) the investigative interview(s) of the child and family. The first two steps (also discussed in Chapters 7–10) are usually performed by a physician, nurse practitioner, or physician's assistant, sometimes aided by a social worker who helps develop the social history. Investigative interviews (described in Chapters 3 and 4) are usually carried out by a social worker, psychiatrist, or other mental health professional experienced in talking to children who may have been maltreated. All clinicians, however, should be aware of the ground rules for performing investigative interviews so that they know which questions to ask and which to avoid.

INITIAL MEDICAL HISTORY

The goals of the initial history are to establish immediate treatment needs and to start formulating a level of suspicion of abuse. Unfortunately, in real abuse cases the medical history is often misleading or false. Improbable or inconsistent stories are important elements of diagnosing abuse, but they they do not help uncover a child's immediate medical problems. In some cases, such as those that actually involve difficult-to-diagnose abdominal trauma, for example, overreliance on a misleading history frequently leads to dangerous delays in treatment. A careful physical exam is mandatory the moment one suspects that the history may be unreliable.

Hearsay

Any history given must be carefully recorded. Because explanations that change with repetition are suggestive of abuse, clinicians involved in the case later will want to check what they have heard with what was told to other observers. Initial statements by parents or children may also have importance as courtroom evidence. In most judicial proceedings, a witness is not permitted to give accounts of what he or she has been told by others. These accounts are usually considered hearsay and cannot be admitted as direct evidence that something has happened. There are, however, a number of exceptions to hearsay rules that may apply to clinical encounters and thus may allow consideration of crucial evidence about a case (Myers, 1986). The extent to which these exceptions are allowed varies from jurisdiction to jurisdiction and from judge to judge. They are much more likely to be made in juvenile or family court cases, where rules of evidence are often ill defined, than in criminal courts, where evidentiary standards are much more strict. Some states have enacted laws that specifically create hearsay rule exceptions to be used in abuse proceedings so that children will not have to testify directly (for example, the so-called tender years exception in Maryland [Md. Cts. & Jud. Proc. Code Ann. Sect. 9-103.1], which applies to children's testimony in criminal prosecutions of child abusers).

So-called excited utterances, or statements made at a time of stress and crisis such as when abuse is initially disclosed or evaluated in an emergency medical setting, may be admitted as evidence if they have been accurately recorded. Their admissibility as evidence is based on the theory that they are spontaneous statements made without time for reflection. (Although the notion of the excited utterance originally applied to statements made immediately after an episode of trauma, in cases involving children courts have sometimes accepted statements made long after an event [Whitcomb et al., 1985]). It is important for the clinician to note whether the statement was spontaneous or the result of a question and whether the affect accompanying the statement suggested stress or excitement. Indications of who was present at the time the statement was made may also suggest whether or not it was made freely.

A related exception to hearsay rules allows consideration of statements made to a physician in the course of diagnosis and treatment. Although it certainly is not always the case in situations involving abuse, there is a certain presumption that individuals tell physicians the truth because they have a direct interest in receiving proper treatment. Therefore, physicians are generally allowed to testify as to the medical history given by a patient and to state the conclusions they have reached based on that history (for example, In re Rachel T., Md. Ct. Special Appeals, No. 400, Sept. term, 1988). Although the limits of this exception are frequently contested, in theory the physician's testimony may include any information gathered from the patient in order to make a diagnosis or develop a treatment plan, even when that same information related simply as part of the child's story would be considered hearsay. For example, in a case of suspected sexual abuse, a clinician may assert that knowing the identity of the abuser is important to deciding what diagnostic tests to use (for sexually transmitted diseases, for example) and to determining whether it is safe for the child to leave the medical facility. When describing the diagnosis and treatment in court, the clinician may then be able to enter the child's identification of the abuser into evidence.

A carefully completed chart can itself be admitted as evidence, possibly sparing the physician the need to testify in person. In many jurisdictions, hospital, physician office, or laboratory records are considered to be documents kept regularly in the course of business (for example, Md. Cts. & Jud. Proc. Code Ann., Sect. 10-101, 1974, 1984 Repl. Vol.). Business records are presumed to be accurate and unbiased, with those who challenge them having the burden to prove otherwise. The major requirement for admissibilty of information under this exception, and the other exceptions to hearsay noted above, is that the information be elicited and documented because it was germane to treating a medical condition. A brief case history can illustrate how hearsay exceptions can work and why documenting them in the medical record can be vital:

An infant was brought to the emergency room by his mother. The mother was tearful and had bruises on her face. She told the examining physician that her boyfriend had come to her apartment and had become angry with her. In the course of beating her, he also kicked the infant several times before ultimately leaving the apartment. The physician wrote this down as part of his medical history, including the name of the person the mother identified as the assailant. The police and child protective services were notified, and the boyfriend was charged with assault. When the case came to criminal court, however, the mother refused to testify against her boyfriend. She went so far as to deny that she had ever named him as the assailant. The trial judge, however, allowed the emergency room physician to read the medical records in court and to enter into evidence the mother's statement as to what had happened. The boyfriend was convicted.

Obtaining the History

When a child is old enough to give a history, one should always ask to speak to him or her away from the family. This may not be possible if the child is too fearful or if the parents are suspicious and refuse. If a family member must be present when the child is giving the initial history, it is best to seat that person so that there is no eye contact with the child (family member and child side by side facing the clinician is the optimal arrangement).

It is important to establish the source of the information being obtained. When the informant is an adult, determine whether the informant is a regular caretaker for the child and the relationship between them. If the evaluation involves a question of trauma, ask whether the informant was actually a witness or whether the information was obtained secondhand. One must be careful to ask for details of events and not to make assumptions about what has happened or volunteer answers. Questions should be open ended (What do you think happened? What are your concerns? What happened next?) rather than leading (Do you think she could have fallen off of the bed? Are you worried that she might have hurt her head? So next you called the ambulance?). A useful technique for both verifying what has been heard and making a reply that does not lead or suggest is to simply repeat what the parent or child has just said. When inquiring about previous illnesses or treatments, enough information should be obtained so that the history can be verified if necessary (including the name and location of hospitals, clinics, physicians, and schools and approximate dates when the services were used).

The clinician must also be alert for aspects of the history that do not make sense in light of his or her clinical experience. Does the story fit the child's developmental age and abilities? Does the proposed mechanism of injury seem plausible given the nature of the child's injuries? Have other children with similar types of trauma suffered the same degree of injury to the same part of the body? (Comparisons of injury characteristics and expected injury patterns from specific types of trauma are discussed in Chapter 9.) Do the symptoms fit with any fairly common condition, or is it necessary to imagine combinations of unlikely conditions to explain the child's illness?

Although it is not often easy, the clinician should try to remain empathetic and nonaccusatory during the evaluation. In many cases, the clinician will choose not to directly mention a concern for abuse at the outset of a discussion. If asked, however, one should usually be candid about the fact that abuse is one of the diagnoses being considered. In most cases, one can truthfully assure parents that they are not the ones suspected of abuse. Ideally, clinician and parent can form an alliance to determine what has happened to the child. The clinician can further this alliance by being interested in and attentive to both the parents' feelings and the condition of the child.

The Physician's Social History

In most abuse and neglect cases, a social worker is ultimately called on to take a detailed family and social history. A nurse practitioner, physician's assistant, or physician, however, is usually the first person to contact the family. Obtaining social information at this early stage may help determine whether a more thorough evaluation is needed. Several items are important, and asking about them usually takes relatively little time.

INFORMATION ABOUT THE PARENTS

What are the parents' ages, occupations, and extent of contact with the child? Does either of the parents have any major illnesses? If so, what medications might be in the home? Are the parents under any particular stresses, such as financial difficulties, job conflicts, or the recent death of someone close? Is there a history of spouse abuse or other violence in the family? Does either of the parents have a problem with alcohol?

INFORMATION ABOUT CHILD CARE IN THE HOME

Who is the child's primary caretaker and who else (sitters, relatives) has a caretaking role? What other children live in the home, and are there siblings who do not live there? What is the health status of these children? Have any siblings died? If so, from what cause? What type of home does the child live in? Do the parents describe it as adequate, or does it have major safety or crowding problems? Does anyone else live there?

Review of Systems

The standard medical "review of systems" is usually too lengthy to be used in an outpatient setting. Certain questions, however, may reveal specifics germane to the concern for maltreatment.

Where does the child go for maintenance health care? Has the child received basic preventive health care such as immunizations? Have there been difficulties with pregnancy, labor, delivery, or the perinatal period that may have resulted in the child being labeled as sickly? In infancy, were or are there feeding difficulties such as colic, refusal of food, or inadequate weight gain? Have there been difficulties with toilet training or relapses of bed wetting? Are the parents' expectations for these motor or self-care skills appropriate for the child's age and development? The presence of chronic health problems (asthma, a learning disability, cerebral palsy, etc.) that require special medical attention or can impair functioning or interaction may also be markers for families in which there is higher risk of abuse.

Is there a history of trauma, including broken bones, serious falls, burns, cuts, or ingestions? Have there been hospitalizations, especially for difficult-to-diagnose problems? In cases of suspected sexual abuse, is there a history of penile, vaginal, or rectal bleeding, discomfort, or unusual discharge? Has the child ever had a urinary tract infection or a sexually transmitted disease?

Do the parents feel that the child has any behavior problems? Specifically, do they feel that this is a difficult child to care for? Do they feel that they are able to make the child happy? Has there been a change in the child's behavior or functioning, such as an increase in problems with discipline, a decline in performance in school, or a loss of interest in previously enjoyable activities? Have there been more severe behavior problems, such as stealing, running away, violent behavior toward other children, problems with the law, or a suggestion of alcohol or drug abuse?

A variety of parent questionnaires have been developed to screen for children's behavioral problems (Schroeder et al., 1983). Questionnaires can be more efficient than interviews with the parents, although they require careful follow-up. The 35-item Pediatric Symptom Checklist (Jellinek et al., 1988), for example, is one of the shorter instruments available for screening school-age children. Parents are asked to answer "never," "sometimes," or "often" to questions about their child, such as "Is your child down on himself or herself?", "Does your child feel he or she is bad?", and "Does your child not show his or her feelings?" When compared with in-depth, standardized psychiatric interviews, the questionnaire was quite sensitive (95%), but relatively less specific (68%) for detecting children with emotional difficulties. These are potentially acceptable characteristics for a screening test, but they illustrate the need for further evaluation before one labels children who screen positive. Furthermore, most testing of such instruments has been with groups of children making general pediatric office visits. Much less is known about how these instruments perform with more impaired children or families or whether they can be used to identify children who are victims of maltreatment.

PHYSICAL EXAMINATION

The physical examination of a potentially abused child must be therapeutic as well as diagnostic. The child may have very little sense of personal security or control over his or her life. One purpose for conducting the exam is to assure the child that he or she is well, is respected as a person, and has some degree of control over what happens. A first step toward achieving this goal is to find the quietest and calmest setting consistent with the child's level of illness. Privacy and modesty are also of paramount importance, even for very young children. The door to the examination room should be kept closed or a curtain drawn. Drapes and gowns should be used as they would be for adults. Preschool children may appreciate having a choice of which color gown to wear or whether to tie it in front or back.

The physical examination should generally be complete, from head to toe. There are two reasons for this. First, because the history may be misleading, there may be surprise findings. Second, the exam gives the child a chance to experience the clinician's touch and presence before having to expose sensitive or embarrassing areas of the body.

Preparations should be made to document physical findings. Required supplies include a ruler or measuring tape, a good light, and anatomic diagrams on which to mark. Photographs may be deferred until the end of the exam (see Chapter 10). Drawings of major findings should be made and labeled (noting location, size, and color) while the patient is still available.

General Appearance

Observation of the child may give clues about ongoing abuse or neglect. The general body habitus, especially among infants, may give clues to nutritional or emotional status. Plotting the child's height, weight, and (for infants) head circumference on a growth chart is more accurate than estimating adequacy of growth, especially if one does not frequently examine small children. Plotting weight as a function of height may also reveal nutritional problems in children who are formally on the curve but are substantially thinner than their height would suggest. Plotting growth parameters from birth and previous health care visits can help one better interpret the child's present status (see Chapter 12).

Lack of clean clothing and poor personal hygiene are frequently taken as signs of neglect, but they are poor predictors that a child comes from an abusive home (Rosenberg et al., 1982; Balaban and Goldfarb, 1983). Likewise, the fact that a child is inadequately clothed for the prevailing weather may be a sign of neglect but it may also simply be a reflection of poverty. Of more concern is a child with injuries, even minor, that suggest neglect, inattention to simple home first aid, or a delay in seeking medical care.

The child's behavior in the exam room may give clues about abuse or neglect. Anxiety over a physical examination, especially of the genitalia, is difficult to evaluate. Fears may be based on abusive experiences, but they also may be attributable to family taboos, what parents have said about the examination, or previous, unpleasant medical experiences. Behaviors suggesting anxious or avoidant attachment (extreme anxious clinging associated with stress, anger directed at the attachment figure after separation or stress) may be more common in abusive or neglectful families (see Chapter 13), as may indiscriminant affection displayed toward strangers and combative or destructive behaviors with peers or toys. These behaviors, however, are not specific to maltreated children and therefore can serve only as initial indicators warranting further exploration. Behavioral abnormalities in infants who have been severely neglected are discussed in Chapter 12.

The interaction between the parent, child, and other family members may also provide clues to the presence of abuse or neglect. Some observations are nonspecific and suggestive only of general problems with family functioning. Other findings may be more specific to families in which abuse is taking place. Some general observations include the following:

- How do members of the family communicate with each other? Are messages given clearly, or are there discrepancies between the words used and the accompanying vocal tone or visual message? Are other family members able to understand these mixed messages or do they become confused?
- How does the family seem to make decisions that affect more than one member? Is there a great deal of quarreling? Does anyone in the family seem able to negotiate a solution rather than impose one? Is there difficulty in perceiving and assessing options or in seeing a problem from the perspective of other family members? Must the children always adapt to the parents' perspective, or is there evidence that the adults can appreciate a child's different point of view?
- Do the family members seem capable of shar-

ing authority or taking turns and allowing various members to temporarily set the group's agenda?

Patterns of interaction in maltreating families do appear to differ from patterns in families in which maltreatment does not occur, although these differences are mostly of degree and not type of behavior (Wolfe, 1985). Abusive parents are more likely to be negative and abusive with each other, a behavior that may be observed in the medical setting or determined by questioning one of the parents. Abusive parents are not necessarily more negative than nonabusive parents toward their children, but they are less likely to be positive. That is, the overall amount of communication with the child is reduced by a lack of positive interaction, and the predominant tone is therefore negative. Even when the child tries in positive ways to initiate interaction with the parent, the response is likely to be relatively negative. Although the stereotypical abusive parent is one who responds to child misbehavior in harsh or punitive ways, in fact many abusive parents (at least when observed) are more likely to respond in a manner that is simply ineffective. It is perhaps this lack of effective strategies for discipline that eventually leads to situations in which the parent loses control. In some cases, the parent and child actually seem to be egging each other on rather than seeking to terminate a confrontational episode; the child will behave in a provocative way, and the parent will respond inappropriately by in turn trying to provoke the child. In contrast to physically abusive parents, those who are neglectful seem more likely to blunt their reactions to the the child's behavior, whether it is positive or negative. When they do respond, however, such parents are even more likely to be negative than abusers.

Opportunities to observe these sorts of interactions abound in medical settings, especially where children and parents must wait for services. The predictive value of a negative interaction for detecting maltreatment, however, is not known, nor is it certain how reliably such interactions can be detected by clinicians. For example, Starr (1987) showed videotapes of parent-child interactions to a group of health professionals and college undergraduates. Some of the parents were known to have abused their children, and others were control subjects recruited from the wards of an acute care hospital. As a group, neither the professionals nor the students could reliably say which parents were the abusers. The findings of the study may be overly pessimistic, however, for two reasons. First, the control group contained some children who had been diagnosed as having nonorganic failure to thrive. It may be that the parents of these children interacted similarly to those who were physically abusive. Second, the researcher did not document that there were, in fact, observable differences in the interactions of these particular abusive and nonabusive parent-child pairs.

Another study, this one involving observations made by pediatric residents, suggested that physicians base their opinions of parent-child interactions on relatively scant data (Leventhal et al., 1986). The residents were much more likely to form their opinions from the parents' behavioral style in the examining room rather than from observations of specific parenting skills or from interview material about the parents' feelings toward the child.

Bruises and Bites

Bruises and other skin lesions are the most common manifestations of physical abuse. It is important to note their number, location, shape, and color. Children suffer many accidental injuries, and active toddlers and school-age children may have many bruises and abrasions at any given time. These injuries, however, are usually over bony areas such as the shins, knees, elbows, and forehead. Injuries in other areas, especially to soft tissues such as the abdomen, genitalia, buttocks, or mouth, are more worrisome.

Bilateral injuries to the eyes or orbits are unusual in unintentional trauma because the prominence of the nose makes it difficult to strike both sides of the face at the same time. Exceptions include injuries to the nose and basilar skull fractures, both of which can cause bilateral bruising under the eyes. Injuries to the inner aspects of the upper or lower arm may occur when the arms are raised to protect the face from a blow. If the child's upper arm has been forcefully gripped, the upper arm may show round bruises in the shape and distribution of fingertips or shallow, crescent-shaped abrasions from fingernails. Similar injuries may also appear on the legs.

Bruises at multiple sites that appear to be of different ages are also suggestive of abuse. The color of a bruise is a rough indicator of how long ago it was inflicted. Bruises are caused when trauma ruptures blood vessels and blood escapes into the skin. At first, the bruise is dark red or violet; as hemoglobin from the blood is broken down, the bruise turns blue-brown (in about 1–3 days), then yellow-green (by about a week), and finally light brown (after more than a week). Two to four weeks from the time of injury, the bruise is usually gone (Wilson, 1977). The progression of colors in a bruise and the timing of their appearance can be quite variable, however. Deep bleeding may not be apparent immediately and may therefore appear to take longer to change color. The surface appearance may not correspond to the location of the injury. Some bruises that the clinician expects to find may not appear at all, possibly because a child has died or gone into shock before blood reached the surface layers of the skin. In some of these cases, the postmortem examination can reveal bruising at deeper tissue levels, often in the shape of an object used to deliver a blow.

A consequence of this variablility is that bruises are difficult to date in an absolute sense, but for a given child bruises of different colors, especially if they are clustered on one site, imply injuries taking place on more than one occasion. A second consequence is that bruises which are initially indistinct may become better defined as more blood comes to the surface or as the color of the bruises becomes more visible against the background of the child's skin color. Serial observations of bruises are therefore desirable, both to better determine how the bruise was inflicted (as its shape becomes more apparent) and to document color changes that may serve to date the injury. In addition, as described below, some permanent pigment changes in children's skin can be mistaken for bruising. Serial observation can confirm that these markings do not change color or shape and thus are not indicative of recent injury.

Because it is very difficult to describe the color of a bruise in words, photographs should be taken whenever possible. Instant cameras often give poor color rendition but are better than nothing; a camera with color roll film and appropriate lighting (daylight or a flashgun) is better. The picture should include a sample of some known colors and a ruled edge (see Chapter 10).

The shape of an injury may be a clue to its etiology. Some of the few lesions that are virtually diagnostic of abuse fall into this category. A looped cord leaves a characteristic mark in the shape of a large, elongated hairpin. The loop may have a double "railroad track" appearance if it was inflicted with an electrical cord (Fig. 6.1), or it may be abraded if it was inflicted with a rough-surfaced rope. Belt buckles also leave characteristic marks, usually a long band (from the belt itself) terminating in a horseshoe-shaped mark from the buckle (Fig. 6.2). A flat palm with spread fingers also leaves a mark that the examiner can test by superimposing his or her own hand. Half-moon-shaped bruises or abrasions may result from the heel of a shoe that was held in the hand and used as a weapon; marks on the chest or abdomen can occur when a child is trodden on while supine (Fig. 6.3). Restraints on the wrists or ankles may leave circumferential bruises, abrasions, or burns. The skin may be thickened and discolored if the restraints were applied repeatedly or for a long period of time. Similar marks at the corners of the mouth, often paired with linear marks on the neck, result from gagging. Petechial lesions from the neck up, with or without bruising or cord-like lesions on the neck, may be a sign of strangulation, although they can result from coughing or vomiting as well.

Bite marks can be very important findings in cases of suspected maltreatment. Whereas many marks on the skin provide nonspecific evidence of trauma, a bite indicates intentional contact by another individual. In addition, while other marks can sometimes establish that a child has been abused, bites can, in some cases, provide evidence of the identity of the abuser. They also have a dramatic impact on professionals that can help a case get needed services from law enforcement or social service agencies.

Bites usually appear as a elliptical or ovoid abrasions, bruises, or lacerations (Figs. 6.4 and 6.5). Contact with only one of the dental arches (mandibular or maxillary) creates an ellipse or crescent, while an oval lesion represents contact with both arches. A reddened area in the center of the mark may result from the force of sucking or from folding of the skin as it is compressed between the teeth (Jakobsen and Keiser-Nielsen, 1981). When marks from both arches are visible, it may be possible to distinguish them. The central incisors of the upper, maxillary arch

56 **Child Advocacy for the Clinician**

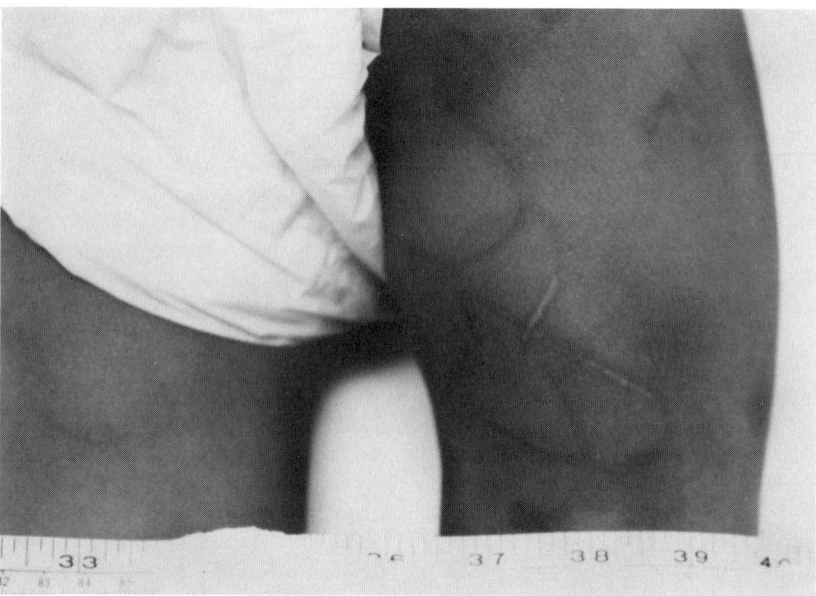

Figure 6.1. Multiple marks on a child's thigh from a looped cord. Some of the marks have the double-lined "railroad track" characteristic of injuries inflicted with two-wire electrical cord.

are wider than the corresponding lower, mandibular teeth. Orienting the bite may help a forensic dentist determine the relative positions of the child and the assailant at the time of the biting. This may help confirm or discredit a history of the event given by either party.

Bite marks are rarely perfect castings of an assailant's mouth. The mechanics of biting are complex and involve sequential motion of the jaw in several directions. Simultaneous sucking or movement of the assailant or victim may distort the shape of the bite or blur the impressions of the teeth. The dimensions of the bite will always be somewhat distorted because the occlusal plane in which the teeth come together is not flat. Therefore, any two-dimensional representation of the bite will be distorted, just as a two-dimensional map distorts differences between points on the curved surface of the earth. In addition, the victim's skin is an elastic and curved surface itself, and its configuration at the time of a bite may well be different from its natural position. Even distorted marks, however, so long as they are relatively clear, can often be unequivocally identified as bites and thus strongly suggest abuse. It is also fairly easy to distinguish human from animal bites. Human teeth are relatively wide and dull and result in crushing and bruising injuries. Animal teeth, in contrast, are sharp and often cause punctures or lacerations. The human dental arch is relatively wide and shallow, 2.5–4 cm across between the maxillary canine teeth (Committee on Early Childhood, Adoption, and Dependent Care, 1986), whereas animal mouths are usually longer and narrower. The diameter of a bite may also suggest that it was inflicted by an adult rather than a child; an intercanine distance of 3 cm or more most likely represents an adult bite.

Biting is apparently rather common in a variety of human encounters. Baker and Moore (1987), in a retrospective study of children seen in an urban emergency room for bites, found that about 60% of the bites were inflicted during fights and about 25% during "play"; 7% were received during sexual activity, and only a handful were acknowledged to have occurred as part of physical abuse. The age distributions of male and female patients were notably different: more than 60% of the girls who were bitten were over 11 years old, compared with only 39% of the boys. About 75% of all the bites were on the face, neck, or trunk.

Biting may also occur as part of some folk medicine traditions. Cases have been reported

Medical History and Physical Exam 57

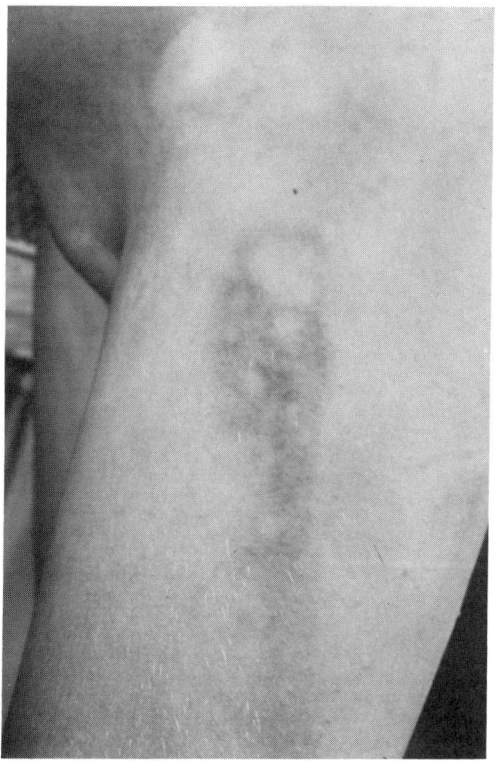

Figure 6.2. Bruise on a child's thigh suggestive of injury with a belt. The long, linear nature of the bruise suggests a belt strap, while the semicircular mark at the top of the bruise suggests a buckle.

in which Chinese parents bit infants who appeared cyanotic in the belief that the resulting pain would stimulate respiration (Leung, 1985).

Perhaps because most bites are inflicted during fighting or sexual arousal, bite marks in cases of suspected child abuse are generally in the same locations as those resulting from other causes. Bites in the context of sexual offenses may be on the breasts, stomach, or genitals; those intended as punishment may be found on the ear lobes, nose, or trunk (Trube-Becker, 1977). In cases seen at our hospital in an urban area of the eastern United States, bites on the wrists or lower arm seem particularly common in cases of neglect and physical abuse.

Specific steps must be taken to preserve the maximum amount of information obtainable from bite marks. If a mark appears relatively fresh, it should be examined repeatedly over a period of days. Because most bites involve bruising, the outline of the dentition may improve as the bruise evolves. Changes in color may also help one date the time of the bite or at least confirm that the lesion was fresh when first seen. Observations should be carefully documented, including the location of the bite, the contour of the skin surface, the size and number of tooth marks visible, and the diameter of the mark or the intercanine distance (if this can be identified). As with any other skin lesion in a case of suspected abuse, multiple bites or bites that appear to be of different ages should be carefully noted. Photographs, when equipment is available, should include color standards and a ruler. Views should include both close-ups of the bite itself and a wider-angle, orienting view that shows the bite in relationship to the rest of the victim's body. To minimize distortion of the mark's apparent dimensions, the camera should be held parallel to the plane of the mark. When possible, serial photographs of the bite should be taken to record its evolution and to provide every chance for correctly assessing its dimensions.

Bites seen within a few hours of the time inflicted should be swabbed for remains of the assailant's saliva. A cotton swab can be moistened with saline and passed over the bite. Because identification may involve testing for blood group antigens in the saliva, it is important to avoid areas of the bite that are abraded so as not to contaminate the swab with the victim's blood. The swab should be dried in cool air and placed in a paper envelope for transfer to a forensic laboratory.

If tooth marks are still embossed in the skin, an examination by a forensic dentist or pathologist offers the best chance of making a precise identification of the assailant. Teeth, like fingerprints, have unique characteristics, and many experts feel that unequivocal identification is possible from a sufficiently clear and well-studied bite mark (Sognnaes, 1977). Proper study of the mark includes careful photography and taking of impressions that can later be compared against experimental bites made from casts of the suspected assailant's dentition (American Board of Forensic Odontology, Inc., 1986; Drinnan and Melton, 1985).

Injuries from Deadly Weapons

The possibility of abuse or neglect frequently arises when children receive firearm or

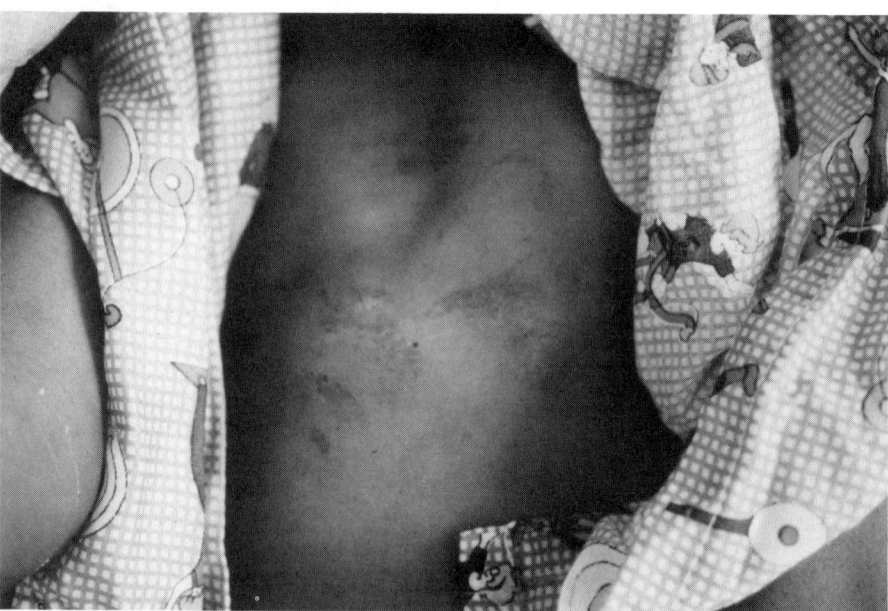

Figure 6.3. Semicircular abraded marks over a developmentally delayed child's sternum and upper abdomen. The child was found to have a duodenal hematoma. It was thought that the marks came from the heel of a shoe, probably when the child was forcefully stepped on while lying on the floor.

knife wounds. Firearms are dangerous items to have in a home. In one study of household firearm fatalities, guns were just as likely to cause "accidental" death as they were to be used in self-defense (Kellerman and Reay, 1986). Suicides outnumbered justifiable homicides by nearly 40 to 1. Children often shoot each other when they find weapons in the home and mistake them for toys or assume that they are not loaded (Wintermute et al., 1987).

The use of deadly weapons is distressingly frequent in domestic violence. The National Family Violence Survey (discussed in Chapter 1) found that about 3–5% of families reported the use or threat of guns or knives in conflicts between siblings and spouses or in force directed at children (Straus et al., 1981). Even when not directly involved in family conflicts, children may be injured as "innocent bystanders" when their parents direct deadly weapons at each other (Nelson, 1984). Children can also be injured when they are literally caught in the crossfire of violent neighborhoods.

A careful examination of gunshot or knife wounds can help substantiate or discredit the explanation offered. Wound characteristics may help identify the type of weapon used, and retained projectiles can sometimes be used to identify a particular weapon and thus its owner. All gunshot wounds, and all knife wounds suspected of being intentionally inflicted, must be reported to law enforcement authorities. The clinician's role is to preserve as much evidence as possible, given the patient's need for urgent care.

A bullet's kinetic energy, primarily its linear velocity and spin, is the predominant determinant of the extent of tissue damage in a gunshot wound. A projectile needs to travel at about 150 feet/second to penetrate skin and about 195 feet/second to break bone (Ordog et al., 1984). These speeds are easily exceeded by the muzzle velocity (the speed with which the bullet leaves the gun) of nearly all handguns and rifles. Small handguns have a muzzle velocity of over 700 feet/second, while even target rifles such as a 22-gauge shoot bullets at over 1000 feet/second. These speeds are essentially constant within about 100 feet of the gun; beyond that, velocity falls off as a function of both distance and the type of bullet used. A 22-gauge rifle with a hollow-point bullet, for example, has a muzzle velocity of about 2700 feet/second. At a distance of 300 feet, the bullet's speed falls by nearly

Medical History and Physical Exam   59

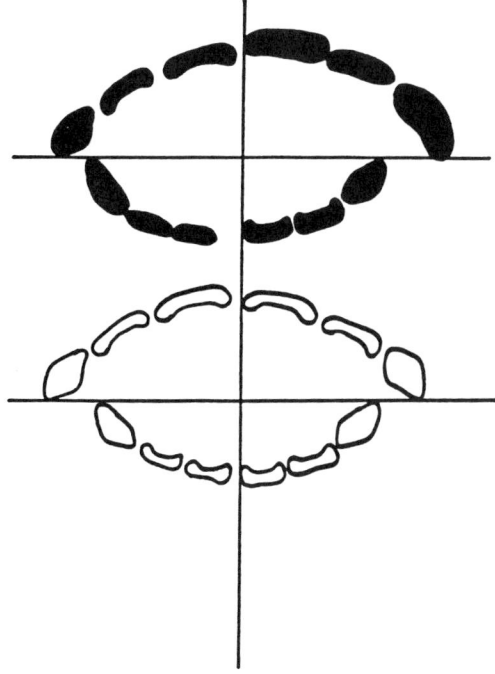

Figure 6.4. Schematic drawing of a human bite mark (*top*) and a dental impression made from the assailant's teeth (*bottom*). The upper crescent would presumably represent the maxillary teeth, as evidenced by the greater width of the central incisors. The drawings have been made to show how the bite may be distorted and result in measurements that do not match the assailant's bite. Only the teeth to the left of the center line match those of the dental impression. (From Rawson RD, Vale GL, Sperber ND, Herschaft EE, Yfantis A. Reliability of the scoring system of the American Board of Forensic Odontology for human bite marks. J Forensic Sci 1986;31:1235–1260. Copyright ASTM. Reprinted with permission.)

60%, to about 1150 feet/second. In contrast, a 300 Winchester Magnum with a much heavier and plastic-pointed bullet has a muzzle velocity of 3400 feet/second. At 300 feet the bullet's speed falls by less than 30%, to about 2430 feet/second (May, 1984). With an identified type of gun and bullet, ballistics specialists can calculate the probable speed of a bullet for a given distance from the gun to the victim. This may allow substantiation of a report that a child was injured by stray shots from a neighborhood altercation.

As with all injuries in potential abuse cases, meticulous documentation is in the best interest of the victim. Even if a bullet cannot be recovered, surgeons or emergency medical personnel may uncover clues about a weapon by noting the extent of injury. Low-velocity projectiles do most damage by crushing tissue in their path or lacerating vital structures. Higher-velocity bullets cause more extensive damage by generating shock waves that disrupt tissues and by producing aerodynamic effects that generate subatmospheric pressures in the wound, resulting in cavitation. Examination of the skin surface may also yield clues. When the patient's condition permits, wounds should be photographed or carefully drawn before local treatment is begun. If a weapon penetrated clothing before striking the skin, the clothing should be carefully removed and placed in a clean paper bag to be turned over to investigating authorities.

Bullet entrance wounds often appear as circular abrasions (Smialek, 1983). If the bullet was fired from close range (within about 3 feet), the skin may be bruised, burned, or marked by gunpowder. Powder marks appear as black soot or a fine tattooing with gray or black speckles. If the bullet passed through clothing before striking the skin, the soot or burn may be present on the cloth rather than the skin. Exit wounds are usually not abraded as are entrance wounds and appear slit-like or stellate. If only one bullet was fired and it is retained within the body, no exit wound will be found. In that case, X rays may be able to document the size, shape, and orientation of the bullet, all of which can contribute to reconstructing the history of the shooting. Shotguns fire masses of pellets rather than a single bullet. Depending on the range and the size of the pellets, a single shotgun wound may appear to have resulted from several conventional bullets. Photographs and drawings are especially critical in these cases.

Knife wounds can also yield valuable information about the weapon used. Elastic fibers cause the skin to retract away from the site of incision, however, distorting the size of the actual wound. Measurements and drawings should be made with the edges of the wound gently approximated.

Differential Diagnosis

Trauma, intentional or accidental, is of course not the only cause of skin lesions. Alternative diagnoses must be carefully considered, both because they may be signs of life-threatening illness and because the accusation of abuse, once made, is not easily retracted.

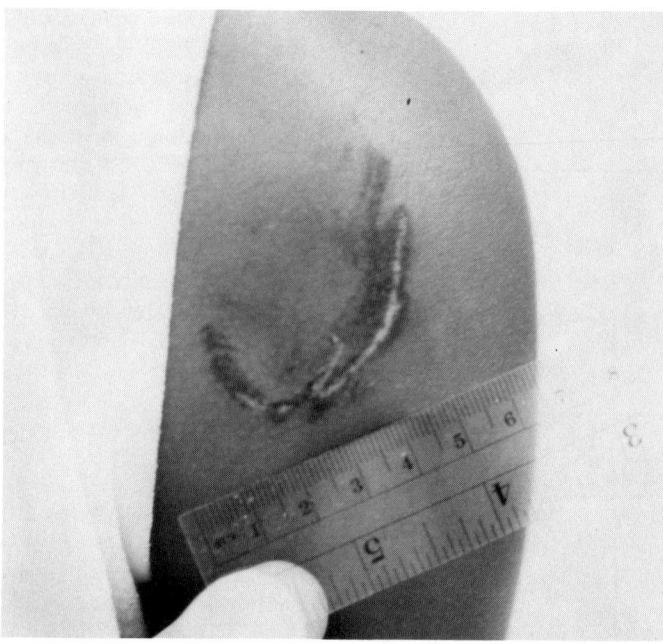

Figure 6.5. Bite mark of the "incised" or "weapon" type (Rawson et al., 1984). This type of bite may have less bruising or crushing than those associated with punishment or sexual activity.

Perhaps the most commonly occurring bruise-like lesions are Mongolian spots, areas of purplish or dark-brown discoloration frequently seen on the buttocks and lower back of many black and Oriental infants and sometimes among members of other racial groups. They may also appear on the trunk, upper extremities, and face. These spots are unrelated to trauma and are usually noted to have been present since birth. The easiest way to distinguish them from bruises is to note that they fail to change color over a period of days. Bruises, on the other hand, change color and eventually fade. Nevi and café-au-lait spots, especially when present in large numbers, may also have the appearance of multiple old bruised areas (Sekula et al., 1986). As discussed in Chapter 16, children who are critically ill or have undergone cardiopulmonary resuscitation may have lesions suggestive of abuse. It is often difficult to determine whether these lesions represent the trauma that caused the child to become so ill, complications of treatment, or agonal changes in circulation. With the administration of drugs to support blood pressure (such as epinephrine or dopamine), there are changes in the peripheral circulation that may result in blotching and blanching. With death, blood pools in dependent areas and may resemble bruising. Frothy, sometimes bloody discharge from the nose and mouth, caused by hemorrhagic pulmonary edema and rupture of mucosal capillaries, may occur after shock or with death.

Thrombocytopenia (from disseminated intravascular coagulation or idiopathic thrombocytopenic purpura, for example), meningococcal disease, and Henoch-Schönlein purpura can all cause bruise-like lesions. The latter can also cause swelling of various parts of the body, including the genitalia (Brown and Melinkovich, 1986). These causes must be considered first (or at least simultaneously with the diagnosis of trauma) when a child presents with altered mental status or seems to be acutely ill. A vasculitis associated with hypersensitivity can also produce streaky ecchymotic lesions on the extremities that look like welts (Waskerwitz et al., 1981). These patients, however, often develop urticaria and other signs of systemic illness.

Erythema multiforme may also begin with circular or irregularly shaped blotches or bruises on the trunk and extremities. Over a period of hours to days, the target lesions more typical of the condition usually appear, but initially the diagnosis of intentional injury may be considered because of the extent and distribution of the ecchymoses (Adler and Kane-Nussen, 1983). Laboratory tests are often normal, and the children may be afebrile at the time the rash appears.

Even if abuse is strongly suspected, it is wise to obtain a platelet count if bruising is the major sign pointing to the diagnosis, especially if the child's parents give a history that the child "bruises easily." Although the clinician may not think that thrombocytopenia is very likely, the platelet count may be useful in proving to a court that alternative diagnoses were carefully considered. (More than one parent of a child with undiagnosed thrombocytopenia has been mistakenly accused of child abuse.) Likewise, it is reasonable to obtain coagulation studies whenever soft tissue bleeding is the major factor suggesting intentional trauma or when it seems that minor trauma may, in fact, have produced an unusual amount of bruising. Hemophilia usually presents as joint or deep soft tissue bleeding, often after minor trauma. Coagulation studies are usually abnormal, although patients who are only carriers of the condition may require determinations of individual clotting factor levels to make the diagnosis. Cases involving known hemophiliacs or their close relatives who may be carriers are not simple to evaluate. Children with hemophilia may also be abused, and perhaps are at higher risk if behavioral problems arise in the care of their chronic illness (Johnson and Coury, 1988). The apparent age of a bruise may still give clues to neglectful or avoidant delays in seeking care; however, once the illness is identified, families and their physicians may decide that not all minor injuries require immediate attention and this may be the source of the delay. Probing for issues related to family functioning and stress may help differentiate unintentional from intentional bruises or bleeds and assist in other aspects of the patient's long-term care.

Folk medicine practices from many cultures may leave cutaneous signs falsely suggestive of abuse (Kirschner and Stein, 1985). Cupping, the application of a heated cup to the skin to draw out an ailment, is practiced by Middle Eastern, Latin American, and eastern European cultures. The procedure may leave circular red lesions, sometimes with petechiae, on the abdomen or other soft tissue area. The skin within the circle may also have been abraded before the cupping. Cao gio (coin rubbing) is a Southeast Asian practice that may leave linear red marks on the back resembling whip or stick welts; the skin on the back is first oiled and then rubbed firmly with a coin.

Burns

Burns are among the most serious manifestations of child abuse. Many authors believe that they are more likely than other physical injuries to represent premeditated acts of violence (Ayoub and Pfeifer, 1979). Scalds account for the majority of the more serious childhood burns, both intentional and unintentional, treated in hospitals in industrialized countries (Libber and Stayton, 1984; Hight et al., 1979). Toddlers and infants appear to be most at risk, and males predominate among both abusive and "accidental" injuries. Less is known about the epidemiology of burns that do not require inpatient care. Any burn that is suspected of having been intentionally inflicted should be carefully evaluated regardless of the severity of the burn itself. Some hospitals have policies of admitting any child with a potentially inflicted burn.

Burns are usually classified as first, second, or third degree according to the degree and depth of tissue damage. First-degree burns are characterized by transient erythema of the skin. The duration of erythema may be brief or prolonged. Second-degree burns involve damage to the upper layers of the dermis. The skin surface may be blistered or weepy. Nerves and vasculature remain intact so that the burn blanches and is very painful when touched. Third-degree burns involve full-thickness destruction of the skin. The burn may appear white or charred and is insensitive to pain. All of these appearances, however, are highly variable. Pressure and heat delivered together, or rapid heating from a very hot object, may result in second-degree burns that initially appear to have an intact, nonerythematous skin surface that later blisters or breaks down to reveal deeper tissue damage. Slower heating may first dilate surface blood vessels and then coagulate the blood. This can result in marked hyperemia that initially resembles a first-degree burn. Blistering may take several hours to develop. Heat sources that transfer energy to deep tissues more than those at the surface (electrical or microwave energy) may cause deep tissue damage without a great deal of obvious surface injury. It is therefore important to observe burns over time before drawing conclusions about their degree and extent. Distinct patterns of burning often are not visible until injuries have been debrided.

Human skin has a relatively narrow range of tolerance for thermal injury (Moritz and Henriques, 1947). There is a great deal of variablity among individuals and skin sites, however. Although studies of children have not been done, studies of adults and animals suggest that children's skin, because it is thinner, may be injured at lower temperatures than adults'. Among adults, contact with liquids or objects below about 45°C (113°F) requires hours to produce a second- or third-degree burn. From about 44°C (111°F) to 51°C (124°F), however, the time it takes to create a second- or third-degree burn falls by half for each degree centigrade of increase in temperature (Fig. 6.6). Thus, at 53°C (127°F) a significant burn occurs in about 1.5 minutes, while at 60°C (140°F) only about 5 seconds is required.

Pain sensation from hot objects is also variable, although there is no evidence to suggest that children have any higher threshold than adults. In one study (Moritz and Henriques, 1947), most volunteer subjects felt discomfort at between 47.5 and 48.5°C (118–119°F), which is safely below the adult threshold for very rapid burns. Some subjects did get burned at these temperatures before reporting a feeling discomfort, however.

Unfortunately, temperatures in the range causing nearly instantaneous burns are frequently attained by household appliances, beverages, and tapwater. Electric hair curlers, for example, commonly attain surface temperatures of over 93°C (200°F), with some having "hot spots" of over 138°C (280°F). Some can attain these temperatures in a matter of minutes, and it can take 15 minutes or more after

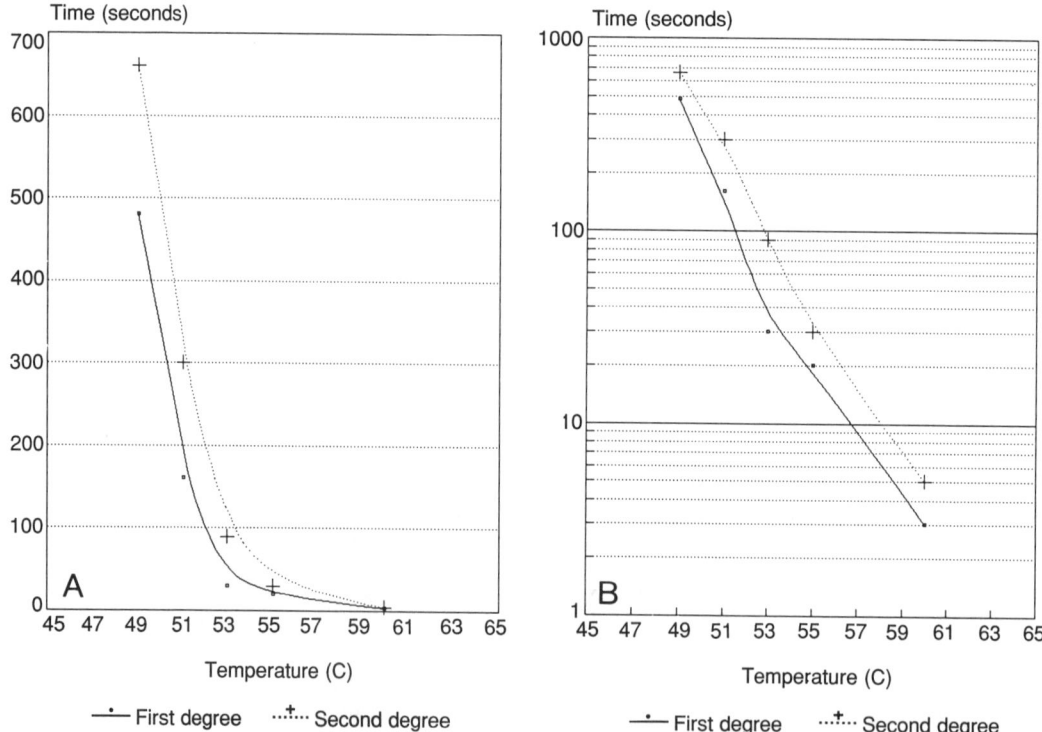

Figure 6.6. Time required to produce first-degree (*solid line*) and second/third-degree (*dotted line*) burns with a hot liquid in the skin of adult human volunteers. **A**, Data with time (*vertical axis*) on linear scale to illustrate change in burn kinetics at about 50°C. **B**, Same data with time plotted on logarithmic scale. Note very short time intervals (less than 10 seconds) required for burns at higher temperatures. (Plots from data in Moritz AR, Henriques FC. Studies of thermal injury: II. The relative importance of time and surface temperature in the causation of cutaneous burns. Am J Pathol 1947;23:710, Table III.)

they are turned off until their hottest areas fall below 38°C (100°F) (E. Groth, Consumers Union, personal communication). Studies of household tapwater have found a high prevalence of temperatures sufficient to scald (Feldman et al., 1978; Katcher, 1987). Most home hot water heaters currently in use are set at 140°F (60°C) or above. Hot beverages prepared from boiling water (100°C) cool to only 70 or 80°C when poured, still hot enough to scald on contact.

The most readily recognizable pattern of intentional scald burn results from forced immersion in hot water. Immersion is often inflicted as punishment for messiness or a lack of bowel control. The resulting burn is usually second or third degree and uniform in depth. There is a sharply demarcated border corresponding to the surface of the water. The burn may have a "glove" or "stocking" distribution when the child's extremities are immersed (Fig. 6.7). If the child is forcibly set in a tub of hot water, there may be sparing of thicker skin on the soles or palms, skin that protruded from the water as the knees and hips were flexed, or skin that was pressed against the cooler surface of the tub (Fig. 6.8). Skin in deep folds around the hips or between the buttocks may also be spared. Repositioning the child may align the borders of the burned areas and demonstrate the water level (Lenoski and Hunter, 1977). Isolated smaller burns from splashed liquid are usually absent. The typical pattern of a forced-immersion burn may be distorted if the child was clothed at the time of the incident. Clothing tends to hold the hot liquid close to the skin for a longer period of time and thus can lead to burns in areas that would otherwise be spared (Fig. 6.9). Outlines of elastic portions of the clothes may also be visible. As mentioned above, in some cases these patterns will be visible immediately, but in others the circumscribed nature of the burns will not be obvious until blistered or otherwise devitalized epidermis is debrided or has sloughed.

Spill or splash burns differ in that they often show a pattern of flow of the hot liquid over the skin. Some areas may be burned more than others as the liquid cools on its way to and over the body. Splash burns often have several "satellite" lesions from drops of liquid, in contrast to the large, smooth-bordered lesions of immersion burns. Splash burns are usually less deep than immersion burns, probably because shorter exposures to heat are involved as the liquid cools on exposure to air and skin. It may be difficult to differentiate unintentional spill or splash scalds from those in which a hot liquid was deliberately poured or thrown at a child. Accidental spills seem more likely to burn the face or chest, while burns to the extremities, perineum, or buttocks are more likely to have been inflicted (Keen et al., 1975). Unintentional burns of the face and oropharynx caused by infant beverages heated in microwave ovens have been reported (Sando et al., 1984). Because microwaves penetrate the surface of an object and heat it unevenly, containers may be relatively cool on the outside but contain liquids capable of causing scalds.

Burns in the shape of hot solid objects are highly suggestive of abuse. Cigarettes, hair curlers, and heating devices or grates are among the more commonly reported objects involved in questionable cases. Often the physician is asked to determine whether such burns occurred by accident or were inflicted. This can be difficult if the object's temperature was so high that a burn would occur with nearly instantaneous contact. Even plastic seats or metal seat belt buckles can be heated to dangerous temperatures if a car is parked in the summer sun. In general, burns in which the object is clearly and uniformly outlined or that are symmetrical (for example, cigarette burns on the knuckles of both hands) are suggestive of inflicted injury. Recent cigarette burns may easily be confused with impetigo, and healed lesions of varicella may leave circular hypo- or hyperpigmented areas that resemble healed burns. In the acute stages, one clue to differentiating impetigo from a burn may come from the depth of the lesion. Impetigo is a superficial skin infection that spares deeper layers. An inflicted cigarette burn will generally be third degree and therefore appear as a relatively painless, deep lesion. Some guidelines for detecting possibly intentional burns, suggested by Feldman et al. (1978) and Hight et al. (1979), include the following:

- Burns of the perineum or buttocks, symmetrical burns on the extremities, or deep burns of what are usually relatively resistant skin surfaces, such as the palms or soles, are suggestive of intentional injury.
- Burns incompatible with the child's developmental abilities are also of concern. For example, immersion burns of the lower extremities are frequently explained by saying that the child "fell into the bathtub," often after turning on the water him or herself. Most children cannot climb until 14–16 months of age, and at that point would most likely go face first over a high

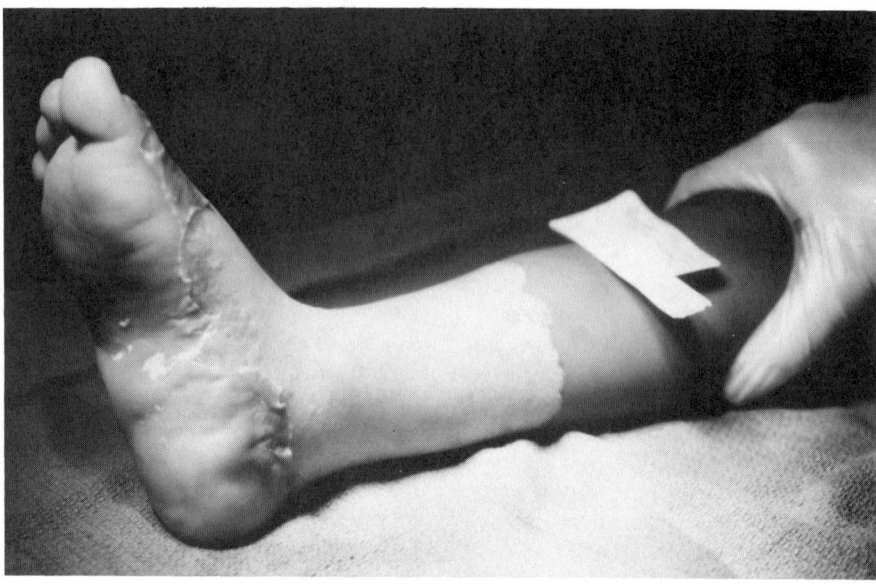

Figure 6.7. Immersion burn in a "stocking" distribution showing sharp, even demarcation between the burned and uninjured skin. Note sparing of the thicker skin on the bottom of the foot. Photograph taken after a whirlpool treatment. Before debridement, the nature of such an injury may not be as obvious.

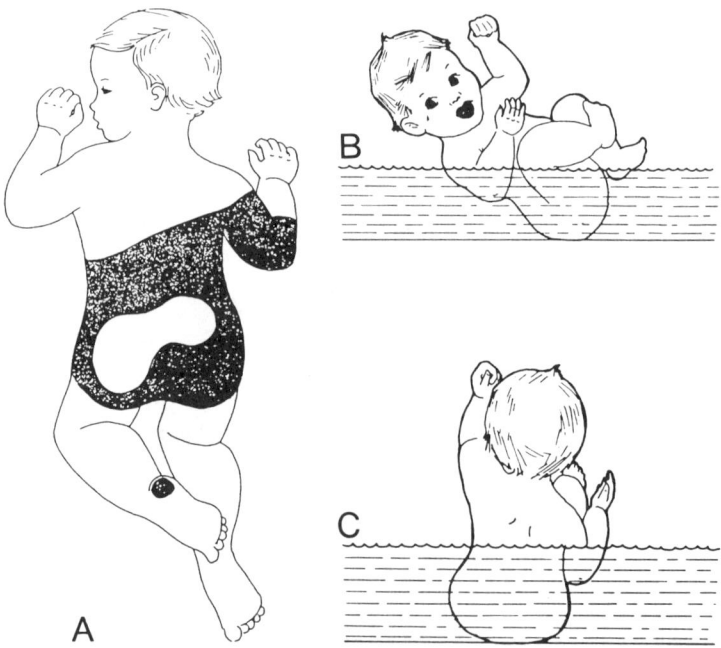

Figure 6.8. **A**, Pattern of burn produced by immersion of an infant in a tub of hot water. **B** and **C**, Presumed placement of the child that results in distribution of burn, showing areas that protrude from water and that are spared because of folds of skin or contact with tub bottom. (From Lenoski EF, Hunter KA. Specific patterns of inflicted burn injuries. J Trauma 1977;17:842–846. Copyright 1977, Williams & Wilkins Co., Baltimore. Used with permission.)

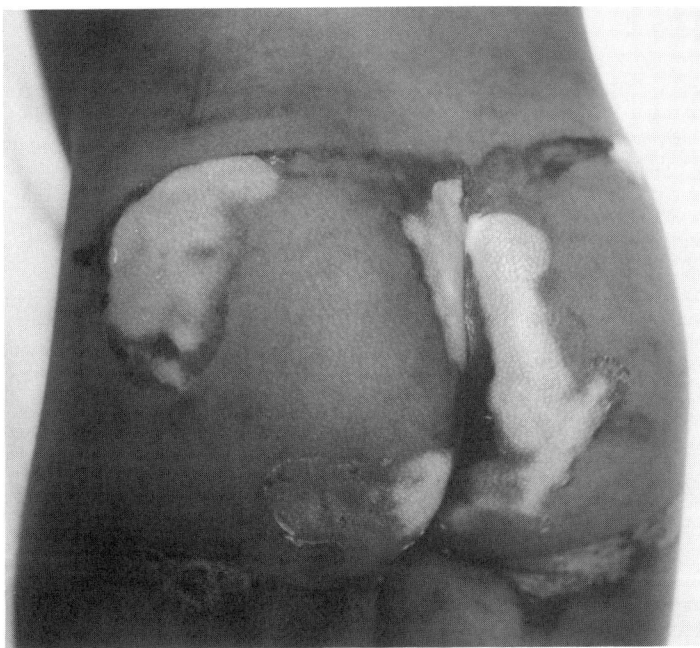

Figure 6.9. Burns on the buttocks of a child who was immersed in hot water while clothed. Note outline of elastic on the underwear and burned area between buttocks where water was trapped by cloth.

tub side (if they could get over it at all). It is only later that they learn to swing their legs up and have a chance to enter feet first.
- Burns attributed to the actions of siblings, that are said to have been unwitnessed, or for which inconsistent explanations are offered are also cause for suspicion.
- Cases in which there was an inappropriate delay in seeking care (keeping in mind that the visible extent of injury may change over time) or the child is brought for care by someone other than the person said to have been present at the time the burn occurred warrant further probing.
- The presence of other injuries or a history of previous burns or unexplained injuries should prompt the clinician to not accept the history at face value.

Microwave ovens, in addition to posing a risk if used for heating beverages, have also been used to injure children intentionally. Fortunately, only a handful of cases have so far been reported (Alexander et al., 1987). The important lesson from these cases is that the victims have burn patterns that do not fit common findings in injuries from surface heating. There may be some areas of well-demarcated second- and third-degree burns in areas that were close to the microwave-emitting source (usually the top of the microwave oven), but there will also be marked damage to deeper layers, notably muscle, caused by the ability of microwaves to penetrate and preferentially heat structures with higher water content. Biopsies of burned areas show a sparing of the fat layer of the skin, sandwiched between damaged dermis and muscle. This pattern would be very unusual in a burn from a conventional surface source of heat.

References

Adler R, Kane-Nussen B. Erythema multiforme: confusion with child battering syndrome. Pediatrics 1983;72:718–720.

Alexander RC, Surrell JA, Cohle SD. Microwave oven burns to children: an unusual manifestation of child abuse. Pediatrics 1987;79:255–260.

American Board of Forensic Odontology, Inc. Guidelines for bite mark analysis. J Am Dent Assoc 1986;112:383–386.

Ayoub C, Pfeifer D. Burns as a manifestation of child abuse and neglect. Am J Dis Child 1979;133:910–914.

Baker MD, Moore SE. Human bites in children: a six-year experience. Am J Dis Child 1987;141:1285–1290.

Balaban DJ, Goldfarb NI. Prediction of child abuse—does it work? [Letter]. Pediatrics 1983;72:437–438.

Brown J, Melinkovich P. Schonlein-Henoch purpura misdiagnosed as suspected child abuse: a case report and review of the literature. JAMA 1986;256:617–620.

Committee on Early Childhood, Adoption, and Dependent Care. Oral and dental aspects of child abuse and neglect. Pediatrics 1986;78:537–539.

Drinnan AJ, Melton MJ. Court presentation of bite mark evidence. Int Dent J 1985;35:316–321.

Feldman KW, Schaller RT, Feldman JA, McMillion M. Tap water scald burns in children. Pediatrics 1978;62:1–7.

Hight DW, Bakalar HR, Lloyd JR. Inflicted burns in children: recognition and treatment. JAMA 1979;242:517–520.

Jakobsen JR, Keiser-Nielsen S. Bite mark lesions in human skin. Forensic Sci Int 1981;18:41–55.

Jellinek MS, Murphy JM, Robinson J, Feins A, Lamb S, Fenton T. Pediatric Symptom Checklist: screening school-age children for psychosocial dysfunction. J Pediatr 1988;112:201–209.

Johnson CF, Coury DL. Bruising and hemophilia: accident or child abuse? Child Abuse Negl 1988;12:409–415.

Katcher ML. Prevention of tap water scald burns: evaluation of a multi-media injury control program. Am J Public Health 1987;77:1195–1197.

Keen JH, Lendrum J, Wolman B. Inflicted burns and scalds in children. Br Med J 1975;4:268–269.

Kellerman AL, Reay DT. Protection or peril? An analysis of firearm-related deaths in the home. N Engl J Med 1986;314:1557–1560.

Kirschner RH, Stein RJ. The mistaken diagnosis of child abuse: a form of medical abuse. Am J Dis Child 1985;139:873–875.

Lenoski EF, Hunter KA. Specific patterns of inflicted burn injuries. J Trauma 1977;17:842–846.

Leung AKC. Pseudo-abusive human bite marks in a Chinese infant [Letter]. Injury 1985;16:503–504.

Leventhal JM, Fearn K, Stashwick CA. Clinical data used by pediatric residents to assess parenting. Child Abuse Negl 1986;10:71–78.

Libber SM, Stayton DJ. Childhood burns reconsidered: the child, the family, and the burn injury. J Trauma 1984;24:245–252.

May HL. The critically injured patient. In: May HL, ed. Emergency medicine. New York: John Wiley & Sons, 1984:231–276.

Moritz AR, Henriques FC. Studies of thermal injury: II. The relative importance of time and surface temperature in the causation of cutaneous burns. Am J Pathol 1947;23:695–720.

Myers JEB. Role of the physician in preserving verbal evidence of child abuse. J Pediatr 1986;109:409–411.

Nelson KG. The innocent bystander: the child as unintended victim of domestic violence involving deadly weapons. Pediatrics 1984;73:251–252.

Ordog GJ, Wasserberger J, Balasubramanium S. Wound ballistics: theory and practice. Ann Emerg Med 1984;13:1113–1122.

Rawson RD, Koot A, Martin C, et al. Incidence of bite marks in a selected juvenile population: a preliminary report. J Forensic Sci 1984;29:254–259.

Rosenberg NM, Meyers S, Shackelton N. Prediction of child abuse in an ambulatory setting. Pediatrics 1982;70:879–882.

Sando WC, Gallaher KJ, Rodgers BM. Risk factors for microwave scald injuries in infants. J Pediatr 1984;105:864–867.

Schroeder CS, Gordon BN, Kanoy K, Routh DK. Managing children's behavior problems in pediatric practice. Adv Dev Behav Pediatr 1983;4:25–86.

Sekula SA, Tschen JA, Duffy OJ. Epidermal nevus misinterpreted as child abuse. Cutis 1986≈ril:276–278.

Smialek JE. Forensic medicine in the emergency department. Emerg Med Clin North Am 1983;1:693–704.

Sognnaes RD. Forensic stomatology (third of three parts). N Engl J Med 1977;296:197–203.

Starr RH. Clinical judgement of abuse-proneness based on parent-child interactions. Child Abuse Negl 1987;11:87–92.

Straus MA, Gelles RJ, Steinmetz SK. Behind closed doors: violence in the American family. Garden City: Anchor Press, 1981.

Trube-Becker E. Bite-marks on battered children. Z Rechtsmed 1977;79:73–78.

Waskerwitz S, Christoffel KK, Hauger S. Hypersensitivity vasculitis presenting as suspected child abuse: case report and literature review. Pediatrics 1981;67:283–284.

Whitcomb D, Shapiro ER, Stellwagen LD. When the victim is a child: issues for judges and prosecutors. National Institute of Justice, Office of Development, Testing, and Dissemination. Washington, DC: US Government Printing Office, 1985.

Wilson EF. Estimation of the age of cutaneous contusions in child abuse. Pediatrics 1977;60:750–752.

Wintermute GJ, Teret SP, Kraus JF, Wright MA, Bradfield G. When children shoot children: 88 unintended deaths in California. JAMA 1987;257:3107–3109.

Wolfe DA. Child abusive parents: an empirical review and analysis. Psychol Bull 1985;97:462–82.

7 Head and Internal Injuries

HEAD INJURIES

The head is a major target of intentional injury in small children, but it is also among the most frequent locations of trauma following unintentional injuries such as falls and motor vehicle collisions. Unfortunately, head trauma caused by abuse is often difficult to diagnose. No history of injury may be given, and the child's real or alleged symptoms may be vague or nonspecific. In addition, clinically important and even life-threatening intracranial injury can occur with little or no external evidence of trauma on the head or face. Therefore, diagnosis requires a high level of suspicion and a relatively liberal use of imaging modalities such as standard skull X rays and computed tomography (CT).

Inspection of the Head

Initial inspection of the head may reveal some signs of injury. The anterior fontanelle (usually open until about 18 months of age) may be used as a rough gauge of intracranial pressure. With the infant sitting up, a normal fontanelle is soft and about even with the rest of the skull. It may be slightly pulsatile. A tense or bulging fontanelle when the child is upright is an abnormal finding usually indicative of increased intracranial pressure. If the pressure increase is long-standing (such as in the presence of chronic subdural hematomas or hydrocephalus), there may also be palpable splitting of the cranial sutures.

Patchy hair loss may be a result of intentional pulling, but there are many other conditions in which it may be noted. Braids or corn rows may be pulled too tightly and result in bald spots. Malnutrition can leave the hair brittle and easy to pull out. Occipital bald or thin spots, once considered a sign of neglect (presumed to reflect an infant left supine in bed for long periods of time), are in fact a fairly common finding in normal infants. Hair may also be lost secondary to fungal infections, but bald areas will usually be accompanied by scaling or oozing. Fungal organisms can sometimes be observed in scrapings or cultured from plucked hairs.

Palpation of the head may reveal boggy areas suggestive of bruises. Large soft or discolored areas may be associated with bleeding under the galea, the fibrous tissue covering the skull (Table 7.1). Subgaleal bleeding may be caused by violent pulling on the hair (Hamlin, 1968) or by blood from an intracranial injury leaking out through a skull fracture. Palpation may also find a "step off" of the skull suggestive of a depressed skull fracture. These may be difficult to feel, however, if the bone defect is under a boggy area of the scalp. Cephalohematoma, a relatively common and benign form of birth injury, may sometimes be mistaken for depressed skull fractures in infants who are a few months old. These lesions often calcify after the initial bleeding has ceased. As the hematoma is resorbed, the calcification collapses, producing

Table 7.1 Layers of the Head (External to Internal)

Scalp
Galea—Aponeurosis (tendenous insertion) of the frontalis and occipitalis muscles; covers most of the skull
Periosteum of the skull
Bones of the skull
Periosteum of the skull—Fused to "true" dura except where layers separate to contain cranial venous sinuses
Cranial venous sinuses—Mostly along the falx (infolding of dura between hemispheres of the brain)
Dura—Tough membrane essentially fused to periosteum of the skull
Subdural space—Normally only a potential space penetrated by cerebral veins carrying blood to the venous sinuses
Arachnoid—"Middle" membrane of brain covering, attached to pia by trabeculae
Subarachnoid space—Filled with CSF
    Cerebral veins and arteries run in this space; veins run up through arachnoid and dura to reach venous sinuses
Pia—Innermost covering of the brain
Cortex of the brain

a relatively circular, raised area on the skull with a central depression. Standard X-ray studies can usually show that the skull itself is intact.

Injuries to the face can be serious but are often subtle. Battle's sign (bruising over the mastoid process behind the ear), raccoon eyes (bilateral ecchymotic areas in the orbits), and blood behind the tympanic membranes may be signs of basilar skull fracture. Injury to the nose may also cause bilateral bruising under the eyes. The mouth, jaw, and teeth should be inspected for signs of trauma. Bernat (1981) suggests the following procedure for a screening examination of the face, jaws, and oral cavity.

First, the examiner stands or sits face to face with the child and looks for asymmetry, bruises, swelling, or scars on the face. The vermilion border of the lips should be smooth and regular. If the child is old enough to cooperate, he or she should be asked to open and close the jaw a few times while the examiner listens for clicks and observes whether the jaw opens smoothly and symmetrically. The motion of the jaw can be examined by placing the first finger of the examiner's hand in the opening of the child's external auditory canal and the other fingers along the mandibular condyle (just below and anterior to the ear) and the angle of the jaw. When the child opens the jaw, the condyle will normally slide out of the glenoid fossa as the jaw lowers. If the condyle does not move or if the jaw deviates to one side while opening, a manibular fracture should be suspected. The zygomatic arches should be palpated from their origins in front of the ears anteriorly toward the orbits, and the orbital rims and bones adjacent to the nose should also be palpated. Any suspicion of pain or irregularity should prompt consideration of a complete skull X-ray series and surgical consulation.

The mouth is examined next. With the mouth closed, the lips can be retracted to expose the anterior teeth and gums. The frenula of the lips are easily torn in trauma to the mouth. Each frenulum, one superior and one inferior, is a small, V-shaped, midline tissue bridge linking the lip with the alveolar ridge. The point of the V attaches to the gums just above and below the grooves between the central maxillary and mandibular incisors, respectively. Tears can occur from direct trauma and from forceful attempts to insert an object in the mouth. Unintentional injuries are unusual before children can sit alone (about 6 months of age) and after toddlerhood, when falls become less frequent.

The teeth can be examined first with the jaw closed and then with it open. The arcs of teeth should be smooth and symmetrical. An apparently missing tooth may be attributable to the child's age (consult a chart of usual times of eruption of deciduous teeth), a complete avulsion, or a traumatic intrusion of the tooth into the alveolar ridge so that it is no longer visible. Any loosening of the teeth raises the concern for trauma except in a child who is 5–6 years old and may be shedding deciduous teeth. Normal shedding may sometimes be differentiated from trauma when only a single tooth is loose or otherwise damaged. Since it is difficult to strike a single tooth, trauma usually results in injuries to several adjacent teeth. Stability of the jaw may again be assessed by putting the thumbs under the chin and the forefingers on the occlusal (biting) surface of the teeth and then gently wiggling the mandible. This can also be done for the maxillary arch by placing the forefinger on the maxillary teeth and the thumbs on the zyomatic arches.

The tongue, floor of the mouth, and palate should all be examined for bruises or ulceration. Forceful thrusting against the palate, as may happen during fellatio, can cause erythema, petechiae, and purpura (Elam and Ray, 1986). Oral ulcers, pharyngeal erythema, and tonsillar exudates may all be caused by sexually transmitted diseases. There are, of course, many other conditions that can cause these findings.

Injuries to the Eye

The eye can be injured both by direct blows and by distant forces transmitted along the vasculature. Retinal hemorrhages are the most commonly reported eye injuries in children hospitalized for abuse (Jensen et al., 1971), probably because the retinal vasculature is very sensitive to the pressure changes caused by increases in intracranial pressure, acceleration and deceleration, and trauma to other parts of the body. Understanding how direct and indirect forces create ocular trauma can help to match findings on examination with explanations offered for the injury.

Direct injury to the globe of the eye can cause several types of damage (Gammon, 1981). Chemical or abrasive injuries can cause damage to the cornea. Direct blows harm the eye by severely distorting the globe and causing disruption of both surface and internal structures. The globe may be ruptured if the force is sufficiently high or if it is lacerated with a relatively sharp object. Some of the major forms of eye injury from blunt trauma include:

- Stretching or tearing the deeper layers of the cornea. These injuries are much more likely to result in visual impairment than superficial abrasions or lacerations.
- Disruption or inflammation of the iris and ciliary body, resulting in decreased production of the aqueous fluid present in the anterior chamber of the eye. Alternatively, bleeding in the anterior chamber can block resorption of aqueous fluid and result in glaucoma.
- Severe distortion of the shape of the globe, rupturing the zonules (suspensory ligaments of the lens) and causing dislocation of the lens.
- Distortion of the vitreous, the contents of the posterior chamber, resulting in avulsion of its attachments to the retina. The result may be bleeding into the vitreous itself, with resulting scars and impairment of vision, or detachment of the retina. The choroid, the nutrient layer of the globe just between the retina and the sclera, may also be disrupted and cause detachment or disruption of the retina.
- The optic nerve itself may be injured, either at the point where it leaves the skull and is tethered relative to motion of the globe, or closer to the globe where it is joined by the retinal artery.

The precise mechanisms by which distant forces act on the eye remain controversial. Most trauma results in a combination of forces, and there are few "pure" injuries to observe. Several authors have suggested classification systems that may be helpful in pairing lesions with the type of trauma that is most likely to have produced them (Marr and Marr, 1962; Duane, 1973).

Valsalva hemorrhagic retinopathy may result from sudden increases in venous pressure. Because the major veins that drain the head have few valves, pressure changes in the abdomen and chest are readily transmitted to the head and eye. When the pressure change is sudden, changes appear to occur in the retinal layers and capillary network closest to the vitreous (Table 7.2). Retinal edema, fluffy superficial transudates, and large blot or boat preretinal hemorrhages are produced (Fig. 7.1). (The term "preretinal" is a misnomer; the hemorrhages are technically within the retina, just under the internal limiting membrane, although they may sometimes rupture into the vitreous.)

Subconjunctival hemorrhages and petechiae of the skin of the head and trunk are sometimes found along with preretinal lesions. It is not certain what types of forces are required to produce this constellation of findings, and its pathophysiology may differ between adults and children. Similar findings have been observed in crush injuries to the chest and abdomen as well as in asphyxia secondary to chest compression. Retinal lesions may be more likely to occur in individuals with underlying retinal vascular diseases (diabetes or atherosclerosis), although these conditions are not common in children.

Prolonged venous hypertension, as may occur with elevated increased intracranial pressure, is also postulated to cause both preretinal and deeper-layer retinal hemorrhages (Lambert et al., 1986). This has been proposed as an explanation for why some children and adults with intracranial bleeding develop retinal bleeding as well (Terson's syndrome). However, observations of children who have increased intracranial pressure for reasons other than trauma will be required to determine whether this is an effect solely of intracranial pressure or whether it results from a combination of trauma and pressure (Giangiacomo and Barkett, 1985).

Because it is at the end of a circulatory loop, the retinal arteriolar network has limited regulatory ability. Chronic arterial hypertension in adults has long been observed to produce exudates and other characteristic changes of the retinal vessels. Acceleration and deceleration of the body produce changes in arterial pressure as well as direct force to the globe. Deceleration is felt to result primarily in angiospasm. Funduscopic findings may be minimal at first, but over a period of days hemorrhages, especially flame and dot lesions, may develop (Table 7.2). Acceleration injuries appear to produce bleeding more quickly, especially flame hemorrhages.

Some abused infants have been noted to have so-called Purtscher's retinopathy, the finding of preretinal and deeper-layer retinal hem-

Table 7.2 Types and Possible Causes of Ocular Hemorrhages

Layer of Eye (Inner to Outer)	Type of Hemorrhage	Appearance and Postulated Cause
Vitreous	Vitreous	Blunt trauma ruptures attachments to retina; may also result from rupture of sublaminar ("preretinal") bleeds
Retina (11 layers in total)		
Internal limiting membrane	Sublaminar ("preretinal")	Large, blot or boat-shaped; may protrude into vitreous; resolves slowly; most likely caused by suddenly increased venous pressure
Nerve fiber layer (contains superficial capillary network)	Flame	Flat, fluted edge, follows orientation of nerve fibers; more common with prolonged elevation of venous pressure elevated intracranial pressure, mixed causes, vaginal birth
Inner nuclear layer (contains deep capillary network)	Dot	Round, small lesions with sharp margins; resolve within days; causes similar to those for flame lesions
Choroid		Bleeds from direct trauma may disrupt retina
Sclera		
Conjunctivia	Subconjunctival	Usually associated with sudden increase in venous pressure rather than direct trauma

orrhages and retinal exudates in association with a history of sudden compression of the chest (Tomasi and Rosman, 1975). Purtscher's findings were originally described in individuals with multiple forms of trauma (such as falling out of a tree and landing on the head), and the exact nature of the retinal findings have been variously described. A finding of several different kinds of hemorrhage along with exudates may therefore suggest the simultaneous occurrence of multiple types of trauma, including acceleration/deceleration, chest compression, and possibly direct trauma to the head.

At the risk of overgeneralizing from relatively scanty case studies, one may make some general statements about causes of injury and retinal findings. (This is an area ripe for further study. The following associations have not been tested.) Isolated preretinal hemorrhages, probably in the absence of exudates, suggest Valsalva forces (sudden increases in thoracic or abdominal pressure). Flame-shaped or dot hemorrhages, when they appear either initially or over a period of days, suggest arterial spasm and acceleration/deceleration injuries. A mixed picture of multiple types of hemorrhages, possibly associated with exudates, suggests multiple mechanisms of trauma or greatly increased intracranial pressure. Serial examinations beginning as soon as possible after trauma are important, since both the timing and appearance of hemorrhages appear to vary with the mechanism. In addition, the diagnostic picture may be confused by increases in intracranial pressure that occur later in the course of treatment.

Retinal findings may often be the only external clue to serious head injury and child abuse. Many authorities suggest that retinal hemorrhages in children other than newborns should be considered diagnostic of abuse until proven otherwise. The list of items in the differential diagnosis is relatively short but, as suggested above, much remains unknown about differentiating various causes related to trauma. Nontraumatic causes include coagulopathies, leukemia, endocarditis and other sources of emboli, brain tumors and other causes of increased intracranial pressure, and malignant hypertension. Retinal hemorrhages have also been found in individuals wearing shoulder belts who were involved in high-speed motor vehicle collisions. Presumably, these persons suffered both deceleration and chest-compressing forces.

The question of whether retinal hemorrhages can be caused by cardiopulmonary resuscitation (CPR), especially by untrained or

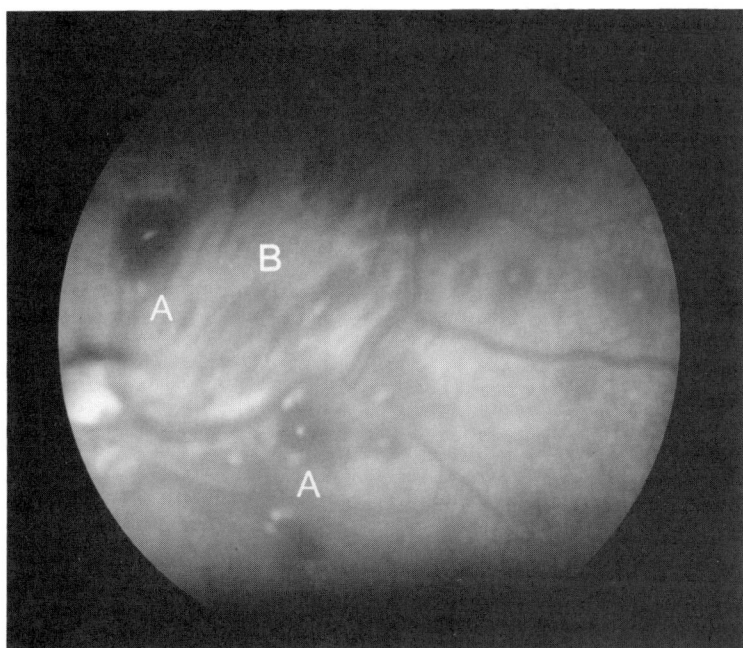

Figure 7.1 Retinal hemorrhages in an abused child. **A**, Preretinal hemorrhages (central white spot is the reflection of the photographic flash). **B**, Flame hemorrhages following nerve fiber layers.

panicking practitioners, remains open. One case report (Bacon et al., 1978) described bilateral nerve fiber layer bleeding in a 2-month-old boy who was found apparently dead at home and was resuscitated by multiple slaps on the back. The resuscitation was not witnessed by medical personnel. Questioning of the family to investigate the possibility of abuse found no grounds for concern. In contrast, Kanter (1986) found retinal hemorrhages in 6 of 54 children who had undergone CPR. All six had conditions that might have accounted for the hemorrhages: four showed evidence of having been physically abused, one had been hit by a car, and the sixth had had arterial blood pressures of 190/120 mm Hg (but no evidence of trauma). The circumstances of CPR were not described, but apparently the procedure was carried out by medical personnel. Kanter interpreted the results as demonstrating that CPR was probably not a likely cause of retinal hemorrhage in children.

By far the most common cause of retinal bleeding in children is normal vaginal delivery. It is hypothesized that compression of the head during passage through the birth canal leads to increased pressure in the central retinal vein and rupture of retinal capillaries (Eller, 1983). The apparent prevalence of retinal bleeding in newborns varies with how long after birth the examination is conducted. At the time of birth, hemorrhages have been found in up to 40% of infants, but by 48 to 72 hours the prevalence is only about 10%. Most hemorrhages are of the dot or flame variety and resolve within a matter of days to 3–4 weeks and have no visual sequelae. A small number, often associated with forceps deliveries and accompanied by other signs of birth injury, may be more severe (of the Purtcher's type) and can lead to visual impairment.

Because retinal hemorrhage may be the only clue to intentional injury as the cause of an infant's illness, an ophthalmologic examination is essential whenever abuse is suspected. Many physicians hesitate to undertake a funduscopic exam of an infant, fearing that it will be a time-consuming and frustrating procedure. It is true that little is usually visible through an infant's mobile, undilated pupil, and even extensive hemorrhages may be missed. After the pupil is dilated, however, the fundus is usually easily visible. Physicians sometimes hesitate to dilate the pupils of seriously injured patients, fearing that they will lose the ability to watch for changes in pupillary reactivity. This is a somewhat less serious problem in infants, in whom the flexibility of the skull and an open fontanelle make brain herniation and its resultant pupillary changes less common. CT scans, which are often obtained very early in an injured child's course of care, can examine the size of the ventricular system and suggest whether intracranial pressure is increased. The fact that the eyes have been dilated should always be immediately noted in the medical chart, however, so that subsequent examiners do not misinterpret the decreased pupillary reactivity.

Skull Fractures

The various types of skull fractures associated with intentional and unintentional injuries are discussed in Chapter 9. Techniques of physical examination for detecting fractures have been discussed above. For most children, with the exception of those who have basilar or depressed injuries, the detection of simple skull fractures has more medical-legal than clinical significance. In cases of suspected abuse, however, fractures may be important clinical clues that prompt a search for other signs of injury. It is reasonable, then, to have a lower threshold for obtaining skull X rays of children who have ill-defined conditions or who are suspected of having been intentionally injured than of children who have apparently straightforward histories of minor household head trauma. One consistent finding has been that CT scans may fail to detect skull fractures that are readily detectable on standard X-ray films (Saulsbury and Alford, 1982). Detection of a fracture may offer an alternative explanation (trauma) for intracranial lesions that were thought to have resulted from spontaneous bleeding or infectious processes. Children suspected of being abused who have positive intracranial findings but a normal skull on CT examinations should have at least a limited conventional X-ray skull series to look for fractures.

Intracranial Injuries

Aside from their obvious and often urgent medical importance, intracranial injuries are significant because they serve as markers for trauma involving much greater force than is normally found in unintentional household mishaps. Evaluations of children hospitalized for head trauma in both the United States and the United Kingdom have found that witnessed minor accidents rarely result in more than a simple, uncomplicated skull fracture or minor concussive symptoms (Hobbs, 1984; Billmire and Myers, 1985). In case studies, the simultaneous occurrence of fracture and concussion, or the finding of intracranial bleeding, is almost always associated with either intentional injury or severe trauma such as involvement in a motor vehicle collision or a fall from a considerable height. Studies of children with documented falls from hospital beds and stretchers (Helfer et al., 1977) and undocumented falls down stairs (Joffe and Ludwig, 1988) have found that simple skull fractures occur infrequently and that concussions are even rarer. Intracranial bleeding was never found in the relatively large groups of children examined.

The head appears to be more vulnerable in early childhood than later in life. Some of the vulnerability results from the child's overall motor abilities: ambulation is difficult, and protective maneuvers such as propping are not well developed or coordinated. There are also differences in the head and brain themselves that increase the likelihood of injury. During infancy, the head is large and heavy in relationship to the rest of the body. The neck muscles are relatively weak and cannot control the head's movements. The infant skull is more pliable than the older child's and more readily transmits force to the brain. The brain itself is softer and more mobile within the skull, making it more vulnerable to injury. The brain may be injured both by direct force and by acceleration/deceleration forces.

The head injury reported to be most commonly found in intentional trauma depends in part on the diagnostic methods used. For example, early reports have suggested that magnetic resonance imaging (MRI) is better than CT for detecting focal injury to the brain parenchyma (Alexander et al., 1986). As a result, some cerebral contusions and tears or intraparenchymal hemorrhages may be missed by currently available studies. At present, the most commonly reported intracranial injury among abuse cases is the subdural hematoma. Subdural hematomas develop when breaks occur in the veins or venous sinuses that drain the cerebral cortex (Table 7.1). Bleeding may come from the cerebral veins themselves or directly from the venous sinuses which are enclosed in the dura.

Blood then enters the potential space between the dura and the arachnoid and creates a mass.

The pressure in the cerebral veins is low and bleeding may be slow, although in some cases blood accumulates quickly enough to compress the brain and cause a rapid alteration in neurologic functioning. The pathophysiology of subdural hematomas is not well understood beyond this acute stage. Some acute bleedings apparently are resorbed and disappear. Some, over a period of days to weeks, develop a membrane around the clotted blood. This membrane acts as a container for fluid which then expands through rebleeding, osmotic pressure, or both. The hematoma is ultimately discovered when it becomes large enough to cause neurologic symptoms. Little is known about the amount of trauma required to produce a subdural hematoma. Adults often report either no history of trauma or only minor falls or blows. As mentioned above, however, intracranial injury appears to be quite rare in children after minor trauma.

Only a small proportion of children with subdural hematomas have associated skull fractures. A higher proportion have long-bone injuries, an observation that formed one of the early clues to what was later named the battered child syndrome (Caffey, 1946; Silverman, 1953). The differential diagnosis of subdural hematomas is relatively limited. Spontaneous bleeding may occur in individuals with congenital malformations (aneurysms, for example) of the cerebral vessels or with bleeding disorders. Dehydration or other causes of decreased brain volume (such as atrophy or shunting off of the cerebrospinal fluid [CSF] to treat hydrocephalus) may predispose to subdural bleeding, possibly by dilating the cerebral veins and allowing more movement of the brain relative to the dura, which is affixed to the inner surface of the skull. Subdural bleeding or nonbloody fluid collections are also sometimes seen as sequelae of purulent meningitis.

In very young infants, the presence of subdural fluid collections may raise the question of birth injury. In the past, subarachnoid and subdural bleeding were felt to be relatively common complications of precipitous or forceps deliveries among large, full-term babies, although their incidence has appeared to decrease with current obstetric practices. Children with these injuries usually come to medical attention at about 4–8 weeks of age with a picture of chronic illness: poor feeding, vomiting, and a head circumference that is increasing too rapidly. In contrast, the mean age for presentation of the shaken baby syndrome (see below) has been reported to be about 8 months, but with a range of 1 month to 2 years (Duhaime et al., 1987). The most difficult cases, then, involve children who present in the first 1–2 months of life with chronic or subacute subdural effusions, normal development, and no history of precipitous or traumatic birth. At present, there seems to be no way to determine from the injury itself whether or not these children have been intentionally harmed.

Intracranial bleeding may also be induced by folk medicine practices. In some Latin American cultures, a sunken fontanelle (caída de mollera), which can result from dehydration or malnutrition, may be seen as a sign that a part of the head has fallen and is resting on the palate, causing an obstruction to eating. One folk remedy for the condition is to hold the infant upside down over a pan of boiling water and pound or slap the soles of the feet. In one reported case, this treatment resulted in subdural bleeding and retinal hemorrhages indistinguishable from those found in battered children (Guarnaschelli et al., 1972).

Subdural bleeding is not always easy to detect. The neurologic symptoms are generally nonspecific and focal findings, when present, do not help to localize the hematoma itself. In acute bleeds, the CSF is usually bloody or xanthochromic, but later it may be normal. Bloody CSF obtained by lumbar puncture should always be centrifuged to differentiate what may be the result of a traumatic procedure from truly bloody CSF. In the former case, the supernatant of the centrifuged fluid will be clear, while in the latter it is likely to be colored from red blood cells that have lysed in the cerebrospinal space. Standard skull X rays and ultra sound are not often useful diagnostic tools because early on there are no calcifications to make the hematoma visible and little shift of the echogenic midline of the brain. On the other hand, X rays may demonstrate splitting of the cranial sutures or a fracture, both of which suggest intracranial injury. CT is the most widely available method for efficient diagnosis, although MRI scanning may ultimately prove more sensitive for small lesions and better able to localize bleeding (Alexander et al., 1986).

One difficulty with CT imaging is that subdural hemorrhages change in density relative to brain tissue as they age (Scotti et al., 1977). Acute bleeds (up to about 1 week old) are more dense than the brain. Subacute lesions (variably defined as from about 1 to 3 weeks old) are likely to be of the same density as the brain and thus potentially invisible to a noncontrast CT scan unless they are large or asymmetrical enough to produce a noticeable mass effect or change in the contour of the brain surface. Older lesions are usually less dense than the brain and therefore may be visible with noncontrast studies.

The location of subdural bleeding may suggest that a shaking injury (see below) rather than another variety of head trauma was responsible. In adults, most subdural bleeding occurs in the parietal areas of the head. In contrast, Zimmerman and colleagues (1979) observed that 15 of 17 children with acute subdural bleeding following abuse had bleeding in the posterior portion of the interhemispheric fissure, a site of bleeding that is unusual in adults. This corresponded to the site of bleeding in experimental animals subjected to whiplash injuries (Ommaya and Yarnell, 1967).

Head trauma may also cause epidural bleeding, a loss of blood into the space between the true dura and the inner periosteum of the skull. This usually occurs when an artery is ruptured in the course of trauma, often at the site of a fracture. Blood may exit the skull through the fracture and form a large, palpable subgaleal collection. Bleeds are most often in the temporoparietal or occipital areas and are more contained than subdural bleeding because the dura is attached to the skull at the skull's suture lines. In adults, epidural bleeding is classically associated with a "lucid interval" after the initial reaction to trauma: the patient may be rendered unconscious or dazed by a blow, recover, and feel relatively well for a few hours, only to again lose consciousness and possibly develop focal neurologic signs as a rapid accumulation of blood compresses the brain. This sequence of events is less common in children, who are more likely simply to develop progressively worsening symptoms soon after the injury.

The Shaken Baby Syndrome

Guthkelch (1971) and Caffey (1972) were among the first to describe the so-called shaken baby syndrome of intracranial injuries, retinal hemorrhages, and long-bone fractures in young infants. Although the precise etiology of the syndrome remains unclear, it represents an important and often difficult-to-diagnose presentation of physical abuse.

As originally proposed, the syndrome was felt to occur when an infant was held by the chest and violently shaken. Flailing of the limbs was said to produce the metaphyseal long-bone injuries characteristic of abuse (see Chapter 9), squeezing of the chest was said to be responsible for rib fractures as well as increased intrathoracic pressure leading to retinal hemorrhage, and shaking of the head was proposed to cause both direct cerebral contusion and shearing of bridging veins leading to subdural bleeding.

One recent study has cast doubt on the mechanism originally proposed to explain the syndrome. Duhaime and colleagues (1987) studied 48 cases of infants suspected of having been shaken. The infants were selected because they had evidence of intracranial bleeding (acute or chronic); 39 of the 48 also had retinal hemorrhages. Some parents admitted shaking their infants, and others said that they had hit them or observed a minor fall. None of the explanations, however, could account for the children's critical state at the time care was sought. Thirteen of the infants died. Of these, all had evidence of blunt head trauma (cranial contusions, fractures, or both), although in only six had evidence of impact been found prior to death. The research team then tested the intracranial forces developed when adult volunteers shook infant-sized dolls equipped with transducers. Shaking alone was not able to generate the amount of force that animal studies had predicted would be necessary to produce subdural bleeding or cerebral contusion. The researchers concluded that a direct blow to the head was probably necessary to cause the extent of injury usually attributed to the shaken baby syndrome.

Regardless of the actual cause of the syndrome, symptoms of brain dysfunction are what usually prompt parents to bring a child for medical care. The child may be seen in the emergency room after seizures or an episode of apnea or may be brought to care because of lethargy, irritability, poor muscle tone, or poor feeding, with or without vomiting. Usually the only history of trauma given is that of a minor fall or relatively mild shaking to end a spell of apnea or cyanosis. There may be a history of colic or other infant temperament, feeding, or sleeping problems that stress caretakers. Sometimes there is a history of previous medical care for unexplained breathing problems or ill-defined seizure-like activity.

Diagnosis of the syndrome is difficult because of the misleading history, lack of external findings, and the fact that the child's condition is also suggestive of meningitis, metabolic diseases, ingestion of a toxin, and a variety of other disorders that present with nonspecific signs. Vital signs and basic laboratory tests may not be useful: blood pressure and heart rate may be unstable and the white blood count may be elevated, suggestive of infection (Ludwig and Warmon, 1984). If the injury happened long enough ago and a large amount of intracranial blood has collected, the hematocrit may be abnormally low. The fontanelle may be full or bulging, and in chronic cases the head circumference may be enlarged and the cranial sutures palpably split.

These difficulties with the initial evaluation underscore the importance of an ophthalmologic exam. Because retinal hemorrhages are part of the case definition for most studies, it is difficult to say exactly how often they would be found if all possible cases were considered. At least among presently recognizable cases, however, they are found more than 80% of the time. A lumbar puncture is often bloody. As mentioned above, bloody specimens should be centrifuged to differentiate a sample obtained by a traumatic tap from true CNS bleeding. Chest films obtained in the course of an evaluation for sepsis or heart failure should be carefully examined for rib fractures (see Chapter 9). CT scanning and skull films are the definitive procedures that establish the diagnosis, but they may be not be obtained initially unless neurologic symptoms predominate or retinal hemorrhages are found.

ABDOMINAL AND RETROPERITONEAL INJURIES

Blunt abdominal trauma, at least to the extent that it is now detected, is among the least common but most lethal forms of physical child abuse. About 50% of patients who require inpatient care die, primarily from massive internal bleeding or septic shock. The finding of blunt abdominal trauma may also be a marker for extremely disturbed families in the late stages of abuse. In one series of patients from two urban hospitals, over half of those children admitted with abdominal injuries were already known to child protective services for previously having been abused (Cooper et al., 1988).

Duodenal hematoma is the lesion most associated with intentional injury. Blunt force compresses the small bowel against the vertebral column, producing bleeding into the duodenal wall and sometimes rupture. In the absence of rupture (and subsequent peritonitis), patients usually have a history of abdominal pain, loss of appetite, and vomiting over a period of 1–5 days (Wooley et al., 1978). They are then brought to medical attention with the onset of obstructive symptoms: persistent bilious vomiting.

When initially seen, a patient with duodenal hematoma may be dehydrated. The absence of diarrhea and the bilious nature of the vomiting help differentiate the condition from gastroenteritis. The variable extent of bleeding, combined with the possibility of dehydration, makes anemia an inconsistent finding. Likewise, serum amylase may be normal if there is no damage to the pancreas. Bruises or abrasions over the abdomen or substernal area (see Fig. 6.3) are the exception rather than the rule. Sometimes an upper abdominal mass is palpable, but the diagnosis is usually made radiographically. A flat plate of the abdomen may or may not show a mass effect, and the obstruction is so high that with the stomach decompressed there may be none of the usual signs of obstruction such as air-fluid levels in dilated loops of bowel. The diagnosis is often made with oral contrast studies, although ultrasound (Orel et al., 1988) may be useful both acutely and to follow the progress of healing. A CT scan is often obtained, even if the diagnosis is already established, to rule out other thoracic, abdominal, or retroperitoneal trauma (Kane et al., 1988). Isolated duodenal hematoma has a low mortality rate, and most lesions resolve spontaneously with bowel rest and intravenous alimentation.

Ruptures of the bowel or stomach and lacerations of the liver, spleen, or major abdominal blood vessels produce symptoms more rapidly than do duodenal hematomas. Peritonitis, with its usual physical findings, is a complication of a ruptured viscus, especially when there is a delay in seeking care and systemic sepsis has begun. Hepatic or splenic injuries often present as shock from massive intracapsular or intraperitoneal bleeding. As with other forms of child abuse, however, misleading histories are common and make prompt diagnosis difficult. In the series of 22 cases of blunt abdominal trauma reported by Cooper and colleagues (1988), not one family gave a history of any sort of abdominal injury. In several cases, accounts of minor head injuries misled physicians into evaluating the child's brain before considering the abdomen. Patients with intra-abdominal bleeding all had varying degrees of tachycardia, hypotension, and anemia; however, the extent of the anemia was not always apparent until fluid resuscitation was administered. Urgent surgical consultation and abdominal paracentesis are required whenever blunt trauma is considered in the differential diagnosis of a patient with unstable vital signs. More stable patients should have emergency CT scans of the abdomen to evaluate the extent of their injuries.

References

Alexander RC, Schor DP, Smith WL. Magnetic resonance imaging of intracranial injuries from child abuse. J Pediatr 1986;109:975–979.
Bacon CJ, Sayer GC, Howe JW. Extensive retinal haemorrhages in infancy—an innocent cause. Br Med J 1978;1:281.
Bernat JE. Bite marks and oral manifestations of child abuse and neglect. In: Ellerstein NS, ed. Child abuse and neglect: a medical reference. New York: John Wiley & Sons, 1981:141–164.
Billmire EM, Myers PA. Serious head injury in infants: accident or abuse? Pediatrics 1985;75;340–342.
Caffey J. Multiple fracture in the long bones of infants suffering from chronic subdural hematoma. AJR 1946;56:163–173.
Caffey J. On the theory and practice of shaking infants. Am J Dis Child 1972;124:161–169.
Cooper A, Floyd T, Barlow B, et al. Major blunt abdominal trauma due to child abuse. J Trauma 1988;28:1483–1487.
Duane TD. Valsalva hemorrhagic retinopathy. Am J Ophthalmol 1973;75:637–642.
Duhaime A-C, Gennarelli TA, Thibault LE, Bruce DA, Margulies SS, Wiser R. The shaken baby syndrome: a clinical, pathological, and biomechanical study. J Neurosurg 1987;66:409–415.
Elam AL, Ray VG. Sexually related trauma: a review. Ann Emerg Med 1986;15:576–584.
Eller AW, Brown GC. Retinal disorders of childhood. Pediatr Clin North Am 1983;30:1087–1101.
Gammon JA. Ophthalmic manifestations of child abuse. In: Ellerstein NS, ed. Child abuse and neglect: a medical reference. New York: John Wiley & Sons, 1981:121–140.
Giangiacomo J, Barkett KJ. Ophthalmoscopic findings in occult child abuse. J Pediatr Ophthamol Strabismus 1985;22:234–237.
Guarnaschelli J, Lee J, Pitts FW. "Fallen fontanelle" (caída de mollera): a variant of the battered child syndrome. JAMA 1972;222:1545–1546.
Guthkelch AN. Infantile subdural haematoma and its relationship to whiplash injuries. Br Med J 1971;2:430–431.
Hamlin H. Subgaleal hematoma caused by hair-pull [Letter]. JAMA 1968;204:129.
Helfer RE, Slovis TL, Black M. Injuries resulting when small children fall out of bed. Pediatrics 1977;60:533–535.
Hobbs CJ. Skull fracture and the diagnosis of abuse. Arch Dis Child 1984;59:246–252.
Jensen AD, Smith RE, Olson MI. Ocular clues to child abuse. J Pediatr Ophthalmol 1971;8:270–273.
Joffe M, Ludwig S. Stairway injuries in children. Pediatrics 1988;82(part 2):457–461.
Kane NM, Cronan JJ, Dorfman GS, DeLuca F. Pediatric abdominal trauma: evaluation by computed tomography. Pediatrics 1988;82:11–15.
Kanter RK. Retinal hemorrhage after cardiopulmonary resuscitation or child abuse. J Pediatr 1986;108:430–432.
Lambert SR, Johnson TE, Hoyt CS. Optic nerve sheath and retinal hemorrhages associated with the shaken baby syndrome. Arch Ophthalmol 1986;104:1509–1512.
Ludwig S, Warmon M. Shaken baby syndrome. A review of 20 cases. Ann Emerg Med 1984;13:104–107.
Marr WG, Marr EG. Some observations on Purtcher's disease: traumatic retinal angiopathy. Am J Ophthalmol 1962;54:693–705.
Ommaya AK, Yarnell P. Subdural hematoma after whiplash injury. Lancet 1967;ii:468–469.
Orel SG, Nussbaum AR, Sheth S, Yale-Loehr, Sanders RC. Duodenal hematoma in child abuse: sonographic detection. AJR 1988;151:147–149.
Saulsbury FT, Alford BA. Intracranial bleeding from child abuse: the value of skull radiographs. Pediatr Radiol 1982;12:175–178.
Scotti G, Terbrugge K, Melançon D, Bélanger G. Evaluation of age of subdural hematomas by computerized tomography. J Neurosurg 1977;47:311–315.
Silverman FN. The roentgen manifestations of unrecognized skeletal trauma in infants. AJR 1953;69:413–427.
Tomasi LG, Rosman NP. Purtscher retinopathy in the battered child syndrome. Am J Dis Child 1975;129:1335–1337.
Wooley MM, Mashour GH, Sloan T. Duodenal hematoma in infancy and childhood. Am J Surg 1978;136:8–14.
Zimmerman RA, Bilaniuk LT, Bruce D, Schut L, Uzzell B, Goldberg HI. Computed tomography of craniocerebral injury in the abused child. Radiology 1979;130:687–690.

8 Injuries to the Genitals and Rectum

INTRODUCTION TO THE EXAMINATION

Clinicians examining children suspected of having been sexually abused are often placed under a great deal of pressure to make positive findings. In the United States, there are no formal requirements for corroborating physical evidence to support a child's allegation of having been sexually abused, but such "proof" is still widely expected by many judges and law enforcement officials. As a result, parents and social service workers may come to a clinician seeking not an objective opinion but confirmation of their own beliefs about what has happened to the child. These sorts of pressures are difficult to resist, especially when a case has political overtones (such as abuse alleged to have happened in a school or daycare setting) or when a child's or parent's story seems particularly compelling. Clinicians must struggle with the desire to control the outcome of the case and, at least for the period of the examination, confine themselves to a disinterested accounting and assessment of the physical findings. Clinicians can also try to educate other child welfare professionals about the proper role of physical findings in the overall evaluation of a case of suspected abuse.

Given these pressures and the risk of bias inherent in the interpretation of subtle findings, clinicians often wish to examine a child without any prior knowledge of symptoms or history. Unfortunately, unless one is following a set protocol for the examination (including routine culturing of all orifices for sexually transmitted diseases), the history is vital to both planning the procedures needed to evaluate the patient and interpreting findings.

The biggest obstacle to getting a medical history is that the child is likely already to have been asked to repeat his or her story several times. As discussed in Chapter 3, there is a risk that the child will interpret the multiple interviews as a sign that the story is not believed. These concerns can be addressed specifically, and the clinician may wish to tell the child that although it would be helpful to hear directly about what has happened, the story need not be repeated if doing so is uncomfortable. If the clinician actively elicits an account of the trauma, the guidelines outlined in Chapter 4 for not leading or influencing the child's history should be followed.

Regardless of whether an account of abuse is elicited, it is important to obtain a history of past or present symptoms that may suggest trauma or infection. Information about pubertal development is important for girls, since the physiology and appearance of the female genitalia change markedly as the child matures (Table 8.1). The minimal information obtained might include:

- Time since the last abusive incident is thought to have taken place.
- Whether abuse is thought to have been chronic or took place on a single occasion.
- If the identity of the perpetrator(s) is known, his or her sex and age, and the nature of medical problems that might pose a risk to the victim.
- Whether the victim has had any oral/pharyngeal, genital, or rectal pain, discharge, bleeding, or infection.
- Whether the victim has had any rashes, ulcers, or other skin lesions, especially in the genital or perirectal area.
- Whether there have been changes in patterns of stooling or urination, including secondary enuresis or encopresis.
- Whether signs of onset of puberty, including onset of breast development or menses, have been noted.
- For older females, a history of signs of pregnancy and contraceptives used.

It is difficult to set absolute guidelines for how soon after disclosure a physical examination must be performed. The chances of finding semen or saliva evidence (see Chapter 10) decrease sharply in a matter of hours, and even fairly marked physical signs of acute injury may be gone in a matter of weeks. As discussed below, the diameter of a dilated hymenal ring may shrink within weeks if no further abuse takes

Table 8.1. Stages of Pubertal Development in Girls[a]

Breast Development	Appearance of Pubic Hair[b]
1. Preadolescent: elevation of papilla only	1. None
2. Breast buds: areola widens, small mound forms under papilla and areola	2. Sparse, downy hair on labia
3. Breasts continue to enlarge and elevate but areola is not elevated above breast mound	3. Hair darker and more coarse but still mostly in midline
4. Areola and papilla form a separate mound projecting from breast mound (menarche usually occurs during this stage)	4. Adult-type hair but covering a smaller area
5. Breasts have adult contour and size, areola again does not project from contour of breast	5. Adult pattern; onto thighs

[a]Adapted from: Copeland KC. Variations in normal sexual development. Pediatr Rev 1986;8:47–55; Copeland KC, Brookman RR, Rauh JL. Assessment of pubertal development. Columbus: Ross Laboratories, 1986.
[b]Generally lags behind breast development by a few months.

place. One possible set of guidelines for obtaining examinations is as follows:

- For a known or highly suspected acute case (within the past 48–72 hours), examine immediately at an emergency facility capable of collecting appropriate forensic specimens.
- For a recent case (within the past, 2–3 weeks) but more than 48–72 hours old, examine immediately if there are any concerns about symptoms (for example, difficulty urinating or passing stool, abdominal discomfort, bleeding, or discharge). If there are no symptoms, attempt to obtain an examination by a specialist on an urgent but not emergency basis. If the delay will be more than a 1 or 2 days, the patient may wish to have a general screening check-up by his or her primary care physician as an interim measure.
- For a vague allegation or disclosure of abuse in the distant past, see the patient urgently if there are any symptoms; otherwise, arrange for a screening examination with the primary care practitioner as soon as possible. Ideally, arrange for the child to be seen by a skilled interviewer or counselor before a specialist examination is performed.

When the child's condition permits, it is usually preferable to have an interview take place before an examination. The discomfort or embarrassment of the examination may lead a child to feel punished for having made a disclosure, and negative findings may be interpreted by family members as a sign that the child should not be believed. There is also a risk that younger children, when subsequently interviewed, may refer to the examination when asked if they have ever been touched or hurt in the genitalia. If the family is not supportive of the child, the interview also gives the child a chance to feel befriended before continuing on with more stressful parts of the evaluation.

Preparation of the parents and child is vital to successfully examination of the genitalia. Even if the child is not initially afraid, a parent may successfully project his or her own fears about the child's "first internal exam" or the need to get "needles." Discussion and opportunities to demonstrate techniques involved in medical procedures can often reduce anxiety and discomfort and increase cooperation. As soon as the examination is scheduled, someone must take responsibility for informing the family of what will be involved. Except in acute cases or when children are known to have symptoms, it is usually fair to say that the examination will involve only "looking" and will not entail use of needles or insertion of objects into the child's body. The clinician can say that any further procedures that may be needed will first be discussed with the parent and child.

It is difficult to make definitive statements about normal reactions of children to examination of the genitalia. Ideally, the clinician has examined enough nonabused children to have some idea of reactions that can be expected given his or her own style. Most children will show no or only mild anxiety about a genital exam that is part of a thorough physical during which they have become used to the examiner. Touching or talking about "down there" is sufficiently taboo in enough families, however, that some degree of extra anxiety should be accepted as normal. Extreme passivity and an ability to "tune out" are at least as worrisome as extreme anxiety.

Some fears can be avoided simply by learning the child's own vocabulary for the genitals and rectum so that an explanation of the exam can be given in language that that the child understands. Vocabulary can be explored by questioning or the use of drawings as described in Chapter 4. One must also be cautious about using the traditional pediatrician's assurances of "it won't hurt" or "please, be a good child and it will be all over soon." These may be the same messages given by an abuser to coax the child into submission. It may help to explain that doctors (or other health care professionals) are trained to examine children and help them, that they touch other people only with permission, and that an assistant is often present to ensure the child's comfort. It may also help to use examination gloves to make the point that this is a special, permitted kind of touching.

The child should never be restrained forcibly during an examination of the genitals or rectal area. It is rare that the examination is so urgent that time cannot be taken for negotiation. When a general exam and review of systems do not suggest serious injury, the child should be allowed to refuse or postpone examination of the genitals. There is the risk that refusal is a tactic to manipulate the clinician or the parents, but it is usually outweighed by the possibility of trauma to the child and revictimization if the clinician persists. This is another area in which the clinician may need to distance himself or herself from the case and accept that the evaluation of suspected abuse does not always follow classic medical tradition. All of these considerations, of course, mean that examining the genitalia can take much longer than would seem warranted. Attempts to conduct an examination when the clinician is rushed or fatigued decrease the chances of success.

Proper documentation is critical in sexual abuse examinations. Careful notation of findings may spare the child a reexamination if a disclosure is challenged in court. Misstatements by the clinician can cause great difficulty for other professionals seeking to help the child.

Special care must be taken not to use words that have specific legal meanings or charged emotional value. For example, physicians may consider "penetration" to mean insertion of an object into the anus or vagina, while in some jurisdictions the term is legally defined as mere placement of the penis on the skin of the anal verge or between the labia. Therefore the conclusion "no signs of penetration" may lead to mishandling of the case by social service or legal authorities. Use of the term can also appear to contradict a victim's statement. Children often experience vulvar coitus or placement of an object between the thighs or buttocks as "having something stuck inside me." The statement "no signs of penetration" gives the impression that the child's account is false; documentation of actual findings, even if the conclusion is "normal examination—does not rule out abuse," allows for alternative explanations of the child's sensations. Other frequently misused words include "intact," "gaping," and "sexual injury." Without supporting descriptive data, these terms turn observations into conclusions that other professionals cannot fully evaluate.

FEMALE GENITALIA

Development

The female genitalia change enormously during infancy and again later during puberty, largely because of the effects of estrogen. Estrogen alters not only the size of the genital structures but also the composition of secretions and the nature of the mucosa. Thus, estrogen alters the nature of the vaginal environment and the normal and pathologic microbial flora that can be found.

At birth, the genitalia are heavily estrogenized from maternal hormone that has crossed the placenta into the fetal circulation. The clitoris and labia are relatively prominent and may be pigmented. Small amounts of white vaginal discharge and in some cases "withdrawal" bleeding can be seen in the first 4–6 weeks of life. By 1–2 months of age, the genitalia gain the usual prepubertal appearance: the labia majora become smaller and the epithelium of the labia minora thins; the vaginal mucosa also thins and appears redder than in the adult, and secretions are usually clear and scanty.

Puberty usually begins at about 10 years of age, initially with an increase in the rate of linear growth and then with breast development (Copeland, 1986). Development of pubic and axillary hair usually lags behind breast development by a few months (Table 8.1). Menarche usually takes place in the later stages of puberty, once breast and pubic hair development is well under way (stage 4). Vaginal secretions may thicken, take on a white color, and increase in volume in the 6–12 months prior to menarche. As puberty progresses, the external genitalia gradually take on their adult appearance: the labia enlarge, and the mucosa thickens and becomes pinker in appearance; the hymen also thickens and may become more scalloped and redundant, making it difficult to determine whether it has been torn.

The age of onset and speed of progression of puberty vary greatly, but the sequence of development is relatively constant. Precocious puberty is defined as the onset of pubertal changes before age 8. Premature thelarche (isolated early breast development) and premature adrenarche (isolated early growth of pubic and axillary hair) are sometimes seen and require evaluation to rule out endocrine or gynecologic problems. Early vaginal bleeding, however, in the absence of other signs of sexual development, is unlikely to represent a hormonal effect. Vaginal trauma or the presence of a foreign body and confusion with bleeding from the urethra or rectum are more likely explanations.

Anatomy

The mons pubis is the mound of largely fatty tissue that lies over the symphysis pubis. From it the labia majora extend posteriorly to surround the openings of the urogenital structures (Fig. 8.1). The labia majora do not meet posteriorly. They end separately in the skin between the vaginal opening and anus, outlining an area known as the posterior commisure. (The point where they fuse with the mons is known as the anterior commisure). Before puberty, the labia majora are relatively flat and unpigmented. With the onset of puberty, they grow and become pigmented and thicker on their outer surfaces. This is the primary site of the first pubic hairs.

Within the area defined by the labia majora, and usually visible only by spreading them, are the labia minora. These thinner folds of tissue encircle the clitoris anteriorly and form its hood. They extend posteriorly to enclose the urethra and the vaginal opening. The band of tissue that joins them posteriorly, known as the frenulum of the labia, forms an area called the posterior fourchette. The frenulum is often tightly stretched when the labia are spread. Even small amounts of tension may cause superficial fissures, usually in the midline. Vulvar irritation or a vaginal discharge can leave the skin in the area of the posterior fourchette very friable. Increased friability has been noted both in prepubertal girls with a history of sexual abuse and in girls with genital complaints (primarily vaginitis, vulvitis, and dysuria) without a known history of abuse (Emans et al., 1987).

Before puberty, the labia minora are covered with a noncornified squamous epithelium that is very susceptible to trauma. After mechanical irritation or vaginitis, the labia may develop adhesions to each other, partially or nearly completely covering the opening of the vagina and urethra. Small adhesions are usually posterior, extending anteriorly from the fourchette. Unless there is obstruction to urine flow, most do not require treatment. Parents and children can be reassured that the adhesion will lyse spontaneously with activity and estrogenation at puberty. Some authorities advocate applications of estrogen creams for short periods until the adhesion is disrupted.

Perhaps most important is distinguishing adhesions from less common but more significant conditions. Vaginal agenesis may at first appear similar to a large adhesion that obscures the opening of the vagina. In this case, however, the labia will be identifiable as not being fused, and the urethra will not be covered. Virilization of a female may result in partial or total congenital fusion of the labia minora. This may be a sign of abnormal sexual differentiation or of congenital adrenal hyperplasia. The latter is especially likely if the fusion is associated with an enlarged clitoris and thickening and hyperpigmentation of the labia majora. An imperforate hymen (see below) may also sometimes have the appearance of an adhesion of the labia minora.

Although it seems logical to expect that labial adhesions would be more common in children who have been sexually abused, this is still a topic of debate. Berkowitz and co-workers (1987) reported finding adhesions in 10 of about 375 girls less than 5 years old referred for evaluation of possible sexual abuse (about 3%). Five

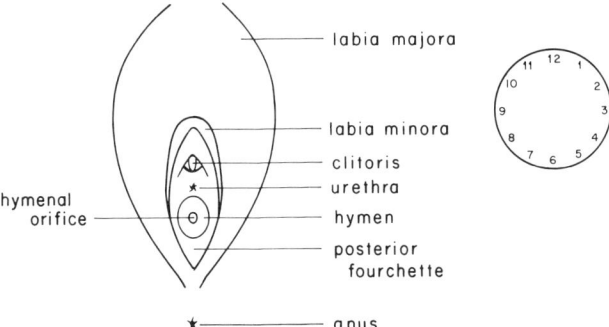

Figure 8.1 Schematic drawing of the prepubertal femal genitalia showing the "face of the clock" method of orientation. (From Seidel JS, Elvik SL, Berkowitz CD, Day C. Presentation and evaluation of sexual misuse in the emergency department. Pediatr Emerg Care 1986;2:157–164, © by Williams & Wilkins, 1986, used by permission.)

of the ten had reportedly given a convincing history of abuse. The 3% prevalence rate was higher than the "normal" rate of 1% or less reported in the literature, but this difference may not have been statistically significant. In a comparative study of asymptomatic prepubertal girls, girls referred for vaginal complaints, and girls who had a history of sexual abuse, Emans and colleagues (1987) found adhesions in 9 of 127 asymptomatic girls (7%), in 4 of 59 girls with vaginal problems (7%), and in 21 of 118 with a history of sexual abuse (18%). There were racial differences in prevalence, however, that altered interpretation of the results. When the results for white girls were analyzed separately, there was no difference in prevalence among the three groups of children (all about 20%). Among black and Hispanic girls adhesions were more common with a history of abuse; however, the number of children examined was small, and most of the comparisons were not statistically significant.

Although the significance of labial adhesions remains unclear, a concern for abuse still seems reasonable given their association with trauma or irritation. As an isolated finding, however, labial adhesions may have no clinical significance. One problem that adhesions do pose is that they sometimes make examination of the hymen impossible, either because they completely cover the vaginal opening or because they limit the degree to which the labia minora may be spread. This is another argument for trying to examine children as soon as possible after a disclosure of abuse has been made.

The vagina is the genital canal that extends from the uterus to the vulva, the external surface of the genital area. The exterior opening of the vagina is often referred to as the introitus. Just inside the introitus are the hymenal ring and the hymen, if present. The placement of anatomic landmarks around the introitus is often described with a face-of-the-clock notation (Woodling and Kossoris, 1981). This form of notation is used in two ways. When one is referring to the entire vulva, an imaginary 9 o'clock–3 o'clock line is drawn horizontally across the vulva just posterior to the urethra, with noon upward toward the symphysis pubis. Tissues above the 9 o'clock–3 o'clock line generally overlie the pubic bone and can easily be crushed, with resultant bruising, in a straddle injury. Tissues below this line are suspended on the perineal musculature: they retract with trauma and are more likely to be injured by anterior-to-posterior penetrating forces such as those encountered during intercourse. The second use of the clock notation is to note the location of structures around the circumference of the introitus or the hymenal ring without regard to the exact placement of the 9 o'clock–3 o'clock line.

Two sets of glands serve to lubricate the urethra and vagina. Skene's glands anteriorly and Bartholin's glands posteriorly. In the pubertal or adult female, these can often be palpated at the edge of the introitus or by inserting one finger and gently squeezing the vaginal wall between that finger and the thumb. They are generally not palpable in prepubertal children;

enlargement may be a sign of infection, possibly with *Neisseria gonorrhoeae*.

It is often possible to see through the hymenal ring to the interior portion of the vagina. Anterior and posterior ridges (columns) run lengthwise, with transverse rugae branching out from them laterally. The length of the vagina varies a great deal with age and among individuals. Just before puberty, it is about 6–7 cm deep along its anterior wall and about 8–11 cm deep posteriorly (Paul, 1986). From birth to about 7 years of age, it is about 4–5 cm long (Cowell, 1981). Penetration with an object larger than a single adult finger will, after only a few episodes, cause the vagina to lengthen and its folds to flatten.

The hymen is a thin membrane that spans the diameter of the vagina just within the introitus. Its normal configuration may vary a great deal among individuals, although congenital absence apparently does not occur except in the case of major genitourinary malformations (Jenny et al., 1987). No standard set of descriptive terms has been developed for the appearance of normal hymens. Pokorny (1987) has proposed the following classification:

- The fimbriated hymen has "redundant, gathered skirts" of tissues with a scalloped rim that attaches to all 360° of the rim of the hymenal ring.
- The circumferential hymen is composed of a "smooth, unfolded skirt" of tissue that also attaches to the full circumference of the hymenal ring.
- The posterior rim hymen appears as a crescent of tissue that runs generally from about 2 or 3 o'clock on the hymenal ring along the posterior edge to a symmetrical location on the opposite side. Partial openings in hymens are usually either central or anterior, probably reflecting how the urogenital sinus and the Müllerian structures join during embryogenesis.
- The hymen may sometimes be imperforate. In that case, its appearance will differ from that of a large labial adhesion in that the urethra will not be covered. The fact that the membrane appears thin instead of thick helps to differentiate an imperforate hymen from agenesis of the vagina. Having the child cough should make the truly imperforate hymen bulge. Children who appear to have an imperforate hymen should be referred to a gynecologist for evaluation. Accumulation of secretions or blood within the vagina and uterus can lead to scarring and later problems with reproductive function.

Inspection of the hymen usually requires gentle spreading of the labia majora to open the hymenal ring and unfold the hymen itself. Before estrogen effects are present, the hymen is usually thin and has a smooth, almost sharp edge. Both thickness and elasticity vary from individual to individual, however. Various characteristics of the hymen have been explored as means of differentiating children who have experienced genital trauma from those who have not.

The size of the opening in the hymen is perhaps the most widely discussed criterion for investigating suspected sexual abuse. The size of this opening depends on two factors: the configuration of the hymen itself and the size of the hymenal ring to which it is attached. Trauma may disrupt the hymen, stretch the ring, or both. Standard texts usually cite some variant of a "1 mm for each year of age up to puberty" rule for the normal upper limit of the diameter of the introitus. Cowell (1981) lists normal "diameters of the hymen" (and thus the ring) as 4 mm in the first 2 months of life, 5 mm from 2 months to 7 years, 7 mm from 7 to 10 years (early signs of estrogen effect), and 10 mm from 10 to 13 years (early puberty).

Cantwell's study (1983) of about 250 girls admitted to a "crisis care unit" because they were suspected of having been abused is one of the most widely cited investigations of the size of the vaginal opening. Children were examined in the supine position by using a tape measure or ruler to estimate the size of the "vaginal opening." The author reasoned that "[n]ormally, the vaginal opening in prepubescent girls is pinpoint to about 3 millimeters (mm)" and so used 4 mm as a cutoff above which abuse might be suspected. All of the girls were less than 13 years old. Some had been admitted explicitly for a history of sexual abuse, whereas others were admitted because of physical abuse or because they had been abandoned or needed temporary shelter. Cantwell compared the vaginal diameter against responses to direct questions about actual or attempted "sexual contact."

A summary of Cantwell's data is presented

in Table 8.2. The results were notable for high specificity and sensitivity as well as good predictive value, given the prevalence of disclosure in the population studied. Criticisms of the study have included the fact that the disclosures and the measurements may not have been made independently and that few details about the possible effects of age and race were provided.

The study by Emans and colleagues (1987) addressed some of these questions by using specific control groups and several examiners, only one of whom conducted interviews. Table 8.3 gives dimensions of the hymenal opening (measured supine) found among children 3–6 years old. Although the asymptomatic children had, on the average, smaller openings, the authors pointed out that only 4 of the 55 children in the abused group had openings larger than the range found in asymptomatic girls. Findings for the abused children and those referred for vaginal complaints were virtually identical.

When the investigators looked only at those children who had been referred for sexual abuse (ages 1–14, $n = 116$), they did find that children who had disclosed vulvar or vaginal trauma had, on the average, larger hymenal openings (5.2 mm) than did those who had been touched or fondled (3.9 mm). Some of this difference was attributable to the fact that the girls in the first group were generally older than those in the latter. The authors concluded that size of the hymenal opening was not a good indicator of whether vaginal or vulvar trauma had taken place, although girls with openings greater than 6 mm in horizontal diameter might be in a group at increased risk if they did not currently have some other vaginal complaint. It was not certain why the girls with vaginal complaints had openings as large as or larger than those of the girls with a history of abuse. The authors speculated that some of the girls may in fact have been abused or that the presence of a larger hymenal opening for some other reason predisposed the children to other vaginal problems. The findings also may have been different if more children in the abuse group had actually suffered vaginal trauma. Only 29 of the 116 reported vulvar coitus, and only 5 reported vaginal penetration.

These studies point out some caveats with respect to measuring the diameter of the hymenal opening. Considerable inter-observer variation is to be expected, if only because making the measurement requires holding a measuring device on the perineum and squinting down the vaginal canal toward the hymenal ring. The hymenal ring itself varies with relaxation and with position; it opens to a greater extent

Table 8.2. Diameter of Vaginal Opening for Girls under Age 13 with and without a Disclosure of Sexual Abuse[a]

Category	Diameter of Opening (mm)[b]	Disclosed Sex Abuse	Did not Disclose
Admitted for sexual abuse	>4	37	
	<4	8	
Admitted for physical abuse	>4	16	6
	<4	2	41
Abandoned	>4	8	4
	<4	3	44
Sheltered	<4	9	2
	>4	0	67
Overall	>4	70	12
	<4	13	152
Total		83	164

Sensitivity (overall) of >4-mm diameter to detect abuse = 70/83 = 0.84
Specificity (overall) of <4-mm diameter to select those who did not disclose = 152/164 = 0.93
Given this prevalence of disclosure (83/247 = 0.34), positive predictive value = 0.85, negative predictive value = 0.92

[a]Adapted from Table 3 of Cantwell HB. Vaginal inspection as it relates to child sexual abuse in girls under thirteen. Child Abuse Negl 1983;7:171–176.
[b]Original data presented as greater than or less than 4 mm.

Table 8.3. Horizontal Diameter of the Hymenal Opening in Girls ages 3–6[a]

Group	n	Mean (mm)	Range (mm)
History of sexual abuse	55	4.0	1–10
Asymptomatic	34	2.9	1–6
Vaginal complaints	19	4.1	2–10

[a]Adapted from Emans SJ, Woods ER, Flagg NT, Freeman A. Genital findings in sexually abused, symptomatic, and asymptomatic girls. Pediatrics 1987;79:778–785.

when the child is in the knee-chest position rather than supine. Care must also be taken that a redundant hymen has completely unfolded so that its true opening can be seen.

There is also evidence that, barring further abuse, a stretched hymenal ring will gradually get smaller. Cantwell (1987) obtained follow-up examinations of some of the children seen in her original study. Twenty children who had reportedly been in safe environments since the time of their first examination were seen an average of 15 months later. Nearly all (19 of 20) had smaller diameters of the hymen. The average amount of reduction was about 4.5 mm (range, 0–12). Using simple linear regression to analyze the data, the reduction in size occurred on the average at a rate of about 0.09 mm/month, although this coefficient was not significantly different from zero ($t = 1.77$, $df = 18$, $P = 0.09$; reanalysis of data presented in the paper). It also seems unlikely that reduction in size as a function of time would be entirely linear; it might be rapid soon after injury and later reach a limit imposed by scar formation or the child's growth.

Several other characteristics of hymens may serve to demonstrate that an individual has a higher likelihood of having been sexually abused. These are well illustrated in the color atlas of prepubertal genital and rectal findings developed by the California Medical Association (Chadwick et al., 1989). Perhaps the most significant is a cleft or tear in the hymen posteriorly, especially at about the 6 o'clock position. Anecdotal reports (Wynne, 1980; Herman-Giddens and Frothingham, 1987) suggest that this is the area most likely to be damaged in violent sexual assault or in attempted penile penetration. In the study by Emans et al. (1987), the presence of a cleft or healed tear in the hymen did not distinguish among abused, asymptomatic, and symptomatic girls. Only three girls, however, had a tear at 6 o'clock, and these were all individuals who had given a history of pain and penetration. Bumps on the hymen in the 3 o'clock–9 o'clock region, adhesions of the hymen to the vaginal wall, attenuation of the hymen (narrowing of the rim), and increased vascularity of the hymen or surrounding tissue have all been found among children with a history of abuse, but Emans and colleagues found them in roughly equal or greater proportion among children with other vaginal complaints. These are all observations based on a relatively small number of studies and patients. Other studies reported to be in progress will certainly add to what is known.

EXAMINATION TECHNIQUES

As mentioned previously, the examination should always begin with an introduction and discussion while the child is still clothed, followed by a complete head-to-toe evaluation before the genitalia are approached. Children who may have been recently assaulted should undress while standing on a clean cloth or paper sheet so that clothing and anything that falls from it can be turned over to the police for forensic testing (see Chapter 10).

When the time comes for the genital examination, prepubertal girls may be comfortable in a modified lithotomy position without stirrups (frogleg), or they may prefer the prone, knee-chest position. The latter offers two potential advantages: first, the internal genitalia fall ventrally, and a good view of the vagina may be obtained through an open hymen; and second, the perirectal area can be examined easily in the same position. The primary disadvantage of the knee-chest position is that it may be more embarrassing for the child. As noted above, the standards that do exist for measurements of hymenal diameter refer to the supine, frogleg position.

Once the child is comfortably positioned, the surface of the vulva can be examined for bruises, lacerations, irritation, or bleeding. The thighs, lower abdomen, and buttocks should also be examined. Venereal warts, erythematous-based vesicles suggestive of herpes infection, or syphilitic chancres may be present, as well as areas that may be semen or other body secretions from the assailant. The latter can be examined with a Wood's light to determine whether they fluoresce; they can then be swabbed for testing (see Chapter 10).

The labia majora may then be spread to examine the vestibule, the area surrounding the introitus. Erythema or bruising around the clitoris or anterior portions of the labia may suggest fondling. Bruises anteriorly in conjunction with posterior tearing of the hymen and circumferential tears of the vestibule strongly suggest forced penetration (Paul, 1977).

As the labia are spread, the area of the posterior fourchette becomes taut. This area may be friable in children who have been abused or have some degree of irritation for another reason; shallow lacerations may be seen if there has been attempted penetration or excessive digital manipulation. Some of these lacerations may be seen with the naked eye, and others can be detected with a magnifying lens. In cases of recent assault or abuse (seen within 48–72 hours), application of a dye such as toluidine blue may highlight superficial lacerations that are otherwise not visible (McCauley et al., 1986). Similar markings may be seen in older women who voluntarily engage in sexual activity.

The opening of the vagina and the hymenal ring are next examined. If the child is in the supine position, gently pulling the labia laterally and slightly downward to the limits imposed by the surrounding tissues will generally open the hymenal ring and allow the configuration of the hymen to be seen. It is reasonable to wait a few moments for the patient to relax, and it may be necessary to open and close the labia two or three times to free redundant folds of the hymen from each other or from the surrounding vaginal wall. If the patient is extremely cooperative and relaxed, a moistened swab may be used to gently free the hymen and test whether it is casually stuck down or actually fused with the vaginal wall. This area is quite sensitive to the touch, however, especially if there is any amount of inflammation.

Good lighting is important to the examination. Many practitioners also use some form of magnification. An otoscope with a bright light, especially the type that has only a cylindrical body and no tapered point when the speculum is removed, works well. This instrument gives a relatively wide field of vision and does not present the child with an intrusive-appearing piece of apparatus. A colposcope (a type of illuminated, binocular operating microscope) gives a variably magnifiable view, excellent lighting, and, depending on its attachments, the ability of to take photographs (Fig. 8.2) or even videotape. These recording devices are ideal for training purposes and may sometimes provide documentation of the findings sufficiently graphic that further examinations can be avoided. Because the colposcope can operate at a foot or so away from the patient, the examiner can maintain more physical distance and thus, perhaps, seem less threatening.

Once the hymen is visible, the findings discussed above can be noted. It may be possible to see through the ring of the hymen into the vagina, in which case the columns and rugae, as well as any suggestion of a foreign body, bleeding, or laceration, can be noted. Concerns regarding the presence of a foreign body may be investigated by palpating anteriorly with a finger inserted in the rectum.

Male Genitalia

The size and appearance of the male genitalia vary considerably with age. Increases in testicular volume and scrotal size, the first stage of puberty (genital stage II), usually take place at 9–13 years of age, before the beginning of rapid gains in height (Table 8.4). Development of pubic hair can lag by as much as 6 months. First ejaculation usually takes place in early to midpuberty, on the average at about 13 years and during genital stage III but before the pubertal growth spurt (Copeland, 1986). The age at which these events begin and the speed of their progression are quite variable, but their sequence is relatively consistent.

Although the testes and scrotum are relatively delicate and certainly sensitive after puberty, the penis is a resilient organ that in the flaccid state is relatively difficult to damage except by significant crushing or use of some lacerating object. The terminal urethra, however, is easily irritated, especially in circumcised males. Mild erythema accompanied by burning at the initiation of urination may be associated with self-stimulatory activity as well as with abuse. A narrowing of the opening of the foreskin so that it is either stretched tightly over the glans or will not open sufficiently to be retracted is called phimosis. Inability to retract the foreskin is not unusual in boys under age 6. Forced retraction can cause painful tearing of the opening and later scarring, with adhesion to the glans. In uncircumcised males, smegma, a cheesy white material composed of sebaceous secretions and epithelial cells, may be present under the foreskin. It may also be present behind the corona of the glans in circumcised boys who have retained some remnants of the foreskin.

A tourniquet syndrome is sometimes seen in males who place some constricting object around the base of the penis (or penis and scrotum) in an attempt to increase and prolong erection. If these objects are rigid or relatively unexpansile they may prove unremovable once

86   Child Advocacy for the Clinician

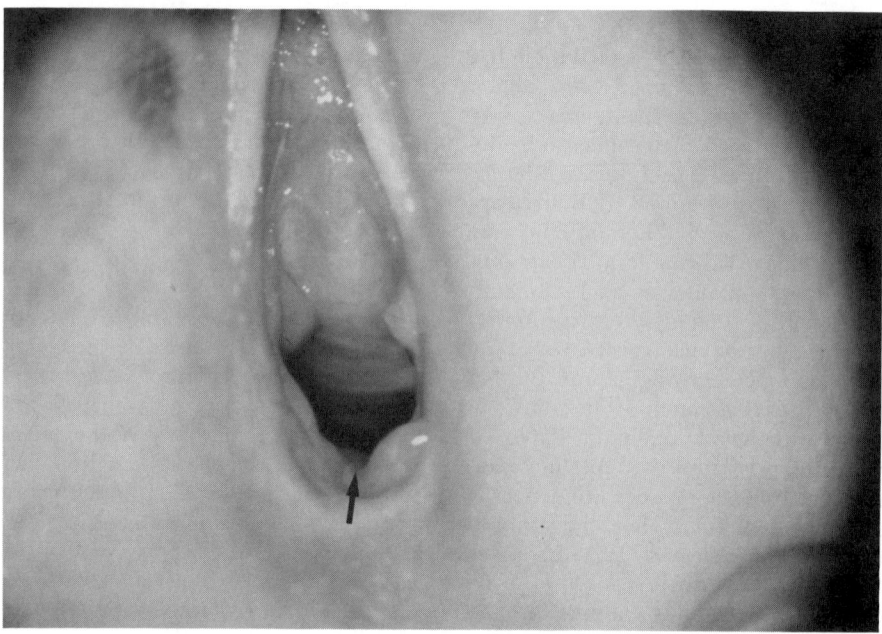

Figure 8.2   Colposcopic photograph of a prepubertal girl's genitalia. The hymen is attenuated, and there is a cleft or interruption at about 6 o'clock. (Courtesy of Dr. T. Doran, Sinai Hospital of Baltimore.)

the penis has become engorged. Rapid removal, with appropriate tools, is required to prevent stasis and infarction of the penis. Small children sometimes develop tourniquet syndrome from a long hair that has come to be wrapped around the penis. Abusers may also place rubber bands or other constricting objects on a child's penis, perhaps as a punishment for wetting.

The penis is vulnerable to "fracture" (actually a rupture of the corpus cavernosum) if it is subjected to trauma while erect. Bleeding is usually local and results in deformity of the penis, sometimes with inability to urinate. Occasionally, bleeding can be extensive and lead to shock. Most fractures apparently can resolve on their own so long as the urethra is not obstructed or lacerated. The result may be a penis with an unusual shape or deviation on erection (Godec et al., 1988). Very little is known about the incidence of this condition, especially among children. Prolonged and possibly rough stimulation of the penis can also cause traumatic lymphangitis, detectable as a nodular cord extending from the corona of the glans back along the shaft of the penis.

Most boys do not resist a genital examination, although many will squirm or be embarrassed. Modesty should be respected, and even school-age boys may prefer that their mother or a female clinician step out of the room. The examination can be conducted with the child supine, sitting, or standing. The temperature of the examiner's hands and the room influence the ease with which the scrotum can be examined. Warmth allows the scrotum to relax and eases evaluation of its contents. Older boys may have an erection during the exam. They can be assured that this is a normal reaction.

The general area of the genitals can first be examined, with notation any bruises, abrasions, bites, or patches suggestive of semen or saliva. The inguinal nodes can be palpated as an aid to diagnosis of sexually transmitted diseases. The shaft of the penis is inspected for bruises, redness, cords, vesicles, or ulcers. The foreskin, if present, can be gently retracted as far as it will easily move. The glans is then inspected for any lesions. Fine vesicles on an erythematous base may be herpetic, while domed, pearly lesions may be molluscum contagiosum. Condyloma acuminatum may present initially

Table 8.4. Stages of Male Pubertal Development[a]

Genital Development	Appearance of Pubic Hair
1. Childhood size	1. None
2. Scrotum and testes (but not penis) enlarge; scrotal skin darkens	2. Sparse downy hair at base of penis; lags scrotal enlargement by a few months
3. Further growth of scrotum and testes; penis starts to elongate	3. Darkening and coarsening of hair; spreads over symphisis
4. Testes and scrotum continue to enlarge; penis elongates and thickens	4. Adult-type hair but over a smaller area; not on thighs
5. Adult size	5. Adult distribution onto thighs
	6. Further spread up midline of abdomen in most but not all males

[a]Adapted from: Copeland KC. Variations in normal sexual development. Pediatr Rev 1986;8:47–55; Copeland KC, Brookman RR, Rauh JL. Assessment of pubertal development. Columbus: Ross Laboratories, 1986.

as individual small papules, but over time it progresses to more flowery or multiple papules that can be on the glans or shaft (see Chapter 10). About 15% of normal males from puberty through young adulthood may have rows of small (1–3 mm) white papules at the margin of the corona. These "pink pearly papules" are unrelated to trauma or sexually transmitted disease (Neinstein and Goldenring, 1984).

The urethral meatus normally appears as a vertically oriented slit in the middle of the glans. Gently squeezing the glans between the thumb and forefinger will open the urethra slightly; the mucosa should be shiny and pink. If no discharge is seen, the penis can be "milked" by gently squeezing the shaft at the base and moving the fingers toward the glans.

The scrotum should be palpated for masses and tenderness. Normally, the testes are sensitive but not painful to the touch. Masses can be transilluminated to help distinguish hydrocoeles (which do transilluminate) from hernias (which generally do not). The epididymis, on the posterolateral surface of the testes, should be sensitive but not tender.

Perirectal Lesions

The prevalence of rectal injury in child abuse may well be underestimated, if only because knowledge of normal variations and the manifestations of trauma is even more scanty than for the genitalia. Serious injury to the rectum seems to be relatively uncommon in prepubertal sexual abuse, possibly because many pedophiles go to great lengths not to inflict trauma so that abuse will go undetected. In addition, the anus is very expansive: many stools are larger than the adult penis and can be accommodated without injury. Healing also appears to be quite rapid, and so minor injuries may be virtually undetectable by 2–3 weeks after a sexual encounter. More serious injuries may be inflicted when the assailant is another child, in the setting of rape, or among adolescents who may be involved with adults practicing some of the more unusual rectal sexual practices such as insertion of hands ("fisting") or foreign bodies. It seems likely that as more sexual abuse victims, especially males, come forward, the true prevalence of anal injuries will be found to be relatively high.

The types of injuries found in children or adults correspond to various aspects of the anatomy of the perirectal area (Paul, 1986; Elam and Ray, 1986). When the buttocks are first parted, the hyperpigmented skin of the anal verge can be seen surrounding the anteriorly-posteriorly oriented slit of the anus itself. The anal verge is roughly circular, and its skin is loosely applied over a thin layer of involuntary muscle and an easily disrupted network of small blood vessels (the inferior hemorrhoidal plexus). The muscle layer normally keeps the skin folded into multiple shallow furrows that fan out from the anus more or less symmetrically in all directions. Penetration with a single finger or other small object, especially if it is well lubricated, may leave no visible mark on the anal verge except possibly a shallow abrasion such as from a fingernail (Paul, 1977). Larger objects, however, especially if no lubricant is used, will tend to draw the anal verge skin inward with them. The fragile blood vessels under the skin may break, causing either localized or circumferential bruising (Hobbs and Wynne, 1986). The skin itself may tear, causing a shallow fissure that may bleed. More extensive tears extending beyond the skin of the anal verge, either onto the adjacent skin of the buttocks or down into the rectal mucosa, are clearly unusual and suggest some nonphysiologic trauma. On the other hand, shallow fissures are indistinguishable from the injuries that can be caused by the passage of a large, hard stool or from the friability and maceration encountered with children who wear diapers or have poor hygiene. Shallow fissuring may leave fine scars that appear to be triangular, with the point of the triangle facing the anal opening, when the skin folds of the anal verge are spread during an examination. Although some authorities have felt that scars created by objects passing out of the rectum look different from those created by objects going in, others (Paul, 1986) feel that these two events generally leave the same markings. The latter opinion is based on the fact that the configuration of superficial rectal scars appears to be determined by the action of the underlying musculature rather than the mechanics of the injury.

Anecdotal reports suggest that unless there is chronic abuse, most minor lesions of the anal verge resolve within weeks. Areas of blue discoloration or hematomas resolve in days, sometimes leaving small skin tags that may persist for an additional 2–3 weeks (Paul, 1977). These can be confused with midline skin tags in or near the anal verge, which are often a normal finding. In those cases, the tag will be noted to have been present since birth. Some observers (Hobbs and Wynne, 1986) feel that increased prominence of the venous markings under the skin of the anal verge, or more pronounced filling and emptying of these vessels, may be a sign of prior trauma. Hemorrhoids may also be found and, since otherwise they are rare in childhood, may indicate prior trauma. Other causes of hemorrhoids include perirectal infections and inflammatory bowel disease.

Chronic abuse does appear to alter the skin of the anal verge. It becomes thickened from repeated abrasion and flattened as the underlying muscle becomes stretched. In extreme cases, the perianal area may take on a funnel-shaped appearance such that the apparent opening of the anus is within the perianal skin, above its normal location at the point where the rectal mucosa begins. Although this finding is said to be rare in children, one group of physicians reported seeing it in 6 of 224 prepubertal children examined for suspicion of sexual abuse (Wright et al., 1987).

The anal canal is the passage that links the lower rectum to the exterior of the body at the anus. It ranges from about 1 cm long in children to 3 cm in adults. The external part of the canal is made up of skin similar to that of the anal verge: delicate and very sensitive to pain, because it in innervated by the somatic sensory system. The internal portion is lined with a mucous membrane that is relatively insensitive to pain because it derives it innervation from the autonomic system. The internal and external portions meet near the so-called dentate line, which gets its name from the appearance of the puckered, longitudinal folds (known as Morgagni's, anal, or rectal columns) of the internal portion. The dentate line is at the level at which the anal canal passes through the levator ani musculature. At the ends of the anal columns are blind folds known as anal valves. The "crypt" within each valve contains glands that lubricate the area and that can be involved in perirectal infections and ultimately in the development of perianal abcesses (Storer et al., 1974).

Both trauma and infection (with chlamydia, gonorrhea, or herpesvirus, for example) may produce erythema and edema of the anal mucosa (proctitis). Symptoms include a burning sensation and pain on defecation. If the irritation is caused by a single episode of trauma and is not associated with infection, it will resolve spontaneously. The anal mucosa may also be lacerated (with or without involvement of the deeper muscle layers), causing pain and bleeding. Laceration may be caused by insertion of the penis, other body parts, or an object of some kind. Care must be taken to ensure that the laceration has not perforated the wall of the anal canal or of the rectum. These are very distensible structures, and perforation suggests either great force or the introduction of a relatively large or sharp object. Perforations may enter either the peritoneal cavity or the perineal tissues. The former type of perforation usually presents rapidly with signs of peritonitis and free air in the abdomen, but the latter may not be readily apparent until cellulitis develops. Initial evaluation can include checking the hematocrit and vital signs to determine the extent of bleeding and an upright abdominal film to search for a foreign body or free air in the peritoneal cavity. Children suspected of having serious acute rectal trauma should be hospitalized for observation, surgical consultation, and possibly proctoscopy.

The anal sphincter is composed of two sets of overlapping musculature, the internal and external sphincters. The internal sphincter, which lies closest to the bowel, is an involuntary muscle innervated by the autonomic nervous system, whereas the external sphincter, which wraps around the internal sphincter and extends the entire length of the anal canal, is a striated, voluntary muscle. The external sphincter has no opposing muscles to force it to open; defecation is possible when the muscle relaxes from its usually contracted position.

Acute stretching of the sphincter may cause it to remain open for a period of hours. If the muscle fibers have not actually been ruptured (sometimes visible at the site of a laceration of the anal skin or mucosa), the injury will be followed by spasm. Injury to the anal area that does not stretch the sphincter may also result in spasm as the muscles attempt to "splint" sensitive tissues and reduce discomfort. After the acute period, unless there has been repeated penetration or tearing, the sphincter will appear normal. Repeated penetration can result in stretching of the sphincter so that it easily accommodates wide objects (several centimeters in diameter) and loses some of its strength (manifested as a decreased "grip" on an examiner's fingers). Scarring from an old laceration or splinting because of an abcess or fissure may produce increases in tone or asymmetry in the shape of the anus when the sphincter is closed.

One of the standard findings in routine physical examinations of children and adults is the so-called anal wink, a reflex tightening of the external sphincter in response to stimulation of the perirectal skin. The reflex is also sometimes triggered by simply spreading the buttocks. It can be abolished by lesions of the sacral segments of the spinal cord or of the pelvic nerves, and individuals can learn to inhibit it if they have experienced frequent stimulation in the perirectal area or if they wish to be cooperative with the examiner. Physicians who perform digital rectal examinations in adults, for example, know that with coaching and relaxation, a patient can relax the sphincter to allow entry of a finger or an instrument. Children who have had repeated rectal examinations or frequent enemas or other instrumentation may also learn to inhibit contraction of the sphincter. It follows that failure to observe a strong wink, or the ability to relax the sphincter during observation or digital examination, is a nonspecific finding that may have many interpretations.

No data exist regarding how far the anus should normally open when the buttocks are spread. Some children tighten the anus when the buttocks are spread, and others relax it slightly, often allowing a small amount of flatus to escape. Both of these reactions are probably normal (Paul, 1986). If traction is applied to the perirectal skin to test the sphincter, the mucocutaneous junction of the anal canal can easily be seen in normal individuals because it is actually just at or below the bottom edge of the sphincter muscles. At present, it is probably best for clinicians to develop their own standards for abnormal dilatation of the anus by carefully examining this area during well-child care. Paul (1986) feels that dilatation of the anus is indicative of chronic abuse only when it is accompanied by thickening and smoothing of the perianal skin and by decreased strength of the sphincter on digital examination.

If the child is willing and able to talk about what has happened, he or she should be asked in an open-ended, nonleading way about discomfort or pain associated with the incident. Anal penetration is usually painful both initially and on withdrawal. This pain is often sharp, and children sometimes will report that the assailant "put a knife in my rear." This may in fact be the case, but it is important to ask whether the child actually saw a knife or other sharp object. The discrepancy between this type of account and a finding of only minor or no lasting trauma often serves to discredit the child's statement erroneously. Clinicians can help by explaining the probable source of the child's perception. There is usually a dull aching sensation after anal penetration or, if there has been more extensive trauma, continued sharp pain. Even with minimal trauma there may be pain on defecation for 2–3 weeks, sometimes accompanied by a change in bowel habits.

If it is not appropriate to ask about the incident of abuse, or if no such event has been disclosed, it is still important to inquire about other rectal symptoms such as burning or pain on defecation, passing of blood, or problems with large, hard stools or chronic constipation. These questions can be put as they would be normally, by asking about the frequency of defecation and medications or enemas that may have been administered. Changes in bowel habits are also of potential significance, as are episodes of encopresis after toilet training or apparent leakage of stool.

The perirectal examination must be more than a quick look. Relaxation and good lighting are vital. The child should initially be assured that the exam will be totally external and not painful. He or she may be comfortable in a variety of positions, including supine, bent over prone (standing or on a special proctoscopy table), or on the side. The knee-chest position also offers good visibility but may be the most embarrassing.

When the child is relaxed, the buttocks can be spread gently and the configuration and reaction of the anus observed. As discussed above, either a reflex tightening or gentle relaxation is probably normal. If there is any doubt about the competency of the sphincter, the perirectal skin can be stimulated to provoke a wink, but a negative response in a relaxed child may not have great meaning. The anus itself should be a relatively uniform anterior-posterior slit surrounded by a symmetrical area of hyperpigmented skin. The buttocks themselves should be examined for bruises and scars.

The perirectal skin should be examined for redness, scars, hemorrhoids, skin tags, fissures, ulcers, and warts. Irritation may be secondary to poor hygiene or pinworm infection. The folds of the anal verge can be gently spread tangentially to look for shallow fissures or scars that may not be immediately visible. Inspection and gentle palpation of the skin around the anal verge, especially anteriorly, may reveal bulging or tenderness suggestive of a perirectal abcess or fistula. Finally, traction on either side of the anal verge allows inspection of the most distal portion of the anal canal, possibly revealing other hemorrhoids either external or internal (if they have prolapsed).

For most children with a normal examination or with no findings suggestive of chronic abuse, no further inspection may be required. A digital examination is not likely to yield any further information unless there is reason to suspect a vaginal foreign body that might be felt through the anterior wall of the rectum. If there is reason to suspect serious acute or complicated chronic injury (perforation, fistula, or foreign body), a specialist should be consulted for an examination with an appropriate instrument, probably under anesthesia.

When chronic abuse is suspected but no acute injury is present, a digital examination may be the easiest way to determine the extent of stretching and decrease in strength or, alternatively, the extent of scarring. The digital exam is best performed with a gloved, lubricated finger (Seidel et al., 1987). Gentle pressure should be exerted with the ball of the finger, not the tip. Older children can be asked to bear down as if they were going to the bathroom. They should be warned that they may feel as if they are about to defecate but that they will not do so. As the sphincter relaxes, the finger can be rotated forward so that the tip enters first. If relaxation fails to occur or there is tightening, waiting for a moment with the finger in place and reassuring the child may help. Once the finger is inserted, it can be rotated gently to assess first the uniformity of the superficial portion of the external sphincter and then the deep portion of the sphincter and the wall of the rectum.

References

Berkowitz CD, Elvik SL, Logan MK. Labial fusion in prepubescent girls: a marker for sexual abuse? Am J Obstet Gynecol 1987;156:16–20.

Cantwell HB. Vaginal inspection as it relates to child sexual abuse in girls under thirteen. Child Abuse Negl 1983;7:171–176.

Cantwell HB. Update on vaginal inspection as it relates to child sexual abuse in girls under thirteen. Child Abuse Negl 1987;11:545–546.

Chadwick DL, Berkowitz CD, Kerns DL, McCann J, Reinhart MA, Strickland SL. Color atlas of child sexual abuse. Chicago: Year Book Medical Publishers, Inc, 1989.

Copeland KC. Variations in normal sexual development. Pediatr Rev 1986;8:47–55.

Cowell CA. The gynecologic examination of infants, children, and young adolescents. Pediatr Clin North Am 1981;28:247–266.

Elam AL, Ray VG. Sexually related trauma: a review. Ann Emerg Med 1986;15:576–584.

Emans SJ, Woods ER, Flagg NT, Freeman A. Genital

findings in sexually abused, symptomatic, and asymptomatic girls. Pediatrics 1987;79:778–785.

Godec CJ, Reiser R, Logush AZ. The erect penis—injury prone organ. J Trauma 1988;28:124–126.

Herman-Giddens ME, Frothingham TE. Prepubertal female genitalia: examination for evidence of sexual abuse. Pediatrics 1987;80:203–208.

Hobbs CJ, Wynne JM. Buggery in childhood—a common syndrome of child abuse. Lancet 1986;ii:792–798.

Jenny C, Kuhns MLD, Arakawa F. Hymens in newborn female infants. Pediatrics 1987;80:399–400.

McCauley J, Gorman RL, Guzinski G. Toluidine blue in the detection of perineal lacerations in pediatric and adolescent sexual abuse victims. Pediatrics 1986;78:1039–1043.

Neinstein LS, Goldenring JG. Pink pearly papules: an epidemiologic study. J Pediatr 1984;594–595.

Paul DM. The medical examination in sexual offences against children. Med Sci Law 1977;17:251–258.

Paul DM. 'What really did happen to baby Jane?'—the medical aspects of the investigation of alleged sexual abuse of children. Med Sci Law 1986;26:85–102.

Pokorny SF. Configuration of the prepubertal hymen. Am J Obstet Gynecol 1987;157:950–956.

Seidel HM, Ball JW, Dains JE, Benedict GW. Mosby's guide to physical examination. St. Louis: CV Mosby, 1987:471–489.

Storer EH, Goldberg SM, Nivatvongs S. Colon, rectum, and anus. In: Schwartz SI, ed. Principles of surgery. 2nd ed. New York: McGraw-Hill Book Co, 1974:1109–1166.

Woodling BA, Kossoris PD. Sexual misuse: rape, molestation, and incest. Pediatr Clin North Am 1981;28:481–499.

Wright C, Fraser EM, Denman M, Duke L. Detection of sexual abuse in children [Letter]. Lancet 1987;ii:218.

Wynne JM. Injuries to the genitalia in female children. S Afr Med J 1980;57:47–50.

9

Skeletal Trauma

Bony injury caused by child abuse may present in two general ways. Often, a child is brought to an emergency facility with an obvious injury. When an X ray reveals a fracture, the clinician may be called on to decide whether the injury happened accidentally or was inflicted. Alternatively, children may come with other injuries, and the clinician may decide to look for evidence of bony trauma as a way of corroborating the suspicion of abuse. In either case, it is important to know which bony injuries are most suggestive of abuse and how best to look for them (Leonidas, 1983).

THE SKELETAL SURVEY

As always, the history and physical examination are the primary tools for detecting suspicious injuries. When trauma is the presenting complaint, the mechanism proposed for the injury must be plausible and related in a consistent manner by the child's caretaker. When presenting symptoms are vague, a thorough physical examination may reveal tenderness, guarding, or asymmetry of motion as clues to the presence of a fracture. In either case, the question arises as to whether a systematic search for fractures should be made of the entire skeleton—the skeletal or "trauma X" survey. It is very compelling to search for bony injury in a case of suspected abuse. One is usually dealing with a child too young to give any verbal account of abuse, and the finding of characteristic skeletal trauma may be the only noncontroversial evidence that abuse has taken place. On the other hand, only a small fraction of all abused children have radiologically visible lesions. The expense and radiation exposure involved in skeletal surveys do not justify screening every suspected case.

Bony injuries are most common in abused infants (generally under age 3); it is in this age group that full skeletal surveys are recommended when there is other evidence suggestive of abuse or neglect. The age range can be extended for children with mental or physical handicaps that may make them more vulnerable to physical abuse. The survey consists of exploratory views of the entire body. There will usually be one or more views of the skull, an anterior-posterior and lateral view of the chest, lateral views of the spine, and frontal views of the upper and lower extremities, including the pelvis, hands, and feet. The smaller the child, the fewer images needed to complete the series. Additional films are taken if abnormalities are noted.

At some facilities, bone scans are also used in the evaluation of suspected abuse. In this type of study, radioactively labeled substances are injected into the bloodstream. Different substances are concentrated in various tissues of the body, where their presence can be detected by a camera sensitive to their radioactivity. Bone scans have some advantages over X-ray films, but they have disadvantages as well (Jaudes, 1984; Kleinman, 1987). In skilled hands, scans are probably more sensitive than standard X rays, and they are better than X rays for detecting recent trauma. As discussed below, nondisplaced fractures may not be detectable by X ray for 1–2 weeks, but may be visible to a scan at 24–48 hours after injury. Scans are also good for detecting injuries to the ribs, hands, or feet (if they are asymmetric) that may be hidden or too subtle on X-ray survey films.

Scans have both technical and logistical disadvantages. An area of bone is visible on a scan because of an increase in blood flow to the traumatized tissue. Unfortunately, some of the injuries most characteristic of child abuse occur in areas of bone that already have increased blood flow because they are where the bone is actively growing. Unilateral injuries to these areas may be visible (by comparing the injured with the normal extremity, for example), but bilateral injuries may not be detected. Scans also are more costly than X rays, may require sedation of the child, and may not be available on an urgent basis or outside of larger hospitals. They involve more radiation to rapidly growing tissues than X rays; additional radiation is required if the scan is positive because positive areas must subsequently be examined with X rays to confirm that a fracture is present.

Both X rays and scans sometimes give false negative results when compared with each other.

The absence of a true standard and the significant role of observer variation in interpreting films or scans make it difficult to say that one is clearly superior to the other. A standard X-ray bone survey is the more practical of the two methods and probably the most frequently used. If a survey is negative and the suspicion of abuse remains high, or if the diagnosis must be made immediately after an episode of acute injury, a bone scan may be obtained.

BONE GROWTH AND INJURY IN EARLY CHILDHOOD

Two characteristics of children's bones make it difficult to see the kinds of fractures most related to abuse. First, the bones of young children are not as fully mineralized as they are later in life. Some areas of bone, particularly the epiphyses of long bones, may not be sufficiently mineralized to be visible on X ray. Second, other bones, such as the ribs, are sufficiently flexible that after injury they return to their original shape. An epiphyseal injury or a rib fracture may not be visible by X ray until 1–2 weeks later, when bone is either removed or laid down in the course of healing. Thus, if recent injury is suspected, X rays may need to be repeated at a later date.

Knowledge of how bone heals is important for knowing when X rays are likely to be positive and for estimating the time of injury from the appearance of a fracture, often called "dating" a fracture. Dating of fractures may help define when an episode of abuse occurred. When more than one fracture is present, dating can provide evidence of whether the fractures occurred at the same time. Fractures of differing ages suggest injury on more than one occasion, a finding that increases the suspicion of abuse.

Although the physiology of healing in simple, unintentional fractures is relatively well understood, the healing of abuse-related injuries may vary from the normal pattern (O'Connor and Cohen, 1987). In the case of unintentional injury, an individual suffers trauma and immediately seeks treatment. The injured bone is usually immobilized soon after the trauma takes place and is allowed to heal without disturbance. In cases of child abuse, in contrast, the healing process is often disrupted. The original injury may involve multiple blows or applications of force to a fracture site, increasing the amount of bleeding and associated damage to soft tissue. The fracture may often be reinjured before healing is complete, either from another episode of abuse or because failure to seek care for the child results in use and movement of the injured body part. As a result, healing may take much longer than in cases of unintentional injuries.

The first stage of bone healing is known as induction. It is defined as the period from the time of injury until the appearance of new bone and usually lasts about 10–14 days, although it may be as short as a week in infants. During this time, a nondisplaced fracture may be invisible to standard X rays except, perhaps, for some tissue changes such as displacement of adjacent fat pads. These inflammatory changes usually last only 3–7 days. Inflammation is the major source of pain associated with a fracture. In young children, it may resolve in 1 or 2 days, which may be one reason why children often appear to tolerate nondisplaced rib and long-bone fractures with relatively few symptoms. Their apparent lack of pain or restricted motion is often used as a reason to doubt or deny a diagnosis of abuse.

New periosteal bone is sometimes the first radiologic sign to appear, often as early as 4 days after injury. More often, soft callus appears around the fracture site and is visible on X rays at about 10–21 days. This timing can be delayed if the child's nutritional status is poor or if there is an underlying chronic illness. As callus forms, bone at the fracture site itself is resorbed. In a displaced fracture, where sharply outlined edges of broken bone were originally visible, this reforming results in a loss of definition of the fracture line. In a nondisplaced fracture that was originally invisible, a fracture line may then be seen for the first time.

The soft callus stage of healing normally lasts about 3–4 weeks in adults; the duration can be shorter in children. Then, new bone begins to bridge the fracture line, sometimes visible as a fading of the fracture on X ray. Hard callus ultimately unites the fracture, and remodeling takes place so that the bone comes to regain its original configuration. In infants, fractures may be united in as little as a few weeks; the time increases with age so that children in their teens may require about 3 months. Remodeling may also be very short in infancy or in other cases where there was minimal displacement of the original fracture and no reinjury. By 6 months to 1 year, evidence of most fractures will be gone, although more serious injuries may take years to remodel.

BONE LESIONS HIGHLY SUGGESTIVE OF ABUSE

For the purposes of the clinician involved in assessing cases of suspected child abuse, fractures can be divided into two categories. First, some fractures, such as those of ribs and the metaphyses of long bones, are felt to be essentially diagnostic of intentional injury. When all cases of abuse are taken together, these fractures are not the most commonly found, but their presence is highly significant. In contrast are the many types of fractures that occur commonly in abuse but are also frequently caused by unintentional injury as well. Evaluation of these fractures requires an open mind and a careful assessment of the plausibility of the history given (Table 9.1).

Metaphyseal Injuries

Growing bones can be roughly divided into three sections: the diaphysis, or main shaft of the bone; the metaphysis, or growth plate; and the epiphysis, the area beyond the growth plate. Injuries to the metaphyses of the long bones are among the lesions felt to be most diagnostic of intentional injury. They are thought to occur when the limbs are subjected to pulling and torsional forces as a child is shaken or pulled violently (Caffey, 1972). These injuries appear radiologically as tufts, chips, or arcs of bone ("bucket handles") at the ends of the diaphysis adjacent to the uncalcified and radiolucent metaphysis (Fig. 9.1). They are most commonly seen in the distal femur and proximal tibia, but they can also be seen in the distal tibia and in the long bones of the upper extremity. They may or may not be accompanied by radiologic signs of periosteal injury (Fig. 9.2).

The appearance of these fractures on X-ray films gave rise to the theory that they were caused by avulsion of metaphyseal bone at its attachment to the periosteum. In childhood, the periosteum is most firmly attached at the metaphysis, and it was thought that flexing of the bone during abuse would concentrate force at that location. Histologic studies, however, have suggested a different mechanism behind the radiologic appearance (Kleinman et al., 1986). It appears instead that the actual injury is a fracture through the newly forming bone just under (on the diaphysis side of) the growth plate.[1] This creates a thin disk of bone just under the radiolucent growth plate and epiphysis. The disk is thicker around its circumference (subperiosteally) and thinner in the center. When the disk is projected onto two-dimensional radiographic film from various angles, it takes on the appearance of arc-shaped or corner fractures (Fig. 9.3).

In its earliest stages, this type of injury appears as only a subtle increased lucency adjacent to the thin linear density of bone along the metaphysis. This is not specific to abuse and may occur in chronic disease, especially leukemia. As the injury heals, it takes on the characteristics described above. The results of periosteal injury, if it occurred, may be visible as extensive calcification alongside the diaphysis and later as a thickening of the cortex of the bone along the diaphysis.

Rib Fractures

Rib fractures in young children are usually nondisplaced and are thus visible only once healing has begun. Healing is manifested by the appearance of the fracture line and development of callus, which in the ribs forms a characteristic rounded thickening (Fig. 9.4) that then persists for months while the bone is remodeled.

Rib injuries in cases of child abuse are classically described as occurring posteriorly near the attachment to the spine. As with metaphyseal fractures, there is some controversy as to the mechanism behind these injuries. It may be that they occur either from a direct blow on the back or from squeezing of the sides of the chest, causing bowing in the front and back. An alternative explanation is that anterior-posterior force causes the posterior portion of the ribs to be flexed over a fulcrum formed by the transverse processes of the spine, resulting in a fracture (Kleinman, 1987).

Some studies have found lateral rib fractures, usually in the posterior axillary line, to be more common in cases in which abuse was highly suspected (Thomas, 1977). Both lateral and posterior fractures may be difficult to see on X rays. Since they are frequently asympto-

---

[1] Classic epiphyseal plate injury (Salter-Harris types I–V) can also occur in intentional injury, although such injuries do not appear to be common and do not have the same diagnostic specificity for abuse.

Skeletal Trauma

Table 9.1. Injury Pattern Studies: Sources for Types of Injury Expected in Common Childhood Trauma[a]

Reference	Mechanism	Intentional/ Unintentional	Method to Ascertain Intentional Nature
Pascoe et al. (1979)	Wear and tear (skin lesions)	Both	Assume clinic population is not abused; compare with abuse reports
Robertson et al. (1982)	Wear and tear	Both	Assume clinic population is not abused; compare with inpatient or emergency room abuse cases
Kravitz et al. (1969)	Falls from low surfaces	Unintentional	Self-report by parents at clinic visit
Helfer et al. (1977)	Falls from beds	Unintentional	Record of observed falls on hospital incident reports
Rieder et al. (1986)	Baby walkers	Unintentional	Emergency room cases; self-report by parents
Wellman and Paulson (1984)	Baby walkers	Unintentional	Chart review; emergency room cases assumed unintentional
Joffe and Ludwig (1988)	Falls down stairs	Unintentional	Chart review; self report by parents
Hobbs (1984)	Falls causing head trauma	Both	Inpatient cases plus abuse team reports
Lenoski and Hunter (1977)	Burns	Intentional	Emergency room cases
Feldman et al. (1978)	Tapwater scalds	Both	Hospitalized cases
Ayoub and Pfeifer (1979)	Burns	Neglect and intentional	Abuse team records
Keen et al. (1975)	Burns	Intentional	Abuse team records

[a]The studies cited are given as examples; others are mentioned in the text or can be found in the literature.

matic, they may not be noticed on a film obtained primarily for another reason (for example, to check placement of an endotracheal tube). Lateral fractures may not been seen because they are hidden by the overlapping shadows of the curving ribs, while posterior fractures may be hidden by the shadow of the transverse spinous processes. Oblique views of the chest and a careful examination of the ribs on each side for asymmetry are useful diagnostic tools.

Lateral rib fractures are felt to occur from anterior-posterior compression of the chest. They do sometimes occur in sick premature infants with osteoporotic bones, apparently caused in the course of urgent care or chest physiotherapy. Rib fractures are rare in pediatric cardiopulmonary resuscitation, however (Feldman and Brewer, 1984). In addition, rib lesions with callus, found at the time of an episode of acute illness, cannot possibly be associated with that episode since the presence of callus suggests a healing lesion that is at least 10–14 days old. Aside from the differential diagnosis discussed below, posterior or lateral rib fractures should be considered suggestive of abuse, especially if more than one fracture is present and if these fractures appear to be of differing ages. Fractures of the lower ribs should prompt an evaluation for abdominal injuries such as lacerations of the spleen or liver.

Complex Skull Fractures

Skull fractures present many dilemmas for the physician. Simple, nondisplaced linear fractures of the parietal bone can occur from relatively minor trauma (Helfer et al., 1977), although they can be caused by abuse as well. Skull fractures may be difficult to see on X-ray, and a ra-

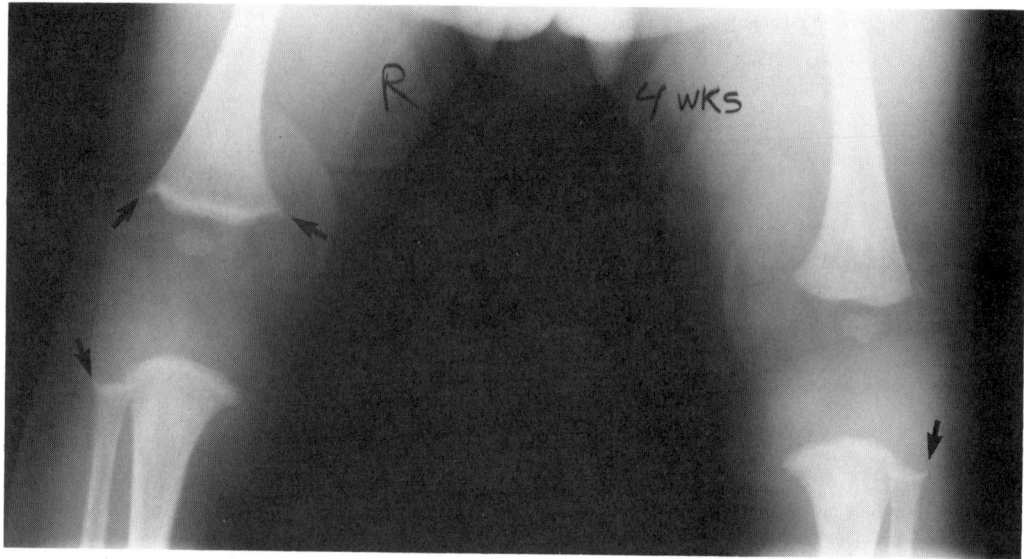

Figure 9.1 Infant's lower extremities showing metaphyseal tufts (*arrows*) of the right distal femur. (Compare the right with the left, where the distal femur appears normal, with a smooth, rounded edge.) Similar lesions are present in the right and left fibula and possibly the right tibia. X ray was taken at about 4 weeks after injury.

diologist's consultation plus additional films may be required to confirm the presence or absence of a lesion. Such consultation is not always available on a timely basis. A radiologist can be asked to look for several features in particular as the film is read (Hobbs, 1984; Meservy et al., 1987). Fractures that are wider than 3 mm, complex (showing branching fracture lines, multiple fractures, involvement of skull suture lines), or bilateral or that occur outside the parietal bone are suggestive of significant force (Fig. 9.5). The cranial sutures may also be widened if there has been an increase in intracranial pressure. The presence of these findings is consistent with an automobile accident, a fall from a considerable height, or a forceful blow to the head. In the setting of minor trauma, or when no explanation is given at all at all, they strongly suggest abuse.

Skull fractures cannot be dated in the manner used for long-bone or rib fractures. They are more likely to be radiologically visible acutely, but their appearance gives no clue as to their age. Children suspected of having suffered head injury often are taken for computed tomography (CT) scans before conventional X rays are performed. CT scans can easily miss fractures, however. The X-ray exposures used in CT scans are not optimal for imaging bone, and the tomographic views taken may not include the area of the fracture. Conventional skull films should be obtained once it is medically safe to do so if abuse is suspected.

Any Combination of Multiple Fractures and Multiple Stages of Healing

Many battered children have fractures in more than one location or fractures that appear to be in different stages of healing. These are unusual findings outside the settings of major trauma or abnormalities of the bones themselves. Again, such fractures are highly associated with abuse but not overly common among abused children. In one series of 189 physically abused children with fractures, for example, about half had only one fracture and only about 30% had three or more (King et al., 1988).

BONE LESIONS SEEN IN INTENTIONAL AND UNINTENTIONAL INJURIES

The long bones of the upper and lower extremities are among the most commonly injured in physically abused children (King et al., 1988). Spiral or oblique fractures of the long bones are frequently cited as being suggestive of abuse. In fact, they may occur in any setting

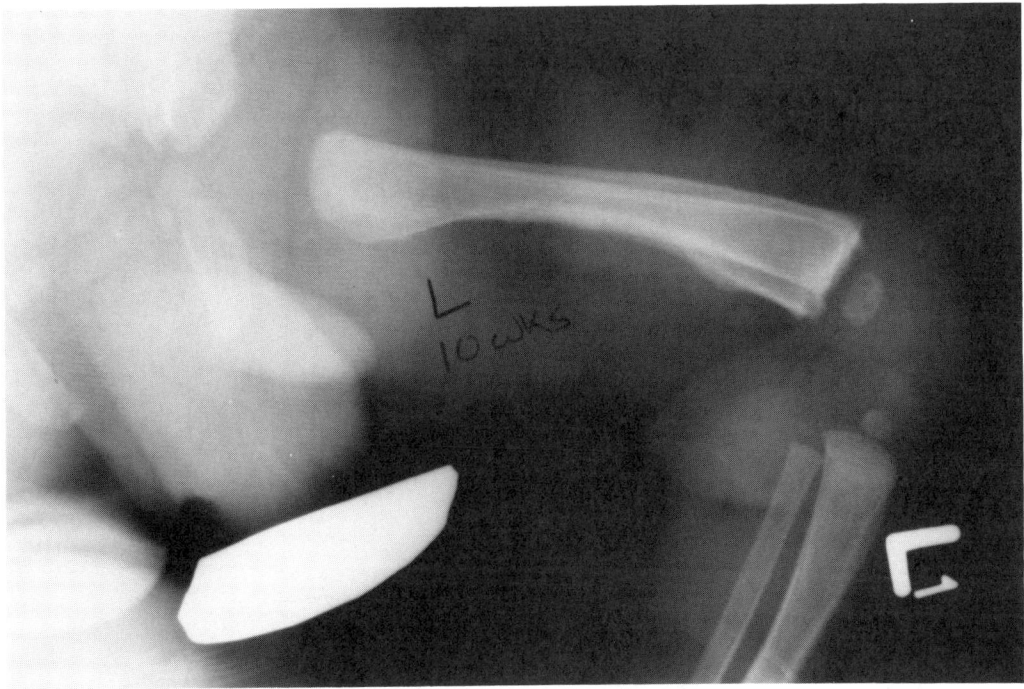

Figure 9.2 Same infant as pictured in Fig. 9.1, film taken about 6 weeks later. The left femur, which appeared normal on the previous films, has extensive periosteal reaction distally.

in which there is rotational force on a bone, although it is thought that a relatively great amount of force is required. Transverse fractures are actually just as common, or more so, as spiral or oblique fractures in cases of abuse. They appear to be caused by direct injury to the bone. Femur fractures of either kind appear to be uncommon in minor household trauma such as falling off a bed (Helfer et al., 1977).

Toddlers may suffer nondisplaced, often spiral-appearing fractures of the tibia. They may appear as only a thin radiolucent line extending down the shaft of the bone. They are felt to occur in the normal course of learning to walk but may also be seen in children with intentional injuries. Likewise, the "nursemaid's elbow" (subluxation of the head of the radius) can occur with or without abuse. These injuries typically occur when toddlers are walking with an adult and are being held by the hand so that the elbow is extended over the child's head. If the toddler trips and the adult holds on, pulling and twisting of the elbow can cause a dislocation. Some children appear to be congenitally susceptible to this injury and will repeatedly dislocate the same elbow.

DIFFERENTIAL DIAGNOSIS

Several conditions may render the bones more susceptible to injury or give radiologic findings that mimic trauma. Some of the less common causes include congenital syphilis, scurvy, infantile cortical hyperostosis, osteogenesis imperfecta, and Menkes's kinky hair syndrome. These have characteristic clinical or radiologic appearances that help to differentiate them from abuse.

Extreme osteoporosis or rickets may be present in sick premature infants or older children who are malnourished or immobilized secondary to physical or mental handicaps. These children may suffer fractures resulting from minor trauma or medical treatments such as cardiopulmonary resuscitation, chest percussion, or physical therapy. The underlying abnormality of the bones is usually readily apparent. Cases have also been reported, however, in which children prescribed passive exercise programs

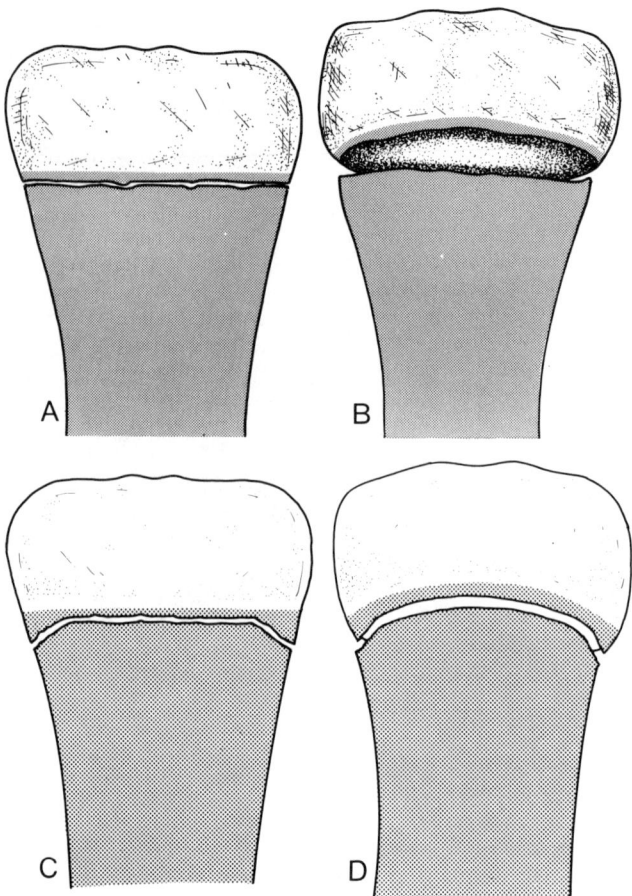

Figure 9.3 Model of the metaphyseal lesion in child abuse, showing variations in appearance as angle of X-ray beam changes relative to the fracture plane. Stippled area represents bone visible on X ray. (From Kleinman PK. Diagnostic imaging in child abuse. Baltimore: Williams & Wilkins, 1987:17. © 1987, the Williams & Wilkins Co., Baltimore. Used by permission.)

had fractures of normal bones (Helfer et al., 1984). These children were felt to have been the victims of excessively forceful "therapy" administered by stressed caretakers. Some of the children had other evidence of intentional trauma. This type of injury supports the observation that children who have or who are perceived as having handicaps are more vulnerable to abuse.

Osteomyelitis, septic arthritis, and malignancies such as leukemia or neuroblastoma may sometimes present radiographic or bone scan pictures that resemble trauma. These diagnoses are often considered when a child presents with a sudden onset of limp or unwillingness to bear weight on one leg. Often only the course of the illness and subsequent laboratory tests allow the diagnosis to be made. If initial suspicions exist or the medical picture is atypical, the social evaluation for maltreatment should be undertaken along with the medical work-up.

Injury during traumatic delivery may also sometimes result in fractures. Periosteal changes in the diaphysis of long bones may be visible and fractures of the clavicle may occur, sometimes in conjunction with brachial plexus injuries. Fractures of the clavicle are common unintentional injuries in older children as well. The usual site is the midshaft of the bone. The mechanism of injury is sometimes a direct blow

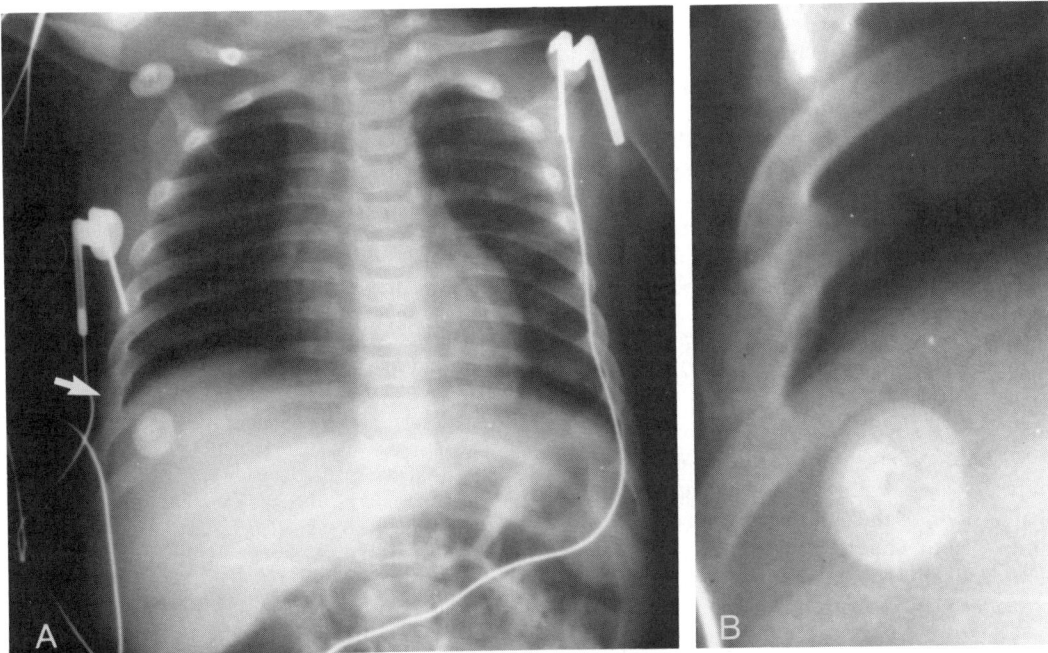

Figure 9.4 A, Chest X ray of a 2-month-old child admitted to an intensive care unit following seizures and apnea. Film unexpectedly showed healing fracture of right seventh rib (*arrow*). B, Enlarged view of fracture site.

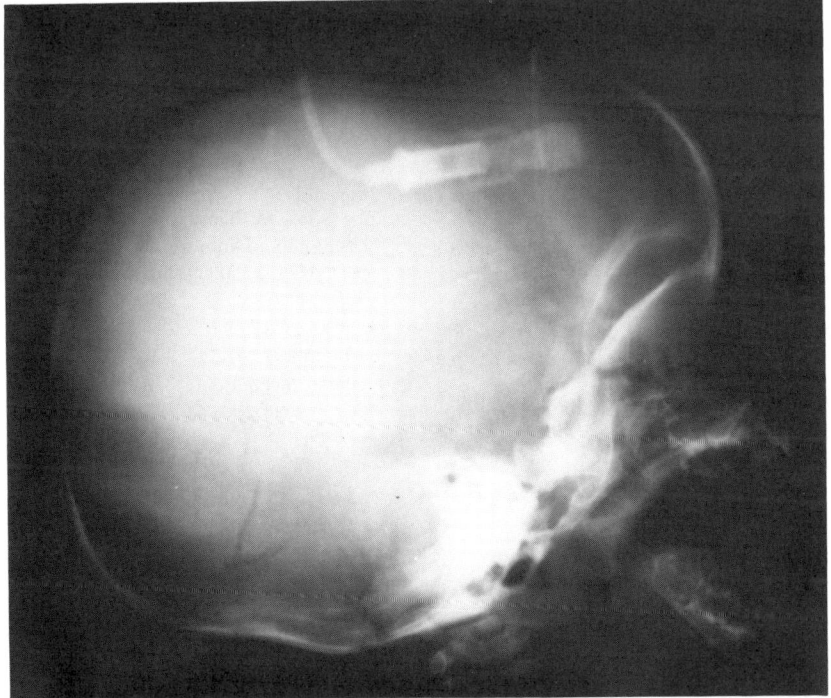

Figure 9.5 Skull fractures in the 2-month-old child with rib fractures shown in Fig. 9.4. Four fractures are visible: three in the parietal-occipital region of the skull that are vertical-oblique, and one in the temporal-parietal region that is horizontal. Widening of the cranial sutures can also be seen: coronal suture is seen as a broad, dark band extending from the orbit to the top of the skull (under the hub of the intravenous connector).

but more often force transmitted from a fall braced by an outstretched arm. The pain of these fractures usually subsides quickly, and it is common for them to go unnoticed. The most troublesome clavicular injuries with respect to abuse are those that occur in children who cannot prop with their arms and who are not ambulatory. Healing clavicular fractures in children under 2 months of age may well have resulted from birth injury, and midshaft fractures in active, ambulatory children may have resulted from unintentional trauma. Between these age groups, however, fresh clavicular fractures or those that seem too recent to have occurred at birth are highly suggestive of abuse (Kleinman, 1987).

Skull fractures at the time of birth are most associated with forceps deliveries, abnormal position of the child in the uterus, and prolonged labor. These fractures are likely to be depressed and have a high incidence of accompanying intracranial injury.

References

Ayoub C, Pfeifer D. Burns as a manifestation of child abuse and neglect. Am J Dis Child 1979;133:910–914.

Caffey J. On the theory and practice of shaking infants. Am J Dis Child 1972;124:161–169.

Feldman KW, Brewer DK. Child abuse, cardiopulmonry resuscitation, and rib fractures. Pediatrics 1984;73:339–342.

Feldman KW, Schaller RT, Feldman JA, McMillion M. Tap water scald burns in children. Pediatrics 1978;62:1–7.

Helfer RE, Slovis TL, Black M. Injuries resulting when small children fall out of bed. Pediatrics 1977;60:533–535.

Helfer RE, Scheurer SL, Alexander R, Reed J, Slovis TL. Trauma to the bones of small infants from passive exercise: a factor in the etiology of child abuse. J Pediatr 1984;104:47–50.

Hobbs CJ. Skull fracture and the diagnosis of abuse. Arch Dis Child 1984;59:246–252.

Jaudes PK. Comparison of radiography and radionuclide bone scanning in detection of child abuse. Pediatrics 1984;73:166–168.

Joffe M, Ludwig S. Stairway injuries in children. Pediatrics 1988;82(Part 2):457–461.

Keen JH, Lendrum J, Wolman B. Inflicted burns and scalds in children. Br Med J 1975;4:268–269.

King J, Diefendorf D, Apthorp J, Negrete VF, Carlson M. Analysis of 429 fractures in 189 battered children. J Pediatr Orthop 1988;8:585–589.

Kleinman PK. Diagnostic imaging in child abuse. Baltimore: Williams & Wilkins, 1987.

Kleinman PK, Marks SC, Blackbourne B. The metaphyseal lesion in abused infants: a radiologic-histopathologic study. AJR 1986;146:895–905.

Kravitz H, Driessen G, Gomberg R. Accidental falls from elevated surfaces in infants from birth to one year of age. Pediatrics 1969;44(Suppl):869–876.

Lenoski EF, Hunter KA. Specific patterns of inflicted burn injuries. J Trauma 1977;17:842–846.

Leonidas JC. Skeletal trauma in the child abuse syndrome. Pediatr Ann 1983;12:875–881.

Meservy CJ, Towbin R, McLaurin RL, Myers P, Ball W. Radiographic characteristics of skull fractures resulting from child abuse. AJR 1987;149:173–175.

O'Connor JF, Cohen J. Dating fractures. In: Kleinman PK, ed. Diagnostic imaging in child abuse. Baltimore: Williams & Wilkins, 1987:103–114.

Pascoe JM, Hildebrandt HM, Tarrier A, Murphy M. Patterns of skin injury in nonaccidental and accidental injury. Pediatrics 1979;64:245–247.

Rieder MJ, Schwartz C, Newman J. Patterns of walker use and walker injury. Pediatrics 1986;78:488–493.

Robertson DM, Barbor P, Hull D. Unusual injury? Recent injury in normal children and children with suspected non-accidental injury. Br Med J 1982;285:1399–1401.

Thomas PS. Rib fractures in infancy. Ann Radiol 1977;20:115–122.

Wellman S, Paulson JA. Baby walker-related injuries. Clin Pediatr 1984;23:98–99.

10 Sexually Transmitted Diseases and Forensic Procedures in Child Sexual Abuse

Of all of the types of child maltreatment, sexual abuse requires the most meticulous collection of laboratory and forensic evidence. Most of this effort is aimed at detecting sexually transmitted diseases (STDs) and other body fluids or tissues that may be transferred from the abuser to the victim during intimate contact. Although this kind of evidence will be found in only a minority of cases, it must be looked for carefully whenever sexual abuse is suspected. When found, it is compelling evidence that abuse has taken place and may at times help identify the abuser.

Only a small proportion of sexually abused children are found to have been infected with an STD. Rimsza and Niggemann (1982) found that about a quarter of sexually abused children under 18 had signs or symptoms of infection at the time of their initial physical examination, and other studies have found smaller proportions. The apparent prevalence of STDs in abused children varies with the nature of the sexual contact, the symptoms present, the length of time from abuse to examination, the diagnostic methods used, and the specific organisms for which tests are performed. Thus, there is no simple rule as to which children should be tested and for what conditions. Some organisms are felt to be relatively certain markers of sexual contact, others seem to be found more commonly with sexual contact but may still be found in presumably nonabused children, and yet others appear to have no relationship to sexual activity at all. The following paragraphs discuss aspects of STD epidemiology and detection as they apply to sexual abuse. Treatment for these conditions will not be discussed in detail. Recommendations are given in the Centers for Disease Control's STD treatment guidelines (Anonymous, 1985), which are updated on a regular basis.

VULVITIS AND VAGINITIS IN PREPUBERTAL GIRLS

The vaginal mucosa and other tissues of the vulva react dramatically to the presence of estrogens. At birth, when maternal estrogens are present, and again at puberty (starting about 6 months to 1 year prior to menarche), the mucosa is thick and secretions are slightly acidic. From about 6 weeks after birth until puberty, the mucosa is thin and the pH neutral. These changes alter both susceptibility to infection and the sites at which organisms will grow. The estrogenized epithelium, for example, is a poor host for the organisms causing gonorrheal and chlamydial infections, which are found, among postpubertal females, in the periurethral glands, cervix, and rectum. *Trichomonas*, in contrast, grows well in the estrogenized vagina. This relationship is reversed in the absence of estrogen effect. Gonorrhea is a truly vaginal infection in prepubertal girls, and *Trichomonas* grows poorly, although it may still be found in the urethra.

Anatomy also plays a role in making the unestrogenized vulva and vagina susceptible to irritation and infection. The skin and mucosa are relatively thin and their surfaces easily disrupted. The labia majora are underdeveloped and offer little protection from mechanical trauma or from potential pathogens. Prepubertal girls are also at risk of relatively poor hygiene either from having to be in diapers, immature personal habits, or self-stimulation. These factors contribute to the fact that vulvitis and vaginitis are common causes of medical consultation among young girls. Sometimes, the presence of vulvar or vaginal irritation prompts a concern for sexual abuse.

Vulvitis is defined as irritation of the external structures of female genitalia (Altcheck, 1984; Emans, 1986). Symptoms include itching, redness, and burning. There may be dysuria, although unless there is also a urinary tract infection, urgency and frequency will not be present. Vulvitis is usually caused by local irritation, either mechanical, chemical, or of a nonspecific infectious nature. Sometimes specific skin lesions, either infectious (herpes, impetigo, condyloma acuminatum) or dermatologic (seborrhea, atopic dermatitis), will be found. Infestations with scabies and pinworms may also be present. If no specific signs of infection are found, cultures of the vagina rarely yield a treatable pathogen. In that case, treatment can be nonspecific (improved hygiene, nonocclusive clothing) or aimed at specific skin conditions. If an STD is found on the vulva, however, vaginal cultures should be obtained for other diseases, regardless of the presence of symptoms.

Vaginitis (usually accompanied by vulvitis) is manifested by a discharge as well as redness or discomfort. Cultures in this case are more likely to yield a specific pathogen, although foreign bodies, congenital anomalies, and nonspecific causes are also common. Table 10.1 lists many (but not all) of the organisms that may be found by culturing or examining the vagina of prepubertal girls.

Perhaps the most controversial organism listed in Table 10.1 is *Gardnerella vaginalis*. *Gardnerella* was once thought to be the causative agent of so-called nonspecific vaginitis (NSV), a well-defined clinical entity characterized by a thin, relatively alkaline vaginal discharge that reacts with potassium hydroxide to release a fishy odor, and clue cells (vaginal epithelial cells coated with bacteria). It is now thought that *Gardnerella* plays only a partial or marker role in NSV and that in small quantities it is part of the normal vaginal flora, at least in postpubertal women. It is regularly found in both sexually active and inactive postpubertal women but more commonly among those who are sexually active (Bump et al., 1986; Shafer et al., 1985). In one study of prepubertal girls (Bartley et al., 1987), *Gardnerella* was found in about 15% of 137 children who were being evaluated for suspected sexual abuse, but only 4% of 119 girls who either were asymptomatic or had vaginal complaints not related to abuse. Detection of *Gardnerella* was unrelated to the presence or absence of symptoms or a discharge. Hammerschlag and colleagues (1985) used clinical criteria (wet preparations for clue cells, the "whiff" test for fishy odor, and measurement of vaginal pH) to diagnose NSV in a group of girls referred for suspected sexual abuse. They also examined a group of girls coming for well-child care. About a quarter had already had the onset of menses, and others had probably experienced the onset of puberty. Of 31 abused children, 8 developed "possible" or "definite" NSV within several days after an acute episode of abuse, while only 1 of the 23 well children developed even "possible" NSV. These studies suggest that *Gardnerella* and NSV may help define groups of children who are more likely than others to have been abused but that they are not absolute indications of abuse.

INFECTIONS WITH SPECIFIC ORGANISMS

Chlamydia trachomatis

Chlamydia trachomatis, an obligate intracellular parasite, is increasingly recognized as among the most common causes of sexually transmitted disease in Western societies. *Chlamydia* has been difficult to detect because it is not readily seen in conventionally stained preparations of clinical materials and because tissue culture techniques are required for its growth in the laboratory. In recent years, however, both rapid diagnostic techniques and tissue culture methods have become widely available.

Chlamydial infection in adults can cause urethritis, cervicitis, pelvic inflammatory disease, and a variety of other conditions, although it may also be present in the absence of any symptoms. When disease appears immediately after contact with the organism, the time from contact to symptoms ranges from about 1 to 3 weeks. Some strains of *Chlamydia* cause lymphogranuloma venereum (LGV), a sexually transmitted disease characterized by small, painless vesicles or ulcers on the genitalia that subsequently disappear and are followed by painful inguinal adenopathy or hemorrhagic proctitis. LGV appears to be most common in Africa, Asia, and South America, although it is occasionally found elsewhere in the world. Only a few pediatric cases have been reported in the United States.

Chlamydia does not grow well in the estrogenized vaginal mucosa but does proliferate in the urethra and cervix. In adults, the presence of *Chlamydia* appears to be highly associated with sexual activity. In a study of teenagers, Shafer and co-workers (1985) found no positive cervical cultures for *Chlamydia* among young women who reported that they were not sexually active. Positive cultures were found in more than 10% of young women who did report sexual activity. In another study of adolescents, Chacko and Lovchik (1984) found positive genital cultures for *Chlamydia* in about 25% of males and females

Table 10.1 Organisms found in the Genital Tract of Prepubertal Girls Beyond the Perinatal Period

Organism	Comments
Flora not associated with sexual activity[a] *Candida* species	Rare to find symptoms except with antibiotic treatment, diabetes, or immunodeficiency; small number of yeasts often found in asymptomatic children
Group A, β-hemolytic *Streptococcus* Pneumococcus *Neisseria meningitidis* *Staphylococcus aureus* *Haemophilus influenzae* *Shigella*	May be associated with symptomatic infection elsewhere; probably transmitted in the same manner as infection of other sites
Diphtheroids *Staphylococcus epidermidis* α-Hemolytic *Streptococcus* *Escherichia coli*	
Normal flora that appear to be more common in children with sexual contact[b]	
Gardnerella vaginalis	Presence in asymptomatic child probably not clinically meaningful; finding organism in association with symptoms suggests NSV; both NSV and asymptomatic colonization appear to be more common in children with a history of sexual contact (Bartley et al., 1987; Hammerschlag et al., 1985)
Lactobacilli *Mycoplasma hominis* *Ureaplasma urealyticum*	
Strong markers of sexual contact[c]	
Chlamydia Condylomata *Neisseria gonorrhoeae* *Trichomonas vaginalis*	
Herpes type 2 Syphilis Molluscum	Demonstrated to have nonsexual transmission to nongenital sites

[a] Although some may cause disease that requires treatment.
[b] Data for *Lactobacilli* and *M. hominis* extrapolated from studies in postpubertal children.
[c] See text for caveats regarding perinatal and possible nonsexual transmission.

who reported having one or no sexual partners but in 8 of 16 individuals who reported having more than one partner. Infection was found more frequently but not exclusively in those with genitourinary symptoms.

Among children, the association of *Chlamydia* with sexual contact is not as well defined as among adults, but it is still strongly suspected beyond the first 1–2 years of life. Studies using good control groups have yet to be done, but the available results have been relatively consistent. Some of the difficulties involved in conducting studies are illustrated by the findings of Hammerschlag and colleagues (1984). They obtained cultures and serologies for *Chlamydia* from 51 children hospitalized for the evaluation of suspected sexual abuse and 43 control children attending a well-child clinic. Five positive cultures were found; however, two were from the hospitalized children and three were from controls. Two of the controls subsequently disclosed that they were victims of incest, but the third, a 7 year old with positive pharyngeal and rectal cultures, gave no history suggestive of abuse. Ingram and co-workers (1986) found positive vaginal cultures for *Chlamydia* in 10 of 124 children who were evaluated for abuse and gave a history of sexual contact but in none of 90 who denied experiencing abuse but were being evaluated for other risk factors. Rettig and Nelson (1981) cultured for *Chlamydia* in 51 prepubertal children who had symptoms of urethritis and vaginitis. Of 31 children found to have gonococcal infections, 9 were also infected with *Chlamydia*, whereas no *Chlamydia* was found in children not infected with gonorrhea. The strong association of gonorrhea with sexual contact suggested that *Chlamydia* was sexually transmitted as well.

Chlamydia can be transmitted at birth. Over a third of infants born to infected mothers have culture-detectable *Chlamydia* in one of their mucous membranes, and over half have serologic evidence of exposure (Schachter et al., 1986). The most commonly recognized perinatal symptoms are conjunctivitis and pneumonitis. The former usually presents at 5–14 days of age. Treatment with topical erythromycin at the time of birth may prevent conjunctivitis but cannot eradicate colonization of other body sites. Pneumonitis usually is diagnosed at about 6 weeks of age, although symptoms (tachypnea, paroxysmal cough, or rales) may have been present and gradually worsening since week 2 or 3.

Longitudinal studies have suggested that once colonization occurs at the time of birth, a substantial amount of either autoinoculation or late growth of organism can occur at a variety of body sites. Cultures at the time of birth are often negative, but subsequently the conjunctiva and nasopharynx become positive, the former in the first month and the latter in the first 3 months (Schachter et al., 1986; Bell et al., 1987). Rectal and vaginal cultures become positive over the following months, even when they have been demonstrated to be negative at these sites earlier in life; in some cases, however, they do appear to become colonized at birth. Colonization of sites other than the conjunctiva and nasopharynx is usually without symptoms. In one study (Schachter et al., 1986), all infants with positive *Chlamydia* cultures became negative by 1 year of age, either because symptomatic infection had been treated or because asymptomatic carriage had cleared spontaneously. The age at which perinatally acquired infection no longer needs to be considered, however, is not known. Latent infections in ophthalmologic disease caused by *Chlamydia* and the relatively high prevalence of asymptomatic infection in adults give reason to suspect that undetected infection may persist longer than 1 year.

Much remains to be learned about the role of *Chlamydia* in diseases of prepubertal children. Serologic surveys and case reports, for example, have suggested that some strains of *Chlamydia* may be associated with respiratory disease beyond infancy. It still seems reasonable, however, to strongly consider the possibility of sexual contact in children who are found to have chlamydial infections beyond age 1–2. Concern for abuse is heightened if there is no maternal history of genital infection or infant history of conjunctivitis or pneumonia.

Studies of both pre- and postpubertal individuals suggest that symptoms are not a reliable indicator of chlamydial infection. In children, pharyngeal and rectal cultures in particular have not been associated with symptoms. The most reliable technique for detection is culture. Cultures appear to be capable of detecting 80–90% of urethral or cervical infections. They would appear to be near 100% specific. Cultures must be obtained and processed carefully. Samples are obtained with synthetic (dacron, calcium alginate, etc.) swabs rather than the cotton-and-wood type. Since the organisms live in epithelial rather than inflammatory cells, the mucosa sampled (vagina in prepubertal girls, cervix in older females) should be gently scraped to obtain material for analysis. Swabs must be immediately placed in special transport medium and either frozen or transferred promptly to culture medium. Cultures take 48–72 hours to grow, longer if apparently negative specimens are passaged blind to a second culture.

Several rapid diagnostic tests using enzyme-linked or direct fluorescence immunoassays have been developed to detect *Chlamydia*. These tests were developed for use in high-prevalence settings, i.e., the assessment of cervical or urethral specimens from symptomatic individuals. Their performance in other settings appears to be problematic. False-positive results have been reported for both types of rapid test (Hammerschlag et al., 1988). The assays use polyclonal antibodies that can cross-react with several bacterial species, including those found normally in the rectum. Direct fluorescence methods offer some protection from this problem because the technician interpreting the test has the opportunity to decide which fluorescent-stained objects seen under the microscope are truly *Chlamydia* elementary bodies and which are artifacts. This can still be a subjective process and one subject to legal challenge as being only presumptive. Standards can be set for the number of elementary bodies that must be counted to make a positive diagnosis, but when counting is done according to the test manufacturer's recommendations, sensitivity may fall considerably. In one study that performed simultaneous cultures and direct immunofluorescence tests, four of eight positive vaginal cultures in sexually abused girls were rated "inconclusive" or "negative" by the rapid method (Fuster and Neinstein, 1987). Thus, the use of presently available rapid diagnostic tests for *Chlamydia* is not recommended in cases of suspected abuse unless cultures are not available or the child has a symptomatic infection of the urethra, vagina (prepubertal), or cervix.

Gonorrhea

Gonorrhea is one of the most common STDs. In adults, its presence is a strong marker for sexual activity. Clinically apparent infections in adults cause urethritis, cervicitis, urethritis, proctitis, pharyngitis, pelvic inflammatory disease, and disseminated infection. Urethritis in males usually develops within a few days of exposure. The incubation period for cervicitis in females is more variable but still usually within 10 days for women who develop symptoms. Because *Neisseria gonorrhoeae* does not grow well in the estrogenized vagina, genital infections in adult females predominantly involve the endocervical canal. In prepubertal children, genital tract infections are primarily vaginal.

N. gonorrhoeae is found fairly frequently among children suspected of having been sexually abused. White and co-workers (1983) found that more than 10% of children seen in a statewide sexual abuse treatment program had positive cultures for the organism. Nonetheless, there remains a long-standing controversy about the possibility of nonsexual transmission of *N. gonorrhoeae* in children. Perinatally acquired disease is well described. Newborns may be infected during passage through the birth canal. Pregnant women may have ascending infection and develop gonococcal amnionitis, and infection of the fetus apparently can take place before the time of birth. For example, some cases of apparent failure of silver nitrate prophylaxis for neonatal gonococcal ophthalmia are associated with prolonged rupture of the amniotic membranes before birth, raising the possibility that infection was established before passage through the cervix and vagina (Gutman and Wilfert, 1984).

Ophthalmologic disease is the most common syndrome associated with neonatal exposure, although it occurs in only a minority of children born to infected mothers. Untreated, it can lead to blindness and requires emergent parenteral antibiotic therapy. Vaginal, pharyngeal, and rectal colonization can also occur at birth, although it appears that symptomatic infection is less likely to develop at these sites. How long this colonization can persist is not known. Two cases of neonatal gonococcal vaginitis reported in the literature involved girls who were about 1 month old (Stark and Glode, 1979; Barton and Shuja, 1981). It may be that colonization does not evolve into symptomatic infection until levels of maternally derived estrogens have fallen and the vaginal mucosa starts to resemble more that of the prepubertal child.

N. gonorrhoeae is very susceptible to drying and low temperatures and consequently does not live long outside the body. Organisms in moist purulent material may remain alive for a few hours, but surveys of public toilets (which might be contaminated with urethral discharge during urination) have not found positive cultures (Gilbaugh and Fuchs, 1979). Studies of cases involving crowded housing conditions, endemic disease, and poor hygiene have suggested that infection may be caused by contaminated bedclothes and other objects (Sore and Winkelstein, 1971), although this type of transmission has not been demonstrated experimentally. Studies in more typical settings still find some unexplained cases among children, but the majority do seem to be related to sexual contact. Farrell and co-workers (1981), for example, studied 46 children under age 12 who were found to have positive cultures for gonorrhea. Of the total, 32 (70%) had a likely source of sexual contact: 19 disclosed sexual abuse or assault, 5 had had genital contact with another child who was infected, and 8 had a mother or female sibling who was infected and who in turn had an infected male sexual partner. The growing realization that disease may be acquired from sexual contact with other children has also served to explain cases that might previously have been attributed to nonsexual contact (Potterat et al., 1986). These contacts are probably more common than is generally believed (see Chapter 18). It is also likely that improved methods of laboratory diagnosis for *N. gonorrhoeae* (see below) will decrease the proportion of false-positive cultures and thus the proportion of otherwise unexplainable cases attributed to nonsexual contact.

OROPHARYNGEAL GONORRHEA

Oropharyngeal gonorrhea is being found with increasing frequency among sexually abused children (McClure et al., 1986). Whereas some persons (usually adults) have symptoms that may include pharyngitis, stomatitis, tonsilitis, and enlarged cervical lymph nodes, the majority of children appear to be asymptomatic (Silber and Controni, 1983). The oropharynx is one of the sites most likely to harbor nonsexually transmitted *Neisseria* species that may give false-positive tests for gonorrhea, so great care must be taken to verify laboratory findings.

ANAL GONORRHEA

Anal gonorrheal infections in children are said to be frequently asymptomatic, although in one study four of five children with positive rectal cultures had reported symptoms of pain or discharge (DeJong, 1986). This high rate of symptoms may have been a characteristic of the population studied, which was composed of children seen at a crisis evaluation and treatment center for sexual assault victims. This type of facility may be more likely to see children who have symptoms or are victims of painful, penetrating abuse. *N. gonorrhoeae* was also cultured from the vagina of one of the symptomatic children. It is postulated that anal infection in females may sometimes result from contaminated vaginal secretions rather than direct anal-genital contact.

VAGINAL AND CERVICAL GONORRHEA

The prepubertal, unestrogenized vaginal mucosa is a ready host to *N. gonorrhoeae*. At puberty, hormonal influences change the vagina so that it no longer supports the growth of the organism; consequently, cervical infections are found instead in older girls. Vaginal gonorrhea in prepubertal children is said to be almost always symptomatic, with discharge, pruritis, a foul smell, and erythema of the external genitalia. DeJong (1986), however, found 5 asymptomatic cases among 15 girls with positive vaginal cultures.

URETHRITIS

Gonorrheal urethritis in boys is usually symptomatic, with dysuria and purulent discharge. In adult males untreated urethritis usually becomes asymptomatic after a period of weeks. Asymptomatic urethral infections have been found in school-age males, in one case as a result of contact tracing from a 5-year-old female playmate who had gonorrheal vaginitis (Potterat et al., 1986).

DIAGNOSIS

Diagnosis of gonorrhea requires a high degree of suspicion and the culturing of multiple sites in children thought to be at risk. Positive cultures are frequently obtained from sites that would not be suggested by the specific history of abuse given at the time of initial evaluation (Rimsza and Niggemann, 1982; DeJong, 1986). Culturing of child contacts of an index case may help identify other victims; culturing adult family members and contacts is an effective way of finding other individuals in need of treatment but not particularly useful for identifying potential perpetrators. First, gonorrhea is a very prevalent disease (the annual incidence among sexually active young adults is estimated to be 1–3/100 individuals); thus, other family members may be positive but not be child abusers. Second, the organism is easy to treat and not always easy to grow in the laboratory. Therefore *not* finding gonorrhea in family members also is of little significance to an investigation of abuse. There is always the risk that those who culture negative will be seen as "cleared" when they may still reasonably be suspected of being perpetrators.

A Gram stain of cervical, vaginal, or urethral discharge may help in the initial diagnosis. *N. gonorrhoeae* has a characteristic appearance: small, gram-negative diplococci found within the cytoplasm of polymorphonuclear leukocytes.

Care should be taken when making a slide that the swab or applicator is simply touched or rolled on the glass rather than rubbed or smeared. The latter maneuvers disrupt white cells and make it more difficult to determine whether the organisms are intracellular. A convincing specimen may be good insurance if cultures are later lost or negative. Characteristics that strongly suggest *N. gonorrhoeae* (as opposed to other similar-appearing, nonpathogenic organisms) include the fact that the sample was from a genital or urethral site, the presence of many polymorphonuclear leukocytes, the observation of few or no other types of organisms on the smear, and the presence of many cells harboring organisms clearly within the cytoplasm. Any slide that is initially read as positive should be so labeled and preserved in the same way as any other piece of forensically important evidence.

The laboratory identification of *N. gonorrhoeae* can be very difficult. False-negative results are common if specimens from a patient (culture swabs, for example) are not placed in appropriate culture or transport media immediately. The major problem concerning child abuse investigation is differentiation of *N. gonorrhoeae* from nonpathogenic *Neisseria* species. Essentially all of the nongonococcal *Neisseria* and several related organisms (*N. meningitidis, N. lactamica, N. cinerea,* and *Branhamella catarrhalis,* for example) are considered to be normal flora in children. Some are associated with disease and some may even at times be sexually transmitted, but they do not at present have the same implications for child abuse as *N. gonorrhoeae*. All can be relatively easily confused with *N. gonorrhoeae* when only simple laboratory tests are performed (Whittington et al., 1988). This is not a merely theoretical consideration. Several cases of mistaken identification have been reported in the literature, many of which triggered inappropriate investigations of possible sexual abuse (Dossett et al., 1985; Whittington et al., 1988).

Difficulties arise because most laboratories accustomed to processing genital or urethral specimens in symptomatic adults make only a presumptive identification of *N. gonorrhoeae*. The organisms are initially grown on selective medium designed to select for a subgroup of the *Neisseria* species, including *N. gonorrhoeae*, that are antibiotic resistant. Given the genital source of the specimen, a characteristic colony morphology, and positive oxidase reaction, an identification is made. This method has a high predictive value for settings in which the prevalence of gonorrhea is high and the chances of finding other organisms relatively low (a cervical specimen from a symptomatic adult female, for example). This is not the case among children, especially those who are asymptomatic or are being cultured from nongenital sites. Unfortunately, even some of the "confirmatory" tests frequently used cannot reliably exclude nongonococcal species, especially those that theoretically do not grow on selective media but sometimes do (Knapp et al., 1984). Several steps can be taken to guard against misidentification:

- Clearly mark all specimens for gonorrhea testing with the body site from which the culture was taken.
- Make sure that the laboratory processing the specimens is aware of the problem of misidentification and takes appropriate steps to check results. Current recommendations are that all identifications be confirmed by two independent methods (for example, an enzyme substrate test and an immunologic method) before a final result is announced.
- Once identification of *N. gonorrhoeae* is made, ask the laboratory to save all worksheets and a subculture of the organism. The subculture must be frozen at $-70°C$ or below or else it will not survive. If a positive culture is obtained in the absence of any other evidence of abuse, or a vigorous defense from the perpetrator is expected, consider sending the specimen to a reference laboratory for confirmation.
- Do not announce preliminary culture results to patients unless clinical findings are strongly suggestive of gonorrhea; to avoid unnecessarily upsetting the patient, always wait until the results are verified. Final determinations are usually made in a matter of days, and treatment of asymptomatic patients is not urgent.

Trichomonas vaginalis

Trichomonas vaginalis is a flagellated protozoan that can cause vaginal and urethral infections in both males and females. Along with chlamydial infections and gonorrhea, it ranks as one of the most common STDs in Western populations. It is one member of a family of protozoans that can colonize humans but appear to have a high degree of tissue specificity. *T. vaginalis* grows in the urethra and vagina but not the rectum or pharynx. In contrast to *Chlamydia* and *N. gonorrhoeae*, it grows well in the estrogenized vagina and less well when estrogen effects are absent.

T. vaginalis appears to have an extremely high rate of transmission when it comes in contact with a favorable environment. It is found in about a third of male contacts of infected women but in up to 70% of those who report contact within the past 48 hours (Rein and Müller, 1984). Most men appear to develop only a self-limited, asymptomatic infection. Women often develop symptoms, but the onset may be delayed, even, apparently, for months. Symptoms may develop or worsen when other infections are present or during or just after menses, when the vaginal pH rises.

Trichomonal vaginitis in adults appears to be almost exclusively associated with sexual contact (Shafer et al., 1985), although there has been widespread speculation about means of nonsexual transmission from sources such as toilet seats and water splashing from contaminated toilet bowels (Burgess, 1963). The organism can survive in warm, moist settings for hours and in purulent material for as long as a day (Burch et al., 1959). As with many other STDs, nonsexual transmission seems somewhat possible but has not been conclusively demonstrated. Casual nonsexual transmission would seem even less likely in prepubertal girls because the unestrogenized vagina is a relatively hostile environment and colonization of the urethra would seem to be logistically more difficult. Neonatal transmission of *T. vaginalis* does occur, although apparently with low frequency. Asymptomatic cases may clear spontaneously once the maternal estrogen effect wanes, although one symptomatic case (vaginitis) was reported to have persisted until the child was 7 weeks of age, at which time it was treated (Al-Salihi et al., 1974).

Classically, trichomoniasis has been diagnosed by finding motile organisms on a wet slide preparation (wet prep) of a vaginal discharge that is relatively frothy and alkaline (pH > 4.5). The organism is ovoid and about 10–20 μm in diameter. Its darting movements and flagella can readily be seen under the microscope and make the live organism easy to differentiate from white blood cells and epithelial cells. Care must be taken that the specimen is not allowed to dry. A drop of saline can be put on a slide before a specimen is collected and the swab then rolled in the drop. Gentle warming can help increase movement of the organism and make it easier to identify. Potassium hydroxide, used to visualize yeasts, kills trichomonads, and therefore a separate preparation is necessary.

The wet prep is highly specific if flagella and motion are seen but unfortunately is not very sensitive. In one series (Fouts and Kraus, 1980), wet preps were positive in only two-thirds of adult patients who had positive cultures (a variety of media are available). Nearly half of the patients who had positive cultures gave a history of discharge, but 20% had no discharge at the time the positive culture was obtained.

These observations suggest some guidelines for detecting trichomonal infections in children suspected of having been sexually abused:

- In prepubertal girls beyond the first few weeks of life, examination of the urine may be the best way to test for the organism in the absence of vaginal symptoms. Reported cases of trichomonal infection associated with sexual abuse of prepubertal girls describe initial detection by microscopic examination of the urine (Jones et al., 1985).
- Regardless of symptoms, a wet prep of any vaginal fluid or discharge should be made for girls suspected of having been abused and who have signs of early puberty (breast or pubic hair development, enlargement of the external genitalia, or thickening of the vaginal mucosa). Alternatively, a vaginal washing using a few milliliters of nonbacteriostatic sterile saline may be performed. A microscopic urinalysis should also be performed.
- Cultures as well as wet preps should be used whenever possible.
- When the infection is found on wet prep and culture is not available, cytopathology specimens may be sent for official reading. This creates a permanent laboratory record of the finding that may be useful for legal proceedings.

Condyloma acuminatum

Condyloma acuminatum (venereal warts) is caused by members of the human papillomavirus (HPV) family, the same group of viruses that cause common skin warts. HPV infections are being reported in increasing numbers in both adults and children and are rapidly joining the ranks of the most common STDs.

There are 50 or more distinct genotypes of HPV. HPV- 1, -2, and -3 are associated with common warts of the hands and feet and are not thought to be sexually transmitted. Types 6 and 11 are the most often found types in vulvar, penile, and perianal warts. Type 11 is also frequently found in laryngeal lesions in young children. In adults, types 16, 18, and 31 are found most commonly in cervical warts but also in malignant lesions of the vulva, vagina, endometrium, and cervix. In one study (Macnab et al., 1986), tissue from 21 of 25 genital tract tumors (84%) contained DNA sequences that hybridized to probes for HPV-16. Although it is not known whether types 16, 18, and 31 actually cause cancer, their presence in lesions suggests that they play some important role. Additional concern has come from the finding that cervical dysplasia, often a precursor of malignant lesions, is also highly correlated with the presence of HPV-16, -18, and -31. In one study, genetic material from HPV was detected in cervical cells of 3% of sexually active adolescents who had normal cervical cytology but in nearly 50% of those who had findings of cervical dysplasia (Martinez et al., 1988).

The various genotypes of HPV appear to be relatively specific for the sites on which they will grow, and the presence of one type of infection does not seem to be related to the presence of another. Individuals with genital warts, for example, are no more likely to have common skin warts than are persons without genital warts. By morphologic identification, only about 1 or 2% of anogenital warts in adults appear to be caused by the viruses that usually cause common skin warts (Bender, 1986). The type 2 (common wart) virus was detected in perianal lesions of one child who also had warts on his hand (Fleming et al., 1987), although in five children with anogenital lesions alone, Rock and colleagues (1986) found only genital types of virus.

Until recently, it was difficult to develop information about the transmission or natural history of HPV infections. HPV has not yet been grown in the laboratory, and until the development of DNA hybridization techniques, gross morphology of lesions and histologic examination of biopsies were the only means of identification. Probes for DNA hybridization identification of HPV types are not yet routinely available in diagnostic laboratories, but they are fairly widely used in research settings. The development of polymerase chain reaction techniques promises to allow detection of HPV DNA in very small samples such as those available from the genital tracts of prepubertal children.

Transmission of HPV appears to require minor trauma to a skin or mucosal surface that allows the infectious material come in contact with deeper tissue layers. In adults, the anogenital HPV genotypes (6, 11, 16, 18, and 31) appear to be transmitted sexually. The time from initial exposure to the appearance of warts is about 4-8 weeks but may be longer or shorter in some cases. Host immunologic factors seem to play some role in this variability, as does the time it takes for infected epithelial cells to mature, a development that may trigger HPV DNA to begin replication and expression. Conditions that depress cell-mediated immunity, such as active infection with the human immunodeficiency virus, are associated with more extensive and difficult-to-control HPV disease. Importantly for transmission to newborns, the immunologic alterations during pregnancy also appear to make active HPV infection more prevalent.

Another area of uncertainty is whether HPV can produce asymptomatic, latent infection and, if so, how long such infection might last. Viral DNA can be detected in histologically normal epithelial cells surrounding laryngeal and genital warts (Ferenczy et al., 1985). Virus in these tissues appears to be capable of causing disease; its presence is highly correlated with recurrence of resected warts. These recurrences occur much more quickly—within 3–6 weeks—than the period required for newly introduced virus to produce symptoms. Viral DNA can also be found in individuals who have no clinically apparent disease. In a study of 530 men 16–85 years old, most of whom were coming to a medical center either to donate blood or for treatment of non-HPV skin disease, HPV DNA was detected in epithelial cell samples from the glans or corona of the penis in nearly 6% (Grussendorf-Conen et al., 1986). The prevalence of viral DNA had a bimodal distribution in relationship to the age of the men: it was high (7–8%) in men 16–35 years old, not detectable in men 46–75, and high again in men over 75 (relatively few elderly men were tested). Similar findings of high prevalence in asymptomatic individuals and peak prevalence during the period of greatest sexual activity have been made for females, including those with normal cervical cytology (de Villiers et al., 1987). These studies, although predominantly cross-sectional, suggest that some or perhaps most individuals infected with HPV, if they do not develop malignant disease related to the virus, gradually lose detectable HPV DNA as they get older (and presumably as the frequency of sexual contact decreases). Whether these individuals can transmit HPV once it is no longer detectable by hybridization is not known. The increase in prevalence of detectable HPV DNA in the elderly suggests that the virus never vanishes and that it can reappear in detectable amounts as immune status changes.

These considerations, plus the fact that many lesions in adult females may be detectable only on cytologic or colposcopic examination, make contact tracing very problematic. Individuals with known genital warts are likely sources of new cases, but new cases with no obvious symptomatic contact are understandably very common. In addition, since vulvar and cervical warts are usually caused by different types of HPV, the presence of visible vulvar warts is a poor predictor of the presence of cervical HPV infection (Martinez et al., 1988).

Genital warts caused by HPV may take on many appearances. On the cervix or in the vagina, they may be flat and visible only with acetic acid rinses (which make the warts appear white). On the external genitalia or perirectally, they may initially appear as small, translucent papules that look like vesicles. They evolve fairly quickly into small, skin-colored, usually multiple lesions that have been compared to the flowerettes on a head of broccoli. These may remain small or coalesce to form larger, exophytic lesions that can become secondarily infected and friable. Discomfort is not usually a problem until the lesions are large or if they interfere with urination. Warts may appear virtually anywhere on the penis, vulva, or perianal area. They may also be present on the buttocks or down the thighs. In adult females, perianal lesions are thought to frequently result as secondary sites from primary genital warts. In men, penile and perirectal warts are thought to occur from separate contacts with an infectious source (Bender, 1986). Perianal lesions may also be associated with warts in the rectum.

The major consideration in differential diagnosis is condyloma lata, a manifestation of secondary syphilis. These lesions are usually flatter, more broad based, and smoother on the surface, and diagnostic tests for syphilis will be positive. In early stages, small lesions may resemble herpetic vesicles, molluscum contagiosum, and benign "pink pearly papules" (see Chapter 8). Herpetic vesicles are usually painful, and condyloma can be differentiated from the other conditions as it changes morphology to become more wart-like.

Nonsexual transmission of the anogenital types of HPV is widely postulated. The virus is extremely resistant to drying and can remain infectious on hands or other surfaces for long periods of time. Perinatal transmission, however, is the only well-documented form of spread outside of genital-to-genital contact. The most commonly recognized syndrome is laryngeal papillomatosis, growth of HPV-related lesions on the larynx and elsewhere in the upper airway. Lesions are usually associated with HPV-11, one of the types related to genital warts in adults. The condition is found more often in children of women known to have condylomata at the time of delivery, and the timing of onset (3–4 months of age at the earliest) is consistent with acquisition at birth. About half of affected children develop symptoms by age 2 and two-thirds do so by age 4, although some cases develop much later (Bennett et al., 1987). Some of this variability is undoubtedly caused by slow growth of the lesions and the time it takes for symptoms to develop; some lesions may also arise from postnatal exposure, possibly sexual. Rare genital lesions have also been noted in newborns (suggesting prenatal transmission) and in an infant who also had papillomatosis (Tang et al., 1984; Hajek, 1956).

The difficulty, then, is determining which HPV-related lesions in a child may be signs of sexual contact. Evidence suggestive of sexual abuse has been found in many cases that have been investigated. The proportion of cases in which abuse is suspected has increased with more recent case studies: in 1982, DeJong et al. reviewed 34 cases of condyloma in children and found 8 to have evidence supporting nonsexual transmission, 8 in which abuse was suspected, and 18 of unknown source. Of the five cases reported by Rock and colleagues in 1986, three of five were suspected to involve abuse. Shelton and colleagues (1986) reported on 30 cases seen over a 14-year period. Of the 14 who were referred to social service agencies, 8 were found to have evidence of abuse. In all of these studies, the diagnosis of nonsexual transmission was one of exclusion: no evidence of social pathology in the family and no apparent source for perinatal acquisition.

At present, it still seems reasonable to consider most new cases of anogenital condylomas in children as reason for concern about sexual contact. If a social evaluation is negative, one might be more comfortable postulating nonsexual acquisition if there is no other evidence of abuse, there are lesions somewhat distant from the anus or introitus, and the child is under 9 months of age when the lesions are first noted (Rock et al., 1986).

Syphilis

Syphilis is not common in sexual abuse, but it is found whenever a large enough group of abused children can be studied. White and co-workers (1983) found 6 cases among 409 abused children under 13. Five of the six were asymptomatic at the time of diagnosis. The risk of contracting syphilis may be increasing, however. Since 1985–86 there has been a sharp increase in the incidence of newly reported primary and secondary cases in the general population. In some urban areas these increases have been dramatic, with near doublings of the number of reported cases (Anonymous, 1988b,c). Incidence rates are generally highest in urban areas (63.5/100,000 in New York City in 1987, compared with 3.4/100,000 in the remainder of the state), with black males at highest risk (144.9/100,000 nationally in 1987). The proportion of newly diagnosed patients who report homosexual or bisexual contact has decreased while reported use of drugs or contact with prostitutes has increased, which suggests that these factors have played a role in the spread of the disease.

Because the increase in the incidence of syphilis is occurring in the heterosexual population, rates of congenital syphilis are also rising. This trend may pose some difficulties in interpreting serologic tests in infants or toddlers suspected of being abused. Positive results must be interpreted in light of results of maternal prenatal testing or any previous medical history suggestive of congenital infection. Particular care must be taken in evaluating condylomatous perianal lesions in infants: the condyloma lata of syphilis may resemble warts caused by papillomaviruses.

Nonsexual transmission of syphilis has been demonstrated through skin contact with contaminated materials and moist lesions or with mucosal membranes of infected persons. Chancres on the genitalia, however, are highly suggestive of sexual transmission. There are two major ways of diagnosing syphilis: by identification of the characteristic skin lesions (morphologic changes in congenital infections; chancres, rashes, condylomata, or epitrochlear adenopathy in primary and secondary stages of postnatal infections) and by serology. Chancres may not appear until 2–3 weeks after exposure, and antibodies may not be detectable for 4–6 weeks. Therefore, it is important that follow-up examinations take place when a patient is seen immediately after an incident of sexual abuse or assault or when the time of possible exposure is not known.

Herpes

Herpes simplex virus (HSV) infections are among the most common infectious diseases among both children and adults. There are two major serotypes: HSV-1 (generally associated with facial and oral infections) and HSV-2 (associated with genital infections). Antibodies to HSV-1 are found in a large proportion of children, and prevalence increases with age. Antibody to HSV-2 is relatively uncommon among individuals who are not sexually active, and its prevalence increases with the extent of sexual activity. Both serotypes, however, can cause infection in either the oral or genital area.

Persons with their first or primary HSV infection of either type often have systemic as well as painful local symptoms. After an incubation period of about 1 week (range, 2–20 days), they may develop fever, chills, and other flu-like symptoms. Painful vesicles and ulcers then appear; in genital herpes, these lesions may be on the internal or external genitalia or the surrounding skin and are usually accompanied by tender inguinal lymph nodes. Dysuria may also be a presenting complaint. Recurrence of lesions is common because HSV is capable of remaining in a latent or dormant state in the ganglia of cutaneous nerves. A variety of stimuli (stress, altered immune function) can cause reactivation of the virus and a reappearance of skin or mucosal lesions. These recurrent lesions are usually painful but are not associated with systemic symptoms. Virus shedding in saliva or genital secretions can occur regardless of whether visible lesions are present, although the amount of virus released is smaller during asymptomatic periods (Corey and Spear, 1986).

Epidemiologic studies strongly suggest that HSV-1 is readily transmitted nonsexually by contact of vulnerable (abraded or otherwise traumatized) skin with infected secretions, including apparent autoinoculation of the fingers or genitalia from oral lesions. Nonsexual transmission of HSV-2, in contrast, has not been demonstrated, although there is evidence that the virus can survive for a period of hours on dry surfaces and thus might be transmitted by other means (Neinstein et al., 1984). Perinatal transmission of HSV-2 is well documented. Transmission appears to take place predominantly at the time of birth and may lead to either localized or disseminated disease. Both may result in either primary or recurrent lesions in the anogenital area, although the occurrence of isolated genital lesions that might be confused with sexual contact does not appear to be common (Brown et al., 1987).

Both HSV-1 and HSV-2 have been found in association with cases of sexual abuse (Gardner and Jones, 1984; Kaplan et al., 1984). Both isolated genital and simultaneous genital and oral lesions (with HSV-1) have been described in cases for which there was other evidence to support the belief that abuse had occurred. The onset of primary oral lesions before genital lesions, however, may support a hypothesis of autoinoculation rather than direct genital contact.

HSV can be detected directly from stained preparations of ulcer or vesicle material (preferably with Papanicolaou [Pap] stain or with Wright or Giemsa stain) or by culture. Serologic testing is also available but not always definitive for the type of virus involved. Many authorities suggest obtaining cultures of suspicious lesions rather than relying on a morphologic diagnosis. Cultures can differentiate lesions caused by HSV from those caused by syphilis or by nonsexually transmitted organisms. Identifying the type of HSV involved may or may not help in determining of means of transmission. Primary genital infections with HSV-2, however, would generally be accepted as strong evidence of sexual contact.

Human Immunodeficiency Virus

The epidemic of human immunodeficiency virus (HIV) infection has raised the question of whether children who are known or suspected to be victims of sexual abuse should be tested for exposure. A small number of cases have been reported in which children were sexually abused by known HIV-seropositive individuals, and in at least one case a child subsequently developed acquired immunodeficiency syndrome (AIDS) (Rubinstein and Bernstein, 1986; Osterholm et al., 1987). The variable and often obscure epidemiology of child sexual abuse makes it difficult to decide which children are at risk and deserve testing.

At the time abuse is disclosed, the identity of the abuser, the nature of his or her medical problems, if any, and the type of sexual contact involved are often not known. The likelihood of genital-to-genital contact varies with the setting of the abuse: in one study of female victims, genital-genital contact occurred in about 20% of intrafamilial abuse cases, about 50% of cases in which the abuser was known to the child but outside the family, and more than 70% of cases involving a stranger (Russell, 1983). The extent of genital-genital or genital-anal contact may be higher among male victims. Similarly, not a great deal is known about other sexual activity among abusers. Many abusers, however, especially young males, may also have been victims of older men who were at risk of carrying STDs. Some pedophiles may also become involved with child prostitutes or other troubled juveniles who are known to have relatively high rates of STDs, including HIV infection.

The prevalence of HIV seropositivity in the adult population is related to several risk factors. Among male military recruits and active-duty Department of Defense employees, the prevalence rate is about 1.3–1.4/1000 persons (Anonymous, 1988a). In one study, about 5% of persons coming for care at a group of urban STD clinics were seropositive (Quinn et al., 1988). Certain STDs were associated with markedly higher prevalence rates: 15–20% of men with syphilis, genital warts, or hepatitis were also seropositive for HIV; similar trends were also observed for female patients. In other studies, 50–60% of individuals in East Coast United States cities who reported using intravenous drugs were found to be HIV seropositive, although the prevalence rate even among drug users appears to be much less in other parts of the country (Centers for Disease Control, 1987).

HIV is more difficult to transmit than are other viruses such as hepatitis B. Among adults, anal intercourse appears to carry the highest risk, although vaginal and, to a lesser extent, oral-genital contacts are well-demonstrated means of transmission. Sexual contact and contact with parenteral fluids appear to be the sole clinically significant means of transmission outside of the perinatal period. These findings suggest one possible set of guidelines for offering HIV testing to victims:

- Test victims who have evidence of any other STD.
- Test males who have been victimized by male offenders (because the likelihood of sodomy and of an extended chain of sexual contact is higher).
- Test victims who were the receiving partner in anal-genital contact.
- Test victims whose abusers are suspected of being in any of the established high-risk groups: intravenous-drug users, homosexuals or bisexuals, and sexual contacts of intravenous-drug users).

Testing for HIV in the context of maltreatment must also follow guidelines for HIV testing in other clinical settings. Patients and their families must have an opportunity to consider the risks and benefits of making the diagnosis, and they must have the opportunity to elect confidential or anonymous testing outside the realm of the abuse investigation. The chance of obtaining false-positive tests in low-risk settings should also be considered (Meyer and Pauker, 1987). Since no postexposure prophylaxis is yet available, it may be reasonable to postpone the decision to test until as many details as possible of the abuse are known and a better assessment of HIV risk can be made. When testing is elected, a commitment to perform adequate follow-up examinations must be made. The time from exposure to seroconversion is variable (about 2–12 weeks); therefore, initial tests, if negative, should be repeated in about 6–8 weeks and probably again in about 6 months. Testing the alleged abuser may be possible or even ordered by a court. A negative test in an otherwise high-risk individual, however, would not replace the need for careful examination and testing of the victim.

The possibility of perinatal exposure to HIV (or of prior sexual contact) must be considered in children who are seropositive when tested immediately after an episode of abuse. The majority of HIV infections in children are now caused by perinatal maternal-child transmission. About 50% of children born to seropositive mothers are themselves infected. The proportion who will ultimately develop AIDS is not known. The majority of those who do develop HIV-related symptoms do so by 3 years of age, although onset as late as 7 years has been reported (Falloon et al., 1989).

Other Infections

HEPATITIS B

Hepatitis B (HBV) virus can be transmitted sexually and by contact of mucous membranes or broken skin with contaminated materials such as blood. The incidence of HBV disease has been increasing, with risk factors similar to those for HIV infection. HBV is more easily transmissible than HIV and and it may be more prevalent outside of commonly assumed risk groups. In one study of white college student blood donors at a major university, the HBV seroprevalence rate was 14% among those who reported having three or more recent sexual partners (Alter et al., 1986). Postexposure prophylaxis with hepatitis B immune globulin (HBIG) is possible. HBIG should be given within 7–14 days of contact (immediately if contact is perinatal). Ideally, the alleged abuser can be immediately tested to determine his or her HBV status, but treatment with HBIG should not be delayed if immediate testing is not possible and the abuser is thought to be in a high-risk group. Testing of victims is most useful in the setting of chronic abuse, where knowledge of HBV status might serve to document the extent of the child's injuries and aid in further medical management. Administration of HBV vaccine should be considered for HBV-seronegative children who may be at future risk of exposure from abuse, from their own sexual behaviors, or from living with adults who are also at high risk (such as intravenous-drug abusers).

MOLLUSCUM CONTAGIOSUM

Molluscum contagiosum is caused by a member of the pox family of viruses. The virus causes smooth, round, 2- to 5-mm papules that are white, translucent, or yellow and have a characteristic central umbilication. Among children, the infection appears to spread by direct contact and fomites; papules appear on the face, trunk, and limbs. In adults, the virus appears to be spread sexually, and lesions may appear on the genitals, thighs, and lower abdominal wall. Genital or lower-abdominal lesions in children may therefore be a sign of sexual contact.

Molluscum is usually diagnosed from the clinical appearance of the lesions and from stained preparations of material expressed from them (looking for viral inclusion bodies). Lesions appear within weeks after contact with the virus and usually resolve spontaneously, although topical treatment may be used.

DETECTION AND EVALUATION OF SEXUALLY TRANSMITTED DISEASES

It is important to have a fairly fixed protocol for diagnosis of STDs in sexual abuse cases. While cultures and specimens must be taken as appropriate to the patient's psychologic condition, history, and symptoms, thorough evaluations of recent cases often find infections that were previously unsuspected. The following protocol is based on this premise and is generally applicable to both recent and more distant (more than 72 hours previously) exposure. Special procedures for recent cases are also mentioned.

Cultures

Cultures for both gonorrheal and chlamydial infections should be obtained from the pharynx, anus, and genitalia (vagina in prepubertal girls, cervix in postpubertal girls if a speculum examination is indicated, and urethra in boys). The site of the specimen should be clearly marked on the label or laboratory requisition. If there are no symptoms and the child is anxious, taking of cultures may be deferred until a follow-up visit a few days later.

Obtaining multiple vaginal cultures and specimens from prepubertal girls may be difficult. The vaginal mucosa is thin and sensitive, especially if there is any degree of inflammation. Small swabs made of synthetic material are better instruments than the standard cotton swabs. If there are secretions, two or more swabs can be bunched together to soak up fluid while gentle pressure is applied to also obtain some epithelial cells. If there are scant or no secretions, the swabs can be moistened with sterile, nonbacteriostatic saline to reduce abrasion and then gently rolled on the vaginal mucosa. Many girls, however, will find this procedure very uncomfortable. An alternative is use of a small dropper (or syringe with a soft, flexible tube attached) to put 2–3 ml of saline into the vagina and aspirate it. The fluid obtained can then be divided among the tests to be performed.

It often seems overly invasive to obtain urethral cultures from asymptomatic males. A first-part voided urine specimen may be an acceptable substitute. The child should be given a sterile container and helped to collect the first few milliliters (no more than 10–15) of urine produced. The presence of 10 or more white blood cells per high-powered microscope field (after centrifugation at $500 \times g$ for 10 minutes) is highly suggestive of urethritis. These children usually then undergo urethral cultures. The presence of 5–10 white cells is considered borderline, and less than 5 cells is considered to be within the range of normal. In one study of adolescent males, cultures positive for gonorrheal or chlamydial infection were found in 21 of 23 patients who had more than 10 white cells in the sediment of a first-part voided sample. Of the 21 positive patients, 11 had had no symptoms or physical findings at the time of examination (Adger et al., 1984). One asymptomatic patient had a negative first-part urine examination but a positive culture for *N. gonorrhoeae*.

The techniques for obtaining rectal and pharyngeal cultures are straightforward, although obtaining a young child's cooperation is not always easy. Care should be taken to minimize contamination of rectal swabs with stool or skin flora from the buttocks as the swab is inserted. The child must be reasonably relaxed; otherwise, even a moistened swab will feel painful as it pushes over the perianal skin. With the child tense, it will also be difficult to judge whether the swab has actually entered the anal canal. Once the swab is in place, it should be left for 30 seconds or so and then gently removed.

Wet Preps, Stained Specimens, and Cytopathology

The techniques used to examine body fluids depend on the age of the child, the amount and location of secretions to be examined, and the tests that are contemplated. Material for examination may be obtained in a variety of ways. (1) If enough material is present, it can be directly aspirated. (2) A swab soaked with the secretions can be put in a sterile tube along with 1–2 ml of saline. The tube can be gently agitated and the fluid examined. Alternatively, the swab can be removed and the fluid centrifuged. The supernatant can be used for chemical analyses, and the pellet can be resuspended and examined under the microscope. (3) A fresh swab can be rolled in a drop of saline on a microscope slide. (4) A vaginal "washing" can be performed as described above. Each technique introduces its own factors of dilution. Since clinicians may vary their techniques to suit individual cases, it is important to develop some personal idea of what normal specimens look like with each method.

When abuse is thought to have occurred at some relatively distant time (more than 72 hours), specimens are examined for signs of infection: smears are air dried and Gram stained for evidence of gonorrhea; saline wet preps are examined for trichomonads and clue cells; and a KOH wet prep can be examined for yeasts or hyphae. If trichomonads (or, unexpectedly, sperm) are found, another slide should be made and immediately placed in or sprayed with the fixative used for Pap smears. This specimen can be sent to a cytopathology laboratory for an official confirmation of the diagnosis. Alternatively, one or more additional smears can be air dried and saved for staining and permanent mounting. When there is a possibility that sexual contact has taken place within the last 72 hours, additional testing must be performed as described below for forensic procedures.

Urinalysis

A urinalysis may reveal evidence of retroperitoneal trauma (blood or heme) or urinary tract infection; contamination of the specimen may help diagnose vaginitis. As mentioned above, *T. vaginalis* infections in prepubertal girls have sometimes been initially diagnosed on urinalysis, presumably because the organism preferentially colonizes the urethra in this age group.

Evaluation of Skin or Mucosal Lesions

Ulcers or vesicles suggestive of herpes infection can be cultured if appropriate transport medium is available. Cytologic examination can also be performed. DNA typing of wart-like lesions is not yet widely available. Lesions can be carefully described in the medical record and/or photographed.

FORENSIC PROCEDURES IN CASES OF SEXUAL ABUSE OR ASSAULT

When abuse or assault has taken place within 48–72 hours, it may be possible to detect materials from the abuser on the victim's body or clothing. This may provide important evidence to demonstrate that abuse has taken place and may sometimes help identify the abuser. Procedures must be carefully followed to adequately collect and preserve available evidence.

Clothing

If the victim is still wearing the clothing worn at the time of the assault, he or she should stand on a large, clean cloth or paper sheet and undress completely. Clothing should be wrapped in the sheet, taking care not to spill any small objects that may have fallen onto it, and the bundle should be labeled and safely stored until it can be submitted to a police laboratory.

Examination for Traces of Semen

Detection of semen on a victim's body or clothing can be strong evidence that sexual contact of some kind took place. The first goal is to demonstrate that semen is present; the second is to isolate genetic markers in the semen that may help identify the perpetrator.

EXAMINATION FOR SEMEN ON SKIN

Victims may have semen from the abuser on the skin, often at sites adjacent to target areas for sexual contact. UV light, which causes semen to fluoresce, can be used to aid detection. After the procedure is thoroughly explained, the room can be partially darkened. A few moments are required for the examiner's eyes to adapt to the dark. The UV light can be used to examine the thighs, buttocks, lower abdomen, chest, and lower face. Secretions may also be found in the hair, especially if the victim has tried to spit out ejaculate. Any positive areas found can be swabbed with saline-moistened swabs, which should be air dried and placed in empty sterile blood-collecting tubes or a clean paper envelope. If sealed tubes are used, the swabs must be totally dry to avoid overgrowth of contaminants. Alternatively, if preferred by the local forensic laboratory, the swabs can be immediately frozen rather than dried. This procedure may help preserve the activity of prostatic enzymes that can be used to identify the material as semen.

Semen is usually identified by looking microscopically for sperm and biochemically for enzymes and other proteins in the ejaculate. Both processes should be applied in all cases since, as discussed below, the factors that influence retrieval of sperm and other seminal components act in a highly variable manner. It is not unusual for sperm to be found in the absence of enzymes or vice versa. (Because some abusers and rapists are impotent, lack of evidence of semen does not rule out genital contact.)

SPERM

Although normal male ejaculate can contain hundreds of millions of sperm, much smaller numbers are recovered from the vagina even immediately after intercourse. In addition, the concentration of sperm in ejaculate may be decreased by elevated testicular temperature, chronic alcohol intake, or procedures such as vasectomy.

Sperm recovered from the vagina shortly after sexual contact may still be motile in wet preparations. The outer limit for finding motile sperm in adult vaginal secretions is often given as 8 hours (Rupp, 1969), although studies report a great deal of variation. Twelve hours appears to be the longest survival generally reported (Bach, 1980). Nonmotile sperm can be found for much longer periods, with reports ranging from 14 to 26 hours (Rupp, 1969; Dahlke et al., 1977; Willott and Allard, 1982). These figures are all for sperm that, while nonmotile, are morphologically intact. Sperm without tails may be identified for considerably longer (Willott and Allard, 1982), but they may be difficult to differentiate from yeasts, debris, or other similar-size objects. Identification of intact sperm is more convincing forensic evidence (Enos and Beyer, 1978).

Sperm may be found in body sites other than the vagina. They can survive in the cervix for up to several days after sexual contact and for hours on the perineal skin. Survival in the anus and rectum is much shorter than in the cervix or vagina; whole sperm can usually be found for only a few hours, although pieces, if they can be properly identified, may be present for up to 2 days (Willott and Allard, 1982). In females, small numbers of sperm found in the anus or perirectal area may be contaminants from the vagina (Enos and Beyer, 1978). Sperm may also be recovered from the oral cavity and surrounding skin. If the suspicion of oral contact is high, separate swabs should be taken from the perioral skin, the gums, the tongue, and the pharynx. The gums may be an especially good source, for their protected location in the mouth allows sperm to be retained for several hours after contact, sometimes despite the use of mouthwashes or toothbrushing.

A variety of techniques are described for obtaining specimens to examine for sperm. Some clinicians feel that wet preparations are generally not useful (Dalke et al., 1977) because of the variable motility of sperm. Dried, stained smears may be more sensitive, and they have the advantage of creating a permanent record that other observers can examine. Swabs soaked with material to be examined can be immersed in 1–2 ml of saline or distilled water, or a portion of the swab can be cut off and dropped into the fluid so that the rest of the swab can be used for biochemical analysis (Willott and Allard, 1982). The fluid and swab are agitated to release sperm, and then a drop of fluid can be air dried on a slide and either stained (with Giemsa or hematoxylin and eosin) or processed as a cytopathology specimen.

BIOCHEMICAL MARKERS

Semen contains several enzymes and other proteins that can be used to demonstrate its presence in vaginal fluids. The most commonly used biochemical marker for semen is the enzyme acid phosphatase (ACP), which is produced in the prostate. Small amounts of ACP are present in normal adult vaginal secretions but at levels that are 100–1000 times smaller than in semen. ACP is measured in international units (IU), with 1 IU equal to the amount of enzyme required to metabolize 1 μmol of substrate in 1 minute. Several quantitative methods are available to measure ACP activity.

Given the excess of ACP in semen compared with vaginal secretions, it would seem simple to use analysis of ACP in vaginal fluids to detect recent intercourse. Unfortunately, ACP activity diminishes rapidly in the vagina, although it is relatively stable on dry materials such as cloth if the materials are kept cool, dark, and relatively acid (Findley, 1977). In the vagina, activity related to prostatic ACP may not be distinguishable from normal vaginal enzyme after about 72 hours following intercourse.

Establishing cutoff values for inferring the presence of prostatic ACP and determining the rate at which activity decays so that the time of coitus can be estimated have been hampered by the fact that various collection and assay methods yield different dilutions of specimens and thus different values for "normal." In addition, normal adult vaginal ACP levels do not have a Gaussian (bell-shaped) distribution. The distribution of activity levels is log normal; that is, most women have relatively low levels of activity, but a small proportion have relatively high levels. Pooling data from several studies, Sensabaugh (1979) calculated that the 99% upper confidence limit for normal vaginal ACP activity is about 6.6 times a laboratory's average normal vaginal level, using a consistent collection technique. For example, if the average ACP activity in adult females is 25 IU/liter, a level of about 165 IU/liter represents a 99% confidence upper limit of normal. ACP levels higher than this point would be presumed to be caused by the presence of prostatic enzyme. Sensabaugh also calculated multipliers to obtain 99% confidence intervals for estimated ACP activity for various time periods between coitus sampling.

Other Tests Potentially Useful for Identifying Assailants

The following procedures may not be required in many cases and some can usually be postponed until after the initial examination. The clinician should consult with a police laboratory official or a designated sexual assault center to decide whether collection is necessary.

It may be useful to search for abuser's hair that has adhered to the patient's body. If the patient has pubic hair, it can be gently combed onto a piece of clean filter paper that is then carefully folded and placed in a labeled envelope for delivery to the police. If the patient struggled with and scratched the assailant, scrapings from under the fingernails may contain tissue useful in identifying the assailant or corroborating details of the struggle. Collection of blood or saliva from the patient may also be useful in differentiating his or her secretions from those of the assailant.

Identification of specific abusers from hair, blood, or semen samples has until recently been a difficult and often frustrating task. Most currently available testing is based on a search for polymorphisms in blood group markers and serum proteins. Although several markers and proteins can be examined (fewer for semen than for blood or other tissues), patterns of variation cannot uniquely identify individuals. It can often be said that only one person in 100 or 1000 would have a similar pattern of polymorphisms, but these odds are frequently not low enough to serve as sole evidence linking a particular individual with a particular crime (Tribe, 1971). This situation has been radically altered by the availability of genetic "fingerprinting" techniques based on detection of polymorphisms in human DNA (Gill et al., 1985). Human DNA molecules have many regions for which no genetic purpose has yet been identified and which show extreme variability from individual to individual. When DNA is hybridized with probes for short, repetitious nucleotide sequences that occur in these regions, one can detect distinctive patterns that occur across an individual's somatic and germline cells and appear to be unique to that individual. When even only one probe is used, it is calculated that the probability of another individual having the same pattern (unless he or she is an identical twin) is less than 1 in 10^{-10}.

Early procedures using this technique were limited by the amount of DNA needed to perform the assays: about 5 μ of semen or 60 μ of blood. The development of polymerase chain reactions to amplify minute amounts of DNA promises to lower this threshold considerably. DNA is degraded by light, moisture, heat, and bacterial action, so the extent to which usable specimens can be obtained from body cavities or surfaces after a period of days is not yet known. In addition, although these tests have been successfully used in several United States court cases (Johnson, 1988), their ultimate acceptance as scientific evidence remains to be seen. The availability of the technique at both commercial and law enforcement laboratories suggests that widespread acceptance is likely.

The Chain of Evidence for Medico-Legal Specimens

It is vital that a chain of evidence be maintained for STD and other laboratory specimens associated with a case of suspected child abuse of any kind. The chain is a written record ensuring that the specimen which arrived in the laboratory for analysis was the specimen taken from the patient. Even though a medical facility's standard procedures are usually adequate for social service and juvenile court proceedings, they may be challenged and provide a handy defense for an abuser should a case be heard in a criminal court.

The intent of the chain can be met in many ways. A slip that accompanies each specimen can have spaces for the name and signature of each person handling the specimen (person collecting, transporting, and evaluating), along with the date and time handled. Alternatively, the clinician may describe the specimens collected in the medical record, carry them to the laboratory, and ask the technician to sign the record stating that the specimens were received and noting the laboratory number that may be assigned to them. Specimens collected for the police laboratory may be placed in a locked cabinet. The police representative who comes to collect the box should be asked to cosign a slip describing the box's contents and the date and time of transfer.

Photographic Record

Photographs of skin lesions, foreign bodies, and laboratory specimens that cannot be preserved can be important to later social service and legal action. They powerfully convey the basis for the medical opinion that abuse has taken place. In most jurisdictions, consent of a parent is not required for photography of lesions suspected of being related to child abuse. The following description outlines ideal procedures; less exact procedures may suffice for informal social service or juvenile court hearings. It should also be remembered that photographs do not take the place of a detailed written description and anatomic diagrams. Photographs always need interpretation of precisely what they show; moreover, they may not turn out well or they may fade or be misplaced. The written medical record is still the primary source of description.

CAMERA

Instant cameras have the advantage of showing immediately how well lesions have been reproduced. They also avoid the problem of taking a few pictures and then having to either waste a roll of film or wait until it has been used for other photos. In general, however, pictures taken with instant cameras have less resolution and poorer color rendition, and they cannot easily be copied. A 35mm camera with either high-speed color film or a flash attachment usually provides the best results. A macro telephoto lens allows one-to-one imaging of lesions without the need for the photographer to get close to the patient. A medical or police photographer may have the best equipment and obtain the best photographs, provided he or she can be shown which lesions need to be recorded.

PHOTOGRAPHS

It is generally recommended that the series of photographs include at least one that shows the face of the victim and enough of the rest of the body and setting to establish where the photos were taken and that the other close-up shots are in fact of this patient. Included in each close-up should be a small card (a piece of a ruler or a 3 × 5-inch index card) marked in inches or centimeters and the patient's name or history number. If one is photographing bruises and expects that the case may hinge on their color, it is wise to include on the card some sample of known colors; small swatches of red, blue, and green from the colored tapes used for coding medical records can be placed along the edge of the ruler or card. Ideally, a color standard card (from a photo supply shop) can be included in some of the frames so that color-corrected prints can be made.

Instant pictures should be immediately labeled with the name of the patient, the date, the name of the person who took the picture, and what the picture is intended to show (for example, "bruise on leg"). These pictures should be fastened in the medical record and become a part of it. Pictures taken on roll film should be accompanied, either in the medical record or in the photographer's notebook, by a list of the exposures and what they were intended to show.

References

Adger H, Shafer M-A, Sweet RL, Schacter J. Screening for *Chlamydia trachomatis* and *Neisseria gonorrhoeae* in adolescent males: value of first-catch urine examination. Lancet 1984;ii:944–945.

Al-Salihi FL, Curran JP, Wang J-S. Neonatal *Trichomonas vaginalis*: report of three cases and review of the literature. Pediatrics 1974;53:196–200.

Altcheck A. Pediatric vulvovaginitis. J Reprod Med 1984;29:359–375.

Alter MJ, Ahtone J, Weisfuse I, Starko K, Vacalis TD, Maynard JE. Hepatitis B virus transmission between heterosexuals. JAMA 1986;256:1307–1310.

Anonymous. 1985 STD treatment guidelines. MMWR 1985;34(Suppl):75S–108S.

Anonymous. Prevalence of human immunodeficiency virus antibody in U.S. active-duty military personnel, April 1988. MMWR 1988a;37:461–463.

Anonymous. Syphilis and congenital syphilis—United States, 1985–1988. MMWR 1988b;37:486–489.

Anonymous. Relationship of syphilis to drug use and prostitution—Connecticut and Philadelphia, Pennsylvania. MMWR 1988c;37:755–764.

Bach CM. Medical-legal consultation. Seattle, Washington: Harborview Medical Center, August 1980.

Bartley DL, Morgan L, Rimsza ME. *Gardnerella vaginalis* in prepubertal girls. Am J Dis Child 1987;141:1014–1017.

Barton LL, Shuja M. Neonatal gonococcal vaginitis [Letter]. J Pediatr 1981;98:171.

Bell TA, Stamm WE, Kuo C-C, Wang S-P, Holmes KK, Grayston JT. Delayed appearance of *Chlamydia trachomatis* infections acquired at birth. Pediatr Infect Dis J 1987;6:928–931.

Bender ME. New concepts of condyloma acuminata in children. Arch Dermatol 1986;122:1121–1124.

Bennett RS, Powell KR. Human papillomaviruses: associations between laryngeal papillomas and genital warts. Pediatr Infect Dis J 1987;6:229–232.

Brown ZA, Vontver LA, Benedetti J, et al. Effects on infants of a first episode of genital herpes during pregnancy. N Engl J Med 1987;317:1246–1251.

Bump RC, Sachs LA, Buesching WJ. Sexually transmissible infectious agents in sexually active and virginal asymptomatic adolescent girls. Pediatrics 1986;77:488–494.

Burch TA, Rees CW, Reardon LV. Epidemiological studies on human trichomoniasis. Am J Trop Med Hyg 1959;8:312–318.

Burgess JA. *Trichomonas vaginalis* infection from splashing in water closets. Br J Vener Dis 1963;39:248–250.

Centers for Disease Control. Human immunodeficiency virus infection in the United States: a review of current knowledge, MMWR 1987;36(Suppl S-6):2.

Chacko MR, Lovchik JC. *Chlamydia trachomatis* infection in sexually active adolescents: prevalence and risk factors. Pediatrics 1984;73:836–840.

Corey L, Spear PG. Infections with herpes simplex viruses. N Engl J Med 1986;314:686–691.

Dahlke MB, Cooke C, Cunnane M, Chawla J, Lau P. Identification of semen in 500 patients seen because of rape. Am J Clin Pathol 1977;68:740–746.

DeJong AR. Sexually transmitted diseases in sexually abused children. Sex Transm Dis 1986;13:123–126.

DeJong AR, Weiss JC, Brent RL. Condyloma acuminata in children. Am J Dis Child 1982;136:704–706.

de Villiers E-M, Wagner D, Schneider A, et al. Human papillomavirus infections in women with and without abnormal cervical cytology. Lancet 1987;ii:703–706.

Dossett JH, Applebaus PC, Knapp JS, et al. Proctitis associated with *Neisseria cinerea* misidentified as *Neisseria gonorrhoeae* in a child. J Clin Microbiol 1985;21:575–577.

Emans SJ. Vulvovaginitis in the child and adolescent. Pediatr Rev 1986;8:12–19.

Enos WF, Beyer JC. Spermatozoa in the anal canal and rectum and in the oral cavity of female rape victims. J Forensic Sci 1978;23:231–233.

Falloon J, Eddy J, Wiener L, Pizzo PA. Human immunodeficiency virus infection in children. J Pediatr 1989;114:1–30.

Farrell MK, Billmire ME, Shamroy JA, Hammond JG. Prepubertal gonorrhea: a multidisciplinary approach. Pediatrics 1981;67:151–153.

Ferenczy A, Mitao M, Nagai N, Silverstein SJ, Crum CP. Latent papillomavirus and recurring genital warts. N Engl J Med 1985;313:784–788.

Findley TP. Quantitation of vaginal acid phosphatase and its relationship to time of coitus. Am J Clin Pathol 1977;68:238–242.

Fleming KA, Venning V, Evans M. DNA typing of genital warts and diagnosis of sexual abuse in children [Letter]. Lancet 1987;ii:454.

Fouts AC, Kraus SJ. *Trichomonas vaginalis*: reevaluation of its clinical presentation and laboratory diagnosis. J Infect Dis 1980;141:137–143.

Fuster CD, Neinstein LS. Vaginal *Chlamydia trachomatis* prevalence in sexually abused prepubertal girls. Pediatrics 1987;79:235–238.

Gardner M, Jones JG. Genital herpes acquired by sexual abuse of children. J Pediatr 1984;104:243–244.

Gilbaugh JH, Fuchs PC. The gonococcus and the toilet seat. N Engl J Med 1979;301:91–93.

Gill P, Jeffreys AJ, Werrett DJ. Forensic applications of DNA "fingerprints." Nature 1985;318:577–579.

Grussendorf-Conen E-I, de Villiers E-M, Gissman L. Human papillomavirus genomes in penile smears of healthy men [Letter]. Lancet 1986;ii:1092.

Gutman LT, Wilfert CM. Gonococcal diseases in infants in children. In: Holmes KK, Mårdh P-A, Sparling PF, Wiesner PJ, eds. Sexually transmitted diseases. New York: McGraw-Hill Book Co, 1984:238–242.

Hajek EF. Contribution to the etiology of laryngeal papilloma in children. J Laryngol Otol 1956;70:166–168.

Hammerschlag MR, Doraiswamy B, Alexander ER, Cox P, Price W, Gleyzer A. Are rectogenital chlamydial infections a marker of sexual abuse in children? Pediatr Infect Dis J 1984;3:100–104.

Hammerschlag MR, Cummings M, Doraiswamy B, Cox P, McCormack WM. Nonspecific vaginitis following sexual abuse in children. Pediatrics 1985;75:1028–1031.

Hammerschlag MR, Rettig PJ, Shields ME. False positive results with the use of chlamydial antigen detection tests in the evaluation of suspected sexual abuse in children. Pediatr Infect Dis J 1988;7:11–14.

Ingram DL, White ST, Occhiutti AR, Lyna PR. Childhood vaginal infections: association of *Chlamydia trachomatis* with sexual contact. Pediatr Infect Dis J 1986;5:226–229.

Johnson K. DNA "fingerprinting" tests becoming a factor in courts. New York Times 7 Feb 1988:1, 46.

Jones JG, Yamauchi T, Lambert B. *Trichomonas vaginalis* infestation in sexually abused girls. Am J Dis Child 1985;139:846–847.

Kaplan KM, Fleisher GR, Paradise JE, Friedman HN. Social relevance of genital herpes simplex in children. Am J Dis Child 1984;138:872–874.

Knapp JS, Totten PA, Mulks MH, et al. Characterization of *Neisseria cinerea*, a nonpathogenic species isolated on Martin-Lewis medium selective for pathogenic *Neisseria* spp. J Clin Microbiol 1984;19:63–67.

Macnab JCM, Walkinshaw SA, Cordiner JW, Clements JB. Human papillomavirus in clincially and histologically normal tissue of patients with genital cancer. N Engl J Med 1986;315:1052–1058.

Martinez J, Smith R, Farmer M, et al. High prevalence of genital tract papillomavirus infection in female adolescents. Pediatrics 1988;82:604–608.

McClure EM, Stack MR, Tanner T, Thevenin J Jr, Gofstein RM, Helgerson SD. Pharyngeal culturing and reporting of pediatric gonorrhea in Connecticut. Pediatrics 1986;78:509–510.

Meyer KB, Pauker SG. Screening for HIV: can we affort the false positive rate? N Engl J Med 1987;317:238–241.

Neinstein LS, Goldenring J, Carpenter S. Non-sexual transmission of sexually transmitted diseases: an infrequent occurrence. Pediatrics 1984;74:67–76.

Osterholm MT, MacDonald KL, Danila RN. Sexually transmitted disease in victims of sexual assault [Letter]. N Engl J Med 1987;316:1024.

Potterat JJ, Markewich GS, King RD, Merecicky LR. Child-to-child transmission of gonorrhea: report of asymptomatic genital infection in a boy. Pediatrics 1986;78:711–712.

Quinn TC, Glasser D, Cannon O, et al. Human immunodeficiency virus infection among patients attending clinics for sexually transmitted diseases. N Engl J Med 1988;318:197–203.

Rein MF, Mller M. *Trichomonas vaginalis*. In: Holmes KK, Mårdh P-A, Sparling PF, Wiesner PJ, eds. Sexually transmitted diseases. New York: McGraw-Hill Book Co, 1984:525–536.

Rettig PJ, Nelson JD. Genital tract infection with *Chlamydia trachomatis* in prepubertal children. J Pediatr 1981;99:206–210.

Rimsza ME, Niggemann EH. Medical evaluation of sexually abused children: a review of 311 cases. Pediatrics 1982;69:8–14.

Rock B, Naghashfar Z, Barnett N, Buscema J, Woodruff JD, Shah K. Genital tract papillomavirus infection in children. Arch Dermatol 1986;122:1129–1132.

Rubinstein A, Bernstein L. The epidemiology of pediatric acquired immunodeficiency syndrome. Clin Immunol Immunopathol 1986;40:115–121.

Rupp JC. Sperm survival and prostatic acid phosphatase activity in victims of sexual assault. J Forensic Sci 1969;14:177–183.

Russell DEH. The incidence and prevalence of intrafamilial and extrafamilial sexual abuse of female children. Child Abuse Negl 1983;7:133–146.

Schachter J, Grossman M, Sweet RL, Holt J, Jordan C, Bishop E. Prospective study of perinatal transmission of *Chlamydia trachomatis*. JAMA 1986;255:3374–3377.

Sensabaugh GF. The quantitative acid phosphatase test. A statistical analysis of endogenous and postcoital acid phosphatase levels in the vagina. J Forensic Sci 1979;24:346–365.

Shafer MA, Sweet RL, Ohm-Smith MJ, Shalwitz J, Beck A, Schacter J. Microbiology of the lower genital tract in post-menarchal adolescent girls: differences by sexual activity, contraception, and presence of nonspecific vaginitis. J Pediatr 1985;107:974–981.

Shelton TB, Jerkins GR, Noe HN. Condylomata acuminata in the pediatric patient. J Urol 1986;135:548–549.

Silber TJ, Controni G. Clinical spectrum of pharyngeal gonorrhea in children and adolescents: a report of 16 patients. J Adolesc Health Care 1983;4:51–54.

Sore WB, Winkelstein JA. Nonvenereal transmission of gonococcal infections to children. J Pediatr 1971;79:661–663.

Stark AR, Glode MP. Gonococcal vaginitis in a neonate. J Pediatr 1979;94:298–299.

Tang C, Shermetta DW, Wood C. Congenital condyloma acuminata. Am J Obstet Gynecol 1984;148:912–913.

Tribe LH. Trial by mathematics: precision and ritual in the legal process. 84 Harvard Law Rev 1329, 1971.

White ST, Loda FA, Ingram DL, Parson A. Sexually transmitted diseases in sexually abused children. Pediatrics 1983;72:16–21.

Whittington WL, Rice RJ, Biddle JW, Knapp JS. Incorrect identification of *Neisseria gonorrhoeae* from infants and children. Pediatr Infect Dis J 1988;7:3–10.

Willott GM, Allard JE. Spermatozoa—their persistence after sexual intercourse. Forensic Sci Int 1982;19:135–154.

11 Neglect

Neglect, in all of its manifestations, is probably the single most common form of child maltreatment as well as the most underreported. Although some forms of neglect seem relatively clear-cut, such as abandonment of children or failure to obtain simple, low-risk preventive medical care, observers often disagree about the extent of risk or harm to children that justifies intruding on parental prerogatives or that falls outside the wide range of differing parenting styles.

The purpose of this chapter is to help clinicians make decisions about when neglect is taking place and when intervention may be appropriate. It begins with a discussion of neglect as a manifestation of more pervasive parent attitudes, as may occur in failure to thrive (see Chapter 12) or overall inattention to a child's physical and social needs. It concludes with a more legalistic view of neglect: the consideration of treatment refusal and a discussion of the so-called Baby Doe law.

PARENTAL FACTORS

Although this book gives relatively little information about the causes of maltreatment in general, some discussion of the etiology of neglect is relevant to making diagnoses. One of the central questions in evaluating a case of suspected neglect is: "Beyond this incident, is there evidence of a more general pattern of neglectful behavior?" Theories and observations about the cause of neglect help direct the clinician's considerations of whether such a pattern appears to exist.

Polansky and co-workers (1981) see three main forces interacting to create child neglect. First, economic forces may define the range of resources available for a child's care. Although neglect occurs in all socioeconomic groups, low income appears to increase its prevalence. However, the majority of low-income families are able to adequately nurture their children, even if it is without many of the amenities that wealthier families consider necessities.

A second force is the parents' personality. As discussed below, Polansky and colleagues as well as others have found that many neglectful parents display a cluster of distinctive personality traits. The way these parents view the world in general, and the task of child rearing in particular, appears to alter their ability to cope with life's challenges and to create a nurturing environment for their children.

Finally, just as all behavior probably has both personal and environmental components, parental characteristics that lead to neglect may be modified by social or ecologic influences. At times these influences may protect against neglect, such as when good fortune or a relatively undemanding job shelters a parent from stress. Alternatively, a community's tolerance for inappropriate child-rearing practices may perpetuate neglect once it begins. Although neglectful parents may be out of touch with community norms, they may respond to direct messages that what they are doing is unusual. Not all communities send these messages, however, when a child has prolonged absences from school or is seen in the care of an obviously intoxicated adult.

In the view of Polansky and colleagues (1981), clinicians approaching cases of suspected neglect may have difficulty because they try to analyze parental behaviors as neuroses rather than as character disorders. Neurotic individuals are felt to have relatively intact egos and generally standard responses to most of the situations they encounter. Certain relatively circumscribed situations, however, lead neurotic individuals to experience intense conflict and to use maladaptive defense measures. Although these problems are by no means trivial, they tend to be more time-limited and open to insight and rational, common-sense solutions than the problems faced by individuals with character disorders.

The problem with common-sense approaches to neglect, according to Polansky and colleagues, is that most neglectful parents are not neurotic, but instead have more pervasive character problems. Although there is disagreement within the field, character or personality disorders are defined as differences from the norm in world view: perceptions of social rules and truisms are altered, and responses to life situations vary across the board and for long periods of time in comparison with other individuals. Thus, common-sense solutions fail for persons with character disorders because the solutions are not logical within the individual's different view of life.

In studies of mothers referred for suspected neglect, Polansky and co-workers found about 40% to have a personality profile that they called the apathy-futility syndrome. Its primary manifestation was the mother's conviction that she was a bad and essentially worthless individual. Thus, nothing good could ever happen to her, nothing in her life could ever work correctly, and little in life was worth doing. This appeared to be a long-standing conviction on the part of the mothers, and it appeared to have had several consequences as their lives had evolved.

To some extent, the mothers seemed to have had their social development arrested at a very early stage. Because they saw themselves as helpless and incompetent, they tended to cling to superficial and even abusive relationships with other adults. They had a child-like inability to empathize with or understand other people's views or needs and a corresponding inability to articulate their own feelings. Their lack of confidence and social skills appeared to contribute to a vicious cycle of failure. Apparently because they could not face taking social risks, they could not tackle the kinds of problem solving required to deal with their immediate problems or to make long-term plans.

These characteristics went beyond what Polansky et al. felt could be labeled depression, which would imply that either reaction to some situational problem or true depressive illness was the cause. The mothers interviewed appeared to have developed an ability to inhibit their responses to what went on around them and to cut themselves off from social interaction, apparently as a shield against their own feelings of inadequacy. This sort of behavior had devastating consequences for their children, who could then be held too closely and yet not nurtured. The mother's loneliness and clinging could deny a child the chance for independence while placing him or her in the role of caretaker for the parent. The mother's inability to empathize with the child's needs could lead to a failure to provide both material and emotional supports and blind the mother to the consequences of her own behavior. Some mothers lost interest in their children once they had grown beyond infancy, perhaps because the children, even with the first signs of independence and individuality, evoked the mother's own fears of loneliness and rejection.

This type of neglectful parent can become immensely frustrating for clinicians. The parents interviewed in Polansky's work had a remarkable ability to induce feelings of futility in anyone with whom they came in contact. Their inability to discuss their feelings and their sense of hopelessness thwarted attempts to provide logical, medically oriented solutions to their problems. The clinician's frustration seemed as if it might even be a positive reinforcement, since it served as one more validation of their hopeless world view.

The apathy-futility model did not fit all of the mothers in the study cited above. About a quarter of the mothers appeared to have some form of impulse disorder, characterized by a low tolerance for frustration, an inability to plan, and poor or hasty judgment. Other parental characteristics associated with neglect included mental retardation, depression, substance abuse, and, less commonly, acute or chronic psychoses.

MEDICAL OBSERVATIONS

Although neglect is often characterized by emotional, behavioral, or school problems, physicians and nurses may encounter medical conditions that suggest inadequate care by a child's parents. Growth patterns that deviate from the norm can be a sign of inadequate nutrition or an abnormal psychosocial environment (see Chapter 12). Plotting growth parameters or calculating growth percentiles from tables is an important part of any pediatric assessment, regardless of the suspicion of maltreatment.

Injuries or conditions for which the parents appear to have delayed seeking treatment may also be signs of neglect or of a disorganized household in which the children's needs are not promptly perceived. This is an area, however, in which clinicians must move cautiously. Even experienced physicians may be surprised at the speed with which some conditions develop and the lack of symptoms caused by others. For example, social service workers may ask a physician whether a child's apparently severe diaper rash could be a sign of neglect. Making such a judgment depends on a consideration of any underlying skin condition (such as eczema), on the presence of some other illness (for example, diarrhea), on the nature of the rash itself (a rapidly spreading yeast infection versus a chronic irritant), and perhaps on response to treatment (superficial yeast infections clear more quickly than deeper erosions caused by continual irritation and bacterial infection). In older children, delayed care for simple fractures may not always indicate parental avoidance or inattention. These fractures may produce only subtle symptoms, such as pain limited to direct pressure over the fracture or barely perceptible changes in the way the child uses an extremity. Before deciding that care for an acute problem has been delayed or neglected, it is important to find out who was caring for the child when the problem developed and how promptly the person now seeking care responded once he or she was aware of the situation.

Delays in seeking preventive care pose both medical and legal dilemmas; failure to obtain well-child care, for example, may not fit local legal definitions of neglect if the child is not yet harmed by the omission. Clinicians must be able to substantiate the need for the care they are proposing. Supporting evidence for many preventive measures is not available in the medical literature. Some clinicians suggest as minimal standards that basic immunizations for life-threatening diseases (diphtheria, tetanus, pertussis, and polio) be completed before 2 years of age and that there be at least two health maintenance visits within the first year, with at least one within the first 2 months (Schmitt, 1981).

Physical neglect may include the failure to provide basic food, shelter, and clothing. There are no satisfying definitions of "basic," but these requirements may be taken to mean food with calories and nutrients sufficient for normal growth, shelter that is safe, sanitary, and adequately ventilated and heated, and clothing that is in good repair and appropriate for the weather. Polansky et al. (1981) found wide agreement across social classes as to the necessity of providing a supervised and physically sustaining environment.

Injuries resulting from falls, motor vehicles, burns, poisonings, and other presumed accidents are the leading cause of death among persons 1–19 years of age (Rivara and Mueller, 1987). Beyond age 4, injuries cause more deaths among children than all other causes combined. Among younger children, many (if not most) injuries occur in or around the home (Matheny, 1987), and many can be traced to hazards that seem to have been avoidable: windows with loose screens (enabling children to fall), tapwater at scalding temperatures, unprotected electrical sockets, improperly stored toxins, and structural designs or damage that failed to protect children from busy roads, deep water, or unforgiving surfaces.

Some authors have called these conditions "culturally condoned child abuse" (Wilson, 1983–85). To a large extent, those guilty of neglect appear to be manufacturers, builders, or landlords who design or maintain inherently dangerous products or dwellings. On the other hand, preliminary research does suggest that certain parental characteristics are associated with an increased chance of injury to children (Matheny et al., 1971; Larsen and Pless, 1988) and that others are related to the increased use of safety devices (Gielen et al., 1984).

Although the link between these attitudes and injuries has yet to be established, several studies have shown that hazards can be reduced (with varying degrees of success) by persuading landlords and parents to make alterations in the home environment (Spiegel et al., 1977; Gallagher et al., 1985; Gorman et al., 1984). At present, however, failure to remove all but the most serious hazards or those that have already caused injury in the past is not generally considered neglectful. There is some indication that societal expectations for child safety have been increasing; as a result, definitions of physical neglect may begin to change. Automobile safety restraint laws, for example, although not explicitly part of abuse and neglect statutes, may provide a new legal basis for establishing neglect in some injury situations. Driving with children while intoxicated and improperly storing firearms in the home (Rivara and Stapleton, 1982) are also coming to be recognized as behaviors with foreseeable adverse consequences and thus possible grounds for allegations of neglect under the category of "reckless behavior" (discussed in Chapter 1).

Children also require adequate supervision, both for their safety and for their emotional well-being. Parents are given the responsibility for ensuring that this supervision is provided, either by themselves or by someone they so designate. Substitute caretakers should have the information necessary to care for the child properly and to enable contact with the parents in the case of an emergency. Preadolescent children are usually not suitable caretakers for younger siblings even on a short-term basis.

MAKING A DIAGNOSIS

While the diagnosis of physical abuse may often be made quickly, concerns for neglect often evolve slowly in the course of interaction with a child and the family. Sometimes it is the medical interaction itself that creates the setting for neglect by prescribing or expecting care that the parents apparently do not wish to provide. As Schmitt (1981) points out, when resistance is encountered, the clinician's first step should be to try to understand the family's perspective, decrease barriers to needed care, and solicit the help of individuals trusted by the family. This may help overcome defenses and increase communication. While this process is going on, however, the clinician may encounter a number of difficulties. Some of these involve the clinician himself or herself, while others involve the family.

As with other forms of maltreatment, perhaps the greatest pitfall for the clinician is developing an overwhelming urge to rescue a child. The need to rescue leads to anger at the parents which, in the case of neglect, is often exacerbated by the parents' apparent resistance and ambivalence to overtures of assistance. Anger has at least two undesirable consequences: it validates the parents' low opinion of themselves and of their view of the impossibility of change, and it leads the clinician to prescribe quick-fix solutions that may not benefit the child.

Perhaps even more serious, anger exacerbates the clinician's own internal conflicts about the situation and makes it even harder to find thoughtful solutions. The desire to rescue the child often coexists with a strong identification with the parents' neediness and with their right to refuse outside interference. This true double bind can make any action seem impossible.

There may be no easy ways to prevent anger or thoughts of rescue, but some tactics may help. First, medical practitioners can follow the lead of mental health professionals and seek case-specific supervision from colleagues. Even if such sessions are informal, the intense feelings engendered by cases of suspected neglect (and child maltreatment in general) may be helped by objective, problem-oriented discussions. Second, clinicians can remind themselves that in many cases the parents' apparent resistance to change is not a conscious challenge to medical authority and the practitioner's competence; in most cases it is truly a part of the "disease" and requires treatment itself. Finally, clinicians facing cases of suspected neglect may have to disregard their usual acute care model of treatment; change in the family is likely to be gradual, and certain conditions will probably be stabilized rather than eliminated.

Even if clinicians are able to resist anger, they may fall victim to the parents' own sense of futility. Although clinicians must set realistic goals for a family, they have to guard against coming to accept a status quo that continues to leave children at serious risk. This can happen fairly easily once the clinician is satisfied that he or she has taken sufficient and appropriate steps (and had them rejected by the family) to assuage his or her own conscience. One approach to avoiding this problem is to set achievable goals early in the course of interacting with the family. Setting goals may take some assessment of the family's material and emotional resources and discussions with colleagues about a position that seems fair and practical. The goals can be periodically reevaluated, but firm time frames for their achievement should be established. Failure to meet the goals should trigger a next level of intervention, perhaps referral to a social service agency. Acting promptly may, paradoxically, help a clinician's relationship with a family more than acquiescing for lengthier periods would. Early intervention can be regarded as a genuine desire to help and a recognition of the urgency of the family's needs, whereas intervention after a long delay can be seen as a betrayal of what the family may have come to consider acceptance of their way of life.

Clinicians may be tempted to use the possibility of social service involvement as a lever to obtain action by a family. Although there are times when this tactic may be necessary, such as when a child is acutely ill and the family refuses consent for urgently needed treatment, in other situations it may be counterproductive. Not only does it serve to reinforce the idea that social service intervention is punitive rather than therapeutic, but it sets up a power dynamic in the clinician-family relationship that plays into maladaptive patterns of behavior. The family gets a legitimate reason to be angry at an authority figure, and clinicians find themselves in a difficult position: if they follow through, they confirm their role as the punishing parent (which at the very least causes some degree of guilt); if they fail to act, on the other hand, they are seen by the family as yet one more person who cannot be counted on to set and honor clear, consistent limits. A preferable tactic is to make a decision about the need for social service intervention on the basis of objective clinical criteria and to humanely but firmly present the decision to the family once those criteria are met.

Polansky et al. (1981) suggest several strategies for helping neglectful families become engaged in care. One is for clinicians to recognize the magnitude of each family's loneliness and near phobia of interaction with other people. Medical settings may offer opportunities for the family to meet the outside world in a supportive environment. Parents can be treated with a respect they may not get elsewhere, and positive aspects of their parenting and their children can be emphasized. This support is not offered in the hope that it alone will resolve the situation, but as a way of amplifying the tenuous opening for communication that the family may have allowed. Some parents will jump at this chance and, while still resisting change, demonstrate their dependency by finding any excuse to call or come for a visit. It may be hard for a clinician to resist becoming angered by a family's needs, but some compromise between the parent's dependency and the clinician's own need to set limits can help to move the family toward seeing relationships in a less frantic and more trusting way.

A corollary of the neglectful family's low skill level and fear of interaction is the tendency to panic when in the face of challenging or threatening situations. Few people think clearly under crisis conditions (see Chapter 5), but neglectful families may see crises where others do not. Clinicians can help by trying to minimize demands that are under their control and by helping families rehearse for potentially stressful situations (such as a meeting with a child's teacher). Clinicians can also help family members better express their feelings and needs. They can echo and try to interpret feelings that are poorly expressed or evident only in body language, and they can encourage people to talk about what they do in certain situations rather than what they may be feeling but cannot express.

Finally, clinicians frequently need to seek help to coordinate the many services needed by neglectful families, such as school counselors, income maintenance and housing workers, in-home aides, and possibly specific medical or mental health services. Help may be available through social workers, Medicaid or health department case managers, or multidisciplinary treatment facilities.

CRITERIA FOR SOCIAL SERVICE INVOLVEMENT

The steps outlined above are designed to develop trust and open avenues of communication so that potentially neglectful families will become more open to receiving help for themselves and their children. Sometimes these steps fail, however, and clinicians feel it necessary to involve outside authorities. Neither laws nor medical or social work practice offer straightforward guidelines for making such a decision. Use of the following considerations offers one possible approach to the problem (Bross, 1982):

- Is there either imminent danger to the child or the risk of some serious future impairment? The purpose of this test is to keep the clinician focused on problems that are serious enough to warrant overriding the parents' freedom to raise their children as they see fit. The emphasis will usually be on physical danger, but reasonably predictable social or emotional impairment may also be grounds for intervention. (Educational neglect, one of the few categories of neglect firmly established by law, is an example of the latter category.)
- Is there evidence that the neglected action would have helped the child or would do so in the future? The important aspect of this test is the clinician's certainty of the effectiveness of the care or treatment he or she is advocating. A problem may be serious (for example, a child's cancer), but if the therapy a parent is purportedly neglecting cannot be said to have some chance of benefiting the

child, intervention may not be justifiable. Obviously, there is no consensus on how great a chance of benefit may be required, although both courts (see below) and ethicists have found it reasonable for even proxy decision makers (such as parents) to refuse care that has only a small chance of success.

- Have the parents disregarded timely and clear information (or what reasonably can be considered common knowledge among parents) that the child would be harmed by the action they have neglected? Parents should not be held accountable for retrospective determinations that a particular action would have been helpful, nor can they be asked to comply with suggestions that they have not had the opportunity to understand.
- Is the neglect part of a more pervasive pattern of parental dysfunction? Is the episode of neglect an isolated event related to a misunderstanding or oversight, or does it reflect a more general attitude of the parents toward the child? Are other needs or aspects of care neglected? Do the parents seem willing to expend the material and emotional resources necessary to raise the child?
- Does the family have the material resources necessary to provide for the child? This test may be even more difficult to use than those cited above. On one hand, some definitions of neglect do not require that parents consciously withhold care from their children (Polansky et al., 1981), and some neglect laws do include parental inability to provide care, for whatever reason, along with parental refusal. Thus, some appear to say that it is the child's state of need, rather than how that state occurred, that is important in determining the need for outside intervention. Under this view, the children of a homeless family might be involuntarily placed until the parents could provide shelter (given the unfortunate circumstance that many agencies are more able to place children than to assist families with housing problems). Other definitions consider the family's resources and try to assess neglect within the scope of what seems possible. Proponents of this viewpoint try to strike a balance between offering children some minimum degree of care and blaming parents who may also be victims of significant injustice and deprivation. Many may say that if good emotional nurturing is present, the risk of emotional trauma from intervention is probably greater than the most severe forms of physical deprivation.

THE SPECIAL CASE OF EDUCATIONAL NEGLECT

In their analysis of data from the first National Incidence Study of Child Abuse and Neglect (US Department of Health and Human Services, 1981), Hampton and Newberger (1985) found that hospital-based professionals reported only 6% of the educational neglect that they encountered, the lowest proportion of reporting for any category of maltreatment. It is not known whether this proportion would be higher among primary care physicians, who have more longitudinal contact with their patients. Concern for adequate school attendance and performance is an integral part of well-child care. Not only is school achievement itself important to a child's development, but behavior and adjustment problems at school may reflect physical or emotional difficulties in other aspects of a child's life. Clinicians are most commonly drawn into school issues when a child has a handicap or chronic illness that requires special educational placement. The Education for All Handicapped Children Act (PL 94-142) requires that public education be provided for handicapped children and specifies that it be offered in the least restrictive setting possible. Children are guaranteed "due process" in the determination of the nature of their handicaps and in the choice of educational resources offered (Palfrey et al., 1978). Physicians and other health care workers are often intimately involved in the diagnostic process and in discussions of how a child's physical and intellectual limitations fit into programs that a school has to offer.

In this setting, neglect issues can arise in several ways. Parents may fail to enroll their children in special programs (which may be provided from age 3 for some handicapped children) or decide not to enroll their children at all (Jaudes and Diamond, 1986). They may also fail to follow through with or participate in school-initiated attempts to seek better diagnoses or placement.

Schools themselves, however, may also be involved with educational neglect. They may fail to identify children in need of special help, or they may not respond promptly or positively to parental requests for evaluation or service planning. Because of PL 94-142, legal measures are often possible in these situations. Referrals to local advocacy groups for the handicapped (some of which may be sponsored by a state developmental disabilities agency) or to publicly available legal resources such as Legal Aid may help hasten a school's actions and connect the family with a wider network of support.

Clinicians can also play a role when schools discriminate against children with certain illnesses. Most recently, discrimination has focused on children with acquired immunodeficiency syndrome (AIDS) (Rubenstein, 1986), but past cases have involved herpesvirus infections (Malcolm, 1985) and hepatitis (Association for Retarded Children v. Carey; Coughlin v. Board of Education; West v. Board of Education. [612 F. 2d 644, 1979]). Protection for these children has been sought both under PL 94-142 and under other federal laws such as the Rehabilitation Act of 1973, which addresses definitions of handicap and issues of workplace discrimination. PL 94-142 has been used to argue against both exclusion from school and overly restrictive placement (Burns, 1985). A recent United States Supreme Court ruling, School Board v. Arline (no. 85-1277), has offered hope that children with asymptomatic human immunodeficiency virus infection would also be afforded protection, at least in schools that receive some form of federal funding. The ruling involved the case of a Florida elementary school teacher who had tuberculosis and was dismissed from her job because of her "susceptibility" to the infection. Florida courts had ruled that the school authorities' duty to protect pupils from infection warranted the dismissal. She countered that her condition, which was under treatment, made her a handicapped individual under the definitions given in the Rehabilitation Act and that the school board was therefore obliged to make some "reasonable accommodation" to her condition rather than just firing her. A federal appeals court agreed with her, finding that the public's significant negative reaction to a condition was sufficient grounds to consider it as handicapping (Arline v. School Board, 722 F. 2d 759, 1985). The appeals court thought it clear that Congress had intended the Rehabilitation Act to "reduce instances of unthinking and unnecessary discrimination" against persons with serious, chronic medical problems. The Supreme Court agreed. Justice Brennan wrote:

> By amending the definition of "handicapped individual" to include not only those who are actually physically impaired, but also those who are regarded as impaired and who, as a result, are substantially limited in a major life activity, Congress acknowledged that society's accumulated myths and fears about disability and disease are as handicapping as are the physical limitations that flow from actual impairment.

There are several ways for clinicians to help children involved in this form of discrimination. Preventive measures can include working with families to decide what information about the child's condition should be divulged and to whom. Clinicians can also help a family realistically assess the medical risks of school attendance, both to the child and to classmates, and then participate in the process of deciding what placement would be most appropriate (Committee on School Health, 1986). These decisions may have to be reviewed periodically as the child's condition evolves. Perhaps most important, clinicians can support families when school or other officials take actions that could inappropriately affect a child's education. Direct contact with school officials or indirect contact via local health authorities may send a signal that the family has an ally and that a discussion based on facts would be in the best interests of all parties.

There are many reasons besides handicap why children do not attend school. Some are truant: they leave home as if to go to school but never arrive. Parents of these children are not considered neglectful so long as they have made a good-faith effort to send their children to school and help remedy the situation once they become aware of the truancy. It may be difficult to tactfully evaluate why some children are allowed to stay home. The family may well have financial difficulties that require older children to remain at home to care for younger siblings while a parent works; low-income parents may be embarrassed to send a child to school without adequate clothing or food. Some children are afraid to go to school because they are threatened by other children or an abusive teacher or because learning difficulties make the classroom experience distressing. Ideally, parents respond promptly to these situations by contacting school authorities.

Prolonged school absence by children who remain at home may be a manifestation of school phobia, a form of separation disorder in which a child develops an unwarranted fear of school or of leaving home. Although formal definitions emphasize only the child's fears of separating from an attachment figure, clinical descriptions recognize the role of the attachment figure, usually a parent, in cultivating and reinforcing the refusal (Rosenberg, 1958; Allmond et al., 1979).

School phobia can occur at any age from nursery through high school. In the typical case, on awakening the child complains of some minor ailment (abdominal pain, headache, nausea) that precludes getting ready or leaving for school. The parents engage in what an outsider would consider disorganized or ineffective attempts to get the child to go, essentially colluding with the child to allow him or her to remain at home. The symptoms usually abate once the threat of going to school has passed for that day.

Frequently, exploration of issues in the child's family finds that the father has taken a physically or emotionally distant stance from both the mother and from day-to-day child care responsibilities. The mother may still be involved in a separation struggle with her own parents. Either because of her own separation problems or as part of a struggle with her husband into which the child is recruited (see Chapter 5), the mother fosters the child's overdependence and fails to help him or her work through the normal separation anxieties associated with going to school. Paradoxically, she may also become angry with the child, either because the overdependence creates behaviors that are particularly annoying or because she transfers to the child hostility that she feels toward other individuals, such as her spouse or parents. The child becomes confused by this combination of overprotective and angry messages, which lays the groundwork for an excessive fear of either upsetting or leaving the mother. Some fairly minor event at school or a brief illness then provides an initial excuse to remain at home, and ongoing refusal to attend school begins.

Making the diagnosis of school phobia is very important for the child and family. The unsuspecting physician can become part of the problem by unquestioningly validating minor symptoms and failing to notice their pattern or frequency. As in Munchausen's syndrome by proxy (discussed in Chapter 15), overresponding to symptoms without considering their psychodynamic relevance can prolong abnormal family interaction and risks iatrogenic harm to the child. There is also a risk that the clinician will unfairly blame the child, without recognizing the parents' role, or label the parent as neglectful when more specific psychologic treatment could be provided. The diagnosis is usually made after discussion with all family members and with the school. A suggestion that the father has a relatively peripheral role and that the mother has a motivation to keep the child close to her may be the first indication that separation problems are occurring. Details of what takes place each morning when the child is supposed to be getting ready to go to school can reveal whether genuine efforts to ease separation problems are being made. Discussion with the child and with teachers can confirm that there are no major learning or social problems at school.

Treatment of school phobia requires an understanding but firm insistence that separation occur and that the child go to school. The parents need to be supported in their resolve, even if it requires helping them explain to the child that the truant officer will have to become involved if attendance does not begin. Sustained attendance sometimes requires therapy for the child but invariably requires help for the parents. Refusal by the parents to seek help, if it results in renewed refusal to attend school, may be grounds for a report of suspected educational neglect.

MEDICAL NEGLECT OF SERIOUSLY ILL OR POTENTIALLY HANDICAPPED NEWBORNS

The case of "Baby Doe," born in Indiana in the spring of 1982, sparked a national political and ethical debate about medical treatment of seriously ill newborns. Baby Doe was a child with Down's syndrome, esophageal atresia, and a tracheoesophageal fistula (Pless, 1983). The esophageal malformation was of the type that did not permit direct passage of food from the mouth to the stomach: the upper esophagus connected only with the trachea, and farther down the trachea there was another connection to the lower esophagus. There were also clinical signs suggestive of a coarctation of the aorta.

The baby's parents chose not to have the esophageal defect repaired or to have intravenous nutrition administered, and the child died 6 days after birth. Treatment during that time involved only medications for pain and "restlessness." The case came to public attention when the administrators of the hospital where the child was born sought legal advice about respecting the parents' decision. Indiana courts agreed that the parents had a right to have treatment withheld.

The problematic nature of this type of case had been recognized early in the history of neonatal surgery and intensive care (Duff and Campbell, 1973). The issues involved included whether a life with certain handicaps constituted a life not worth living, whether provision of food and water was an optional "medical" treatment or a basic necessity of which no individual, however sick, could be deprived, and whether parents who would shoulder financial and emotional burdens of caring for chronically ill children should be allowed to participate in treatment decisions.

For reasons that historians will continue to debate, in May 1982, about a month after Baby Doe's death, the U.S. Department of Health and Human Services issued the first of what came to be known as the Baby Doe regulations. During a tumultuous period in which successive sets of regulations were promulgated, challenged in the courts, and eventually struck down by the Supreme Court (Anonymous, 1986), Congress passed the Child Abuse Prevention and Treatment Act of 1984 (PL 98-457), crystallizing federal policy regarding medical treatment of newborns.

This act had several provisions that were important for other types of child abuse treatment and prevention, but its most powerful clause linked federal funding of state child protection efforts to the establishment of specific state mechanisms for responding to cases of medical neglect, especially those involving the withholding of care from newborns. As elaborated in regulations (45 CFR 1340; Federal Register 1985;50:14878-14901), the Act set major limits on parents, physicians, and social service decision makers.

First, it essentially required that future "quality of life" not be a consideration in making treatment decisions about seriously ill newborns. Treatments were to be considered medically indicated, and therefore not subject to parental or physician discretion, if they addressed a condition that would have an immediate or long-term impact on the child's survival, regardless of level of functioning. There were to be only three circumstances in which these treatments might reasonably be withheld: when the child was "chronically and irreversibly comatose," when treatment would "merely prolong dying" or be unable to address all of the child's life-threatening conditions, and when the treatments would be futile (with respect to the child's survival) and thus inhumane. Failure to give treatment except in these circumstances was defined as medical neglect and grounds for legal intervention.

Second, the act specified that nutrition, hydration, and "medication" were not to be withheld even in the exceptional circumstances listed above. This type of support is, in fact, now usually considered to be part of minimal essential care. In circumstances involving adults, however, arguments have been made that even hydration may constitute a life-sustaining treatment that a reasonable person may wish to have withdrawn on the grounds that it prolongs suffering (Steinbrook and Lo, 1988). Again, failure to provide nutrition and hydration were grounds for a finding of medical neglect.

Early versions of Baby Doe regulations had included provisions requiring hospitals to post large signs stating the obligation to report suspected medical neglect, establishing national hotlines for reporting, and forming rapid-response teams that would be called on to investigate suspected cases. In the final regulations, these requirements were dropped or modified. It was suggested, but not required, that hospitals establish Infant Care Review Committees (ICRCs) that could help parents and physicians make decisions about individual cases and that could assume an educational role within the institution. The ICRCs were not to serve as ethics committees, however; their main task would be to see that appropriate information was provided to decision makers and that parents and physicians retained their prerogatives within the limitations of the regulations.

The full impact of the Baby Doe regulations has yet to be assessed. Hospital ethics and ICRCs have become more prevalent, although in many cases their roles remain to be fully defined (Leikin, 1987). States did respond to the legislation by training protective service workers in issues involving medical neglect and by setting up mechanisms for reporting and investigating cases of in-hospital medical neglect. Critics of the regulations remain embittered that so much emphasis has been placed on treating children with serious birth defects while society has been less willing to fund prevention programs that would reduce the incidence of defects requiring treatment (Lantos, 1987). Baby Doe cases have not been reported to social service agencies in large numbers, but it is not known whether this is because practices have changed or because, in response to the law, physicians and parents have drawn the cloak of privacy around themselves even more tightly.

LEGAL INTERPRETATIONS

Religious Exemptions from Medical Neglect Statutes

All United States child abuse laws, in part because of the Baby Doe issue, consider failure to provide adequate medical care to be a form of child neglect. In the past, adequate care was almost always defined by what a treating physician recommended. Increasingly, however, states have passed laws exempting from neglect statutes parents who refuse some or all standard medical therapies on the basis of religious beliefs. These laws create conflicts between advocates for children's physical and spiritual well-being. They also raise questions about children's rights to equal protection under the law and pit the state's interest in protecting children against the parents' right to religious freedom under the First Amendment to the Constitution (Committee on Bioethics, 1988).

Treatment Refusal on Nonreligious Grounds

In situations where parents refuse to treat children for nonreligious reasons, courts have generally been willing to act only when clear threats exist to a child's life or physical well-being (Williams, 1980). This position parallels that of many pediatric ethicists, who feel that a "clear and probable threat" to the child's health is the only basis for intervention in what otherwise is a private family decision. In this view, parents do, in fact, have a right to make decisions that outsiders might judge not to be in a child's best interests, and only decisions that pose serious threats to the child's health can be overridden (Fost, 1983).

The landmark court case in this area involved Chad Green, a child who developed acute lymphocytic leukemia at 20 months of age and whose parents wished to have him treated with the experimental drug laetrile (In re custody of a minor, 379 N.E. 2d 1053 [Mass., 1978]; 393 N.E. 2d 836 [Mass., 1979]). Chad was originally treated with standard chemotherapy and went into remission. He relapsed, however, when his parents stopped medication without informing his physician. Massachusetts courts first ordered Chad treated on the basis of fact that the chemotherapy was not "extraordinary" treatment and that it offered a substantial chance not just of prolonging life but of curing the disease. Remission was again induced, but Chad's family then proposed using laetrile and other "metabolic" therapies in addition to the standard chemotherapy. The court ordered that these treatments not be given because medical testimony suggested that their toxicities outweighed any potential benefit of administration. By that time, however, Chad's parents had taken him to Mexico, where he died.

In contrast, a New York court refused to order treatment for a 14-year-old child with a cleft palate who, along with his father, felt that "natural forces" and self-healing were preferable to surgery (In re Seiferth, 127 N.E. 2d 820 [N.Y., 1955]) The court felt that the child was old enough to have become convinced of his father's philosophy, that the problem was not life threatening, and that the child's own objections would hinder both treatment and recovery.

Treatment Refusal on Religious Grounds

Parental refusals of treatment based on religious grounds have come from many denominations, including Jehovah's Witnesses and Christian Scientists. Jehovah's Witnesses refuse blood products on the basis of biblical passages (such as Lev. 17:10, "And if any man of the house of Israel or of the strangers who reside among them partakes of any blood, I will set My face against the person who partakes of the blood, and I will cut him off from among his kin." [The Torah. Philadelphia: The Jewish Publication Society of America, 1962]) that are interpreted as forbidding transfusions. Parents who are Jehovah's Witnesses feel that they have a duty to help their children adhere to the precepts of the religion, and transfusions are seen as risking permanent spiritual harm to a child. Christian Scientists avoid all standard medical treatments. They believe in divine healing and consider disease a mental concept that can be dispelled through the introduction of spiritual truth (Mead, 1970).

Most legal cases involving religion-based treatment refusal cite the ruling in Prince v. Massachusetts (321 U.S. 158, 1944), in which Jehovah's Witnesses challenged a Massachusetts child labor law that had been invoked to forbid children from selling religious tracts in the streets. In the case, the court found as follows:

> Parents may be free to become martyrs themselves. But it does not follow that they are free, in identical circumstances, to make martyrs of their children before they have reached the age of full and legal discretion when they can make that choice for themselves.

As a general rule, courts in the United States have ruled that in situations in which child welfare and religious freedom conflict, children have no religious conviction or denomination, regardless of their parents' desire to assign one to them (Rozovsky, 1984). A parent's constitutional right to religious freedom is not felt to include "the liberty to expose children to ill health or death" (Jehovah's Witnesses v. King County Hospital, 278 F. Supp. 488, 1967, aff'd 390 U.S. 598, 1968).

Courts have not uniformly sided with suggestions for treatment, however. As in cases where refusal was based on nonreligious grounds, the need for treatment must still generally involve serious or life-threatening illness. For example, a Pennsylvania court refused to find neglect in the case of a 17 year old whose mother refused consent for surgical treatment of severe scoliosis (In re Ricky Ricardo Green, 307 A. 2d 270 [Pa., 1973]). Refusal was based not only on the possibility that a transfusion was needed (the family were Jehovah's Witnesses) but also on the fact that the child himself refused. Medical testimony convinced the court that the surgery would be beneficial, but the fact that the scoliosis was not life threatening and that the patient himself did not wish to prolong a stay in the hospital led the court to find that this was a decision the family had a right to make.

Christian Scientists and other religious groups that shun all medical contact pose more serious dilemmas than Jehovah's Witnesses. Whereas Witnesses seek care for ill children, objecting only to the use of blood products, Christian Scientists, for example, see any medical contact as a serious breach of faith (Swan, 1983). Thus, children may become seriously ill or die before their conditions come to the attention of persons outside their family or religious group. Reliance on Christian Science or other spiritual treatment alone has led to what may have been preventable deaths from conditions such as meningitis and pneumonia. Most states, however, have adopted laws that specifically exempt treatment by spiritual means alone from the definition of child neglect. These laws have been challenged in the courts, but cases have not been heard at higher levels where widespread precedent might be set. The Ohio law was tested when prosecutors tried to charge the parents of Seth Miskimens, a 13-month-old boy who died of bacterial pericarditis. An Ohio court found the law to be unconstitutional, at least in part because it denied children equal protection under the 14th Amendment to the Constitution (Ohio v. Miskimens et al., 490 N.E. 2d 931 [Ohio Com. Pl., 1984]). In making its ruling, the court pointedly wrote that the statute meant to them that

> . . .you may not violate your parental duties and thereby endanger your child's health or safety unless you and some of your co-worshipers believe you can.

The court still dismissed the charges against the parents, however, making a distinction that offered a compromise between the parents' beliefs and the child's need for more standard medical care. The court wrote:

> Although it is inaccurate and unfair to say that these defendants killed their son, or even that they are bad or evil persons, the evidence has established that the death of Seth Miskimens was a preventable occurrence. . .

The Ohio court ruling applied only within its limited jurisdiction. Many similar laws still stand, some including provisions that exempt treatment based on religious grounds from mandated reporting as well as from prosecution. For child advocates, the most serious issue is how children in Christian Science families or in families with similar beliefs can be brought to medical attention when they have a serious illness. At that point, societal mechanisms for balancing rights can be invoked to seek treatment for the child without any attempt to blame or punish parents. Although revocation of exemption laws would not necessarily accomplish this goal, the presence of such laws sanctions behaviors that can harm a child's physical well-being and limits the ability of the state to intervene.

References

Allmond BW, Buckman W, Gofman HF. The family is the patient: An approach to behavioral pediatrics for the clinician. St. Louis: The CV Mosby, 1979.

Anonymous. Arguments before the court. US Law Week 1986;54:3507–3508.

Bross DC. Medical care neglect. Child Abuse Negl 1982;6:375–381.

Burns S. Fear itself: AIDS, herpes, and public health decisions. Yale Law Policy Rev 1985;3:479–518.

Committee on Bioethics, American Academy of Pediatrics. Religious exemptions from child abuse statutes. Pediatrics 1988;81:169–171.

Committee on School Health, Committee on Infectious Diseases, American Academy of Pediatrics. School attendance of children and adolescents with human T lymphotrophic virus III/lymphadenopathy-associated virus infection. Pediatrics 1986;77:430–432.

Duff RS, Campbell AGM. Moral and ethical dilemmas in the special care nursery. N Engl J Med 1973;289:890–894.

Fost N. Parental control over children. J Pediatr 1983;103:571–572.

Gallagher SS, Hunter P, Guyer B. A home injury prevention program for children. Pediatr Clin North Am 1985;32:95–112.

Gielen AC, Eriksen MP, Daltroy LH, Rost K. Factors associated with the use of child restraint devices. Health Ed Q 1984;11:195–206.

Gorman RL, Charney E, Holtzman NA, Roberts KB. A successful city-wide smoke detector giveaway program. Pediatrics 1984;75:14–18.

Hampton RL, Newberger EH. Child abuse incidence and reporting by hospitals: significance of severity, class, and race. Am J Public Health 1985;75:56–60.

Jaudes PK, Diamond LJ. Neglect of chronically ill children. Am J Dis Child 1986;140:655–658.

Lantos J. Baby Doe five years later: implications for child health. N Engl J Med 1987;317:444–447.

Larsen CP, Pless IB. Determinants and the prediction of injury in a birth cohort of 3-year-olds [Abstract]. Am J Dis Child 1988;142:400.

Leikin S. Children's hospital ethics committees: a first estimate. Am J Dis Child 1987;141:954–958.

Malcolm AH. Experts try to allay fears on herpes. New York Times 12 Jan 1985:6.

Matheny A, Brown A, Wilson R. Behavioral antecedents of accidental injuries in early childhood: a study of twins. J Pediatr 1971;79:122–124.

Matheny AP. Psychological characteristics of childhood accidents. J Soc Issues 1987;43:45–50.

Mead FS. Handbook of denominations. Nashville: Abingdon Press, 1970.

Palfrey JS, Mervis RC, Butler JA. New directions in the evaluation of handicapped children. N Engl J Med 1978;298:819–824.

Pless JE. The story of Baby Doe [Letter]. N Engl J Med 1983;309:664.

Polansky NA, Chalmers MA, Buttenwieser E, Williams DP. Damaged parents: an anatomy of child neglect. Chicago: University of Chicago Press, 1981.

Rivara FP, Mueller BA. The epidemiology and cause of childhood injuries. J Soc Issues 1987;43:13–31.

Rivara FP, Stapleton FB. Handguns and children: a dangerous mix. J Dev Behav Pediatr 1982;3:35–38.

Rosenberg L. School phobia: a study in the communication of anxiety. Am J Psychol 1958;114:712–718.

Rozovsky FA. The medical needs of the child and religious doctrines (North America). In: Carmi A, Zimrin H, eds. Child abuse. Berlin: Springer-Verlag, 1984:66–76.

Rubenstein A. Schooling for children with acquired immune deficiency syndrome. J Pediatr 1986;109:242–244.

Schmitt BD. Child neglect. In: Ellerstein NS, ed. Child abuse and neglect: a medical reference. New York: John Wiley & Sons, 1981:297–306.

Spiegel CN, Lindaman FC. Children can't fly: a program to prevent childhood morbidity and mortality from window falls. Am J Public Health 1977;67:1143–1147.

Steinbrook R, Lo B. Artificial feeding—solid ground, not a slippery slope. N Engl J Med 1988;318:286–90.

Swan R. Faith healing, Christian Science, and the medical care of children. N Engl J Med 1983;309:1639–1641.

US Department of Health and Human Services, Office of Human Development Services. Executive summary: national study of the incidence and severity of child abuse and neglect. DHHS Publ. (OHDS) 81-30329. Washington, DC: US Government Printing Office, 1981.

Williams JC. Power of court or other public agency to order medical treatment for child over parental objections not based on religious grounds. 97 ALR3d 421, 1980.

Wilson MH. Childhood injury control. Pediatrician 1983–85;12:20–27.

12 Failure to Thrive and Psychosocial Dwarfism

INTRODUCTION

Failure to thrive is the name given to a syndrome that includes growth failure (of weight, height, or both) and that may or may not include abnormalities of behavior and development. Growth failure is the result of an inability to either obtain, assimilate, or efficiently use necessary foods. Failure to thrive occurs most often in children under age 2, whereas the related syndrome of psychosocial dwarfism generally occurs in older children.

Failure to thrive has traditionally been divided into two subsets, organic and nonorganic. The former term has been used in cases in which growth failure is associated with other, identifiable illnesses such as cystic fibrosis, congenital heart disease, or bronchopulmonary dysplasia. The latter has been used to describe cases that appeared to involve no illness; in these cases, growth failure was considered to be caused primarily by poor parenting.

Little is known of the incidence of failure to thrive among children who were felt to be healthy at birth. Altemeir and co-workers (1985), in a longitudinal study of 232 infants born to largely low-income mothers, found 21 cases of failure to thrive (6 organic and 15 nonorganic) occurring in the first year of life. Mitchell and co-workers (1980), reviewing the records of 312 children enrolled in a group of rural health clinics, found 7 organic and 30 nonorganic cases occurring in the first 2 years of life.

In contrast to this preponderance of nonorganic cases among birth cohorts or in ambulatory care settings, studies of hospitalized cases usually find that 50–60% of cases are organic. Thus, many children with failure to thrive and no identifiable illness are apparently treated solely as outpatients. Data from the study of Mitchell et al. (1980) also suggest that some of these children may never be diagnosed as having failed to thrive even though their medical records document low heights and weights.

The traditional view of organic versus nonorganic failure to thrive has recently been eroded by challenges to both its theoretical validity and its clinical utility. From a theoretical standpoint, the idea that infants are only passive recipients of their parents' care has yielded to the realization that even newborns play an active role in their own development and nurturing. This role is modified by a wide range of developmental, temperamental, and physiologic differences among infants and by the ability of their parents to cope with these differences. Thus, all children who are failing to thrive may have a variety of organic and nonorganic problems that, in combination, produce inadequate growth.

The clinical utility of the organic/nonorganic distinction has also given way as evidence mounts that the two forms of the syndrome cannot always be differentiated by a response to feeding. Most clinical texts still state that the main diagnostic maneuver in cases of failure to thrive is a trial of feeding under controlled circumstances. In theory, children with no organic cause for growth failure will begin to gain weight, whereas those with an underlying illness will not grow until that illness is specifically treated.

Recent studies, however, have suggested that response to refeeding does not regularly differentiate between organic and nonorganic causes. Berwick and co-workers (1982) found that the majority of children with socioenvironmentally caused failure to thrive (nonorganic cases) did gain weight when they were hospitalized and fed, but that many children with organic causes also gained. Bell and co-workers (1985) also found that children with organic causes of failure to thrive gained weight as rapidly as did children with presumed nonorganic causes.

ETIOLOGIES OF FAILURE TO THRIVE

Identifiable Illnesses

Table 12.1 lists a number of illnesses that are sometimes associated with growth failure.

Table 12.1 Medical Conditions Sometimes Associated with Failure to Thrive

Cardiac conditions
    Congestive failure
    Congenital heart disease

Prenatal influences
    Fetal alcohol syndrome
    Intrauterine growth retardation
    Intrauterine infection (e.g., rubella)

Perinatal conditions
    Neonatal narcotic addiction
    Bronchopulmonary dysplasia

Gastrointestinal
    Malrotation
    Pyloric stenosis
    Short bowel syndromes
    Cleft palate
    Celiac disease

Immunodeficiency (congenital or acquired)

Cystic fibrosis

Urinary tract infection

The prevalence of these conditions among children hospitalized for evaluation of failure to thrive depends on two major influences: the referral patterns at the institution in question and the extent of the search for specific illnesses. Children followed by a primary care provider may have their growth failure evaluated on an outpatient basis, whereas children seen in clinics may be more likely to be admitted. Children referred to tertiary care centers may sometimes come expressly because they have an identifiable illness that requires specialist care or because outpatient evaluation has failed to find a strong suggestion of either organic or social causes. Therefore, hospital-based clinicians need to know about referral mechanisms at their institutions so that they will have an idea of how often specific disease entities will be found. Advances in diagnostic maneuvers, especially for functional gastrointestinal problems such as gastroesophageal reflux, may also lead to a diagnosis in a child who formerly would have been considered not to have an identifiable illness. Berwick and co-workers (1982), reviewing 122 cases of children 1–25 months old admitted to a children's hospital for growth failure, found that about 10% had some specific medical problem (such as intestinal obstruction or chronic infection) and about 20% had functional gastrointestinal problems (reflux or chronic diarrhea).

Temperament

Temperament is most commonly defined as those elements of an individual's behavioral style that are manifested very early in life and that are probably inherited (Buss and Plomin, 1975). The most widely known formulation of temperament comes from the landmark New York Longitudinal Study (NYLS), in which Thomas, Chess, and colleagues (1963) observed the children of 84 mostly middle-class families from age 3 months until adulthood. Using data from interviews with the children's parents, they outlined what they felt were nine distinct aspects of temperament: activity level, rhythmicity, approach/withdrawal, adaptability, intensity, mood, persistence, distractability, and sensory threshold. It was felt that most children fell into one of three temperament categories defined by combinations of these nine factors: easy, difficult, and slow to warm up.

The NYLS concept of temperament has formed the basis for many rating scales used to measure temperament in individuals. Research psychologists, however, have been increasingly critical of whether the scales do this reliably, whether they agree with independent perceptions of a child's interactional style, or whether there is sufficient evidence to support the existence of all nine aspects of temperament (Gibbs et al., 1987). Buss and Plomin (1984), for example, have proposed an overlapping but smaller set of characteristics of temperament that appear to be more strongly supported by experimental work. The three aspects of temperament that they propose are:

- Emotionality—The ease with which fear, anger, elation, depression, and other emotions can be elicited and the intensity with which they are experienced by the individual.
- Activity—An apparent preference for remaining physically active; included are how fast regular activities are performed, whether the individual tends to choose physically active over less active pastimes, and whether the individual tends to keep moving when others are still.

- Sociability—A preference for being with others rather than being alone; included are how hard the individual tries to make contact with others, whether shared or solitary activities are preferred, and whether the individual's first reaction to new people is to make contact or back away.

Whatever formulation is used, most clinicians agree that temperament plays an important role in how well infants are able to adapt to their environments, how well they engage adults in the two-way interactions necessary for nurturing, and how much flexibility may be required of their caretakers. This view logically leads to the hypothesis that some types of temperament, at least when coupled with certain types of parents, may be related to failure to thrive.

Studies of temperament as a cause of failure to thrive are handicapped, however, by the fact that most take place once the child has already failed to thrive and thus when malnutrition itself may also be playing a role in changing temperament. In adults, starvation produces lethargy, decreased attention, and irritability. Children with marasmus (protein-calorie malnutrition) often develop a deep detachment from their surroundings that is coupled with a state of apparent hyperwariness of contact with others. Observation of these changes has become a part of the diagnostic evaluation for failure to thrive (see below), but it has meant that evaluation of temperament as a cause of growth failure has had to rely on parents' reports about their children's behavior before they became ill.

Bithoney and Newberger (1987) found that children who had no apparent medical problems but had failed to thrive were seen by their parents as more distractable and more reactive to visual and auditory stimuli. Some of these children, by extension, may also have had decreased regularity (ability to adopt a consistent pattern of eating and sleeping) and a greater intensity of reactions to day-to-day stimuli. These traits may make it more difficult for parents to have gratifying interactions with their children and especially may make feeding difficult. Experienced parents may be able to overcome these problems and help their children achieve better control and regularity, but others may feel frustrated or rejected and react by withdrawing attention.

Mechanical and Developmental Feeding Problems

Some children may fail to grow because they are unable to suck, chew, or swallow enough food. These children may eat so slowly or sloppily that their caretakers are unable to feed them sufficient amounts of food; some children may tire of eating before a feeding has finished. Some of these problems may be caused by persistence of primitive neurologic reflexes (such as a startle or tongue thrust that makes it impossible for the child to take food in the mouth), abnormal tone (making it difficult for the child to stay in an eating position), a weak or uncoordinated suck, or a structural abnormality of the pharynx (such as a cleft palate). Table 12.2 lists these and other conditions. Most can be diagnosed with a detailed history and physical examination, although some will require follow-up radiologic studies.

These mechanical problems may also have behavioral components. Sometimes the apparent problem, such as a tongue thrust, is a normal condition; it is the parent who is trying to start solid foods before the child is capable of eating them. On the other hand, a supposed mechanical problem may in fact be a manifestation of food refusal brought on by a long-standing conflict over control of the feeding interaction.

Parental Factors

Most of the literature examining the parents' role in causing failure to thrive concerns mothers; fathers enter the picture only to the extent that they either support or undermine the mothers' nurturing efforts. Obviously, this does not mean that fathers cannot parent infants or that mothers are solely responsible for causing failure to thrive. The following discussion, however, will focus largely on mothers simply because they have been the subjects of most of the studies performed to date.

Altemeir et al. (1985) found that neither maternal age, time of registration for prenatal care, nor breast versus bottle feeding could predict which infants would fail to thrive in the first year of life. They did find, however, that the incidence of failure to thrive was correlated with:

- Ongoing social stress caused by frequent arguments between the parents, by separation followed by reconciliation with the father, by

Table 12.2 Observations of the Parent-Child Feeding Interaction[a]

Parent behaviors (positive answers desired)

1. Positioning of child
   Held securely but has full freedom to move arms
   Head is higher than hips
   Trunk is in contact with parent
   Eye contact is possible

2. General interaction with child
   During feeding, generally attends more to child than to other people or things in the room
   Has generally positive affect during feeding, including smiling, praising, playing games
   Talks to child or makes eye contact
   Acknowledges child's distress in positive, comforting manner and by making adjustments to position, feedings, etc.
   Able to vary intensity of stimuli to fit child's needs

3. Interactions specifically related to feeding
   Responds verbally to child's hunger or satiety cues
   Paces feeding to child's cues: does not offer food when child is not attentive, pauses when child turns away or fusses, slows when child seems distracted or sleepy, stops when child falls asleep or persists in refusing food
   Does not interrupt child's eating or switch foods offered before child pauses
   Allows and teaches child how to participate in feeding (hold bottle, self-feed) as appropriate; is not too concerned with mess
   Does not show anger when feeding does not go well

Child behaviors

1. Motor problems
   Inadequate head control for age
   Uncoordinated or ineffective suck or swallow
   Persistent startle reflex or excessive reaction to touch
   Abnormal tone (greater or less than expected for ages) making positioning difficult
   Seems to have difficulty swallowing or has excessive drooling
   Coughs, gags, or has difficulty breathing during feed
   Tongue thrust making taking in of food difficult

2. Feeding behavior problems
   Holds food in mouth instead of swallowing
   Spits food out, vomits, or ruminates
   Turns head or pushes with hands to avoid food

3. Feeding capabilities (positive answers desired)
   Looks at parent, signals readiness to eat and satiety
   Remains alert during feeding
   Responds to parent's communications with vocalization, smile, or change of state
   Movements coordinated and smooth

[a]Adapted from: NCAST (see text); Chatoor I, Schaefer S, Egan J. Non-organic failure to thrive: a developmental perspective. Pediatr Ann 1984;13:829–843;, Lewis JA. Oral motor assessment and treatment of feeding difficulties. In: Accardo PJ, ed. Failure to thrive in infancy and early childhood: a multidisciplinary team approach. Baltimore: University Park Press, 1982:265–295.

the father leaving his job or getting arrested, or by the death of a friend.

- Mother's perception of her own nurturing as a child. Children were more likely to fail to thrive if their mothers reported having had an unhappy childhood, feeling unloved as a child, or not wanting to be like their own mothers.

Kotelchuck and Newberger (1983) also found that a mother's perception of her present support was related to the incidence of failure to thrive. Mothers who perceived their neighborhoods as hostile and unfriendly or who reported limited contact with extended family members were more likely to have children who had failed to thrive. All of these factors may contribute to a decreased tolerance for infant behaviors or a decreased ability to meet an infant's emotional needs. Interestingly, they are very similar to risk factors for intrafamily violence found by Straus and co-workers (see Chapter 22) in a national survey of intrafamilial violence and child physical abuse.

Parental perceptions of the child's health also appear to be a factor in the incidence of failure to thrive. These perceptions seem less related to actual health problems than to unresolved concerns that something is the matter with the child. In the prospective study by Altemeir et al. (1985), infants whose mothers reported trouble feeding them in the newborn nursery or who were discharged with unresolved (although minor) health concerns such as mild jaundice were more likely to fail to thrive.

Early Interactions between Mother and Child: The Development of Bonding and Attachment

Attachment is a phenomenon that has been observed in many lower animal species as well as in humans. It is manifested by a group of behaviors that includes the strong desire to be near the object of attachment (often but not always another person), an increase in this desire with stress or separation, frequent contact with the object when separation does occur, and a greater display of affection toward the object than toward others.

In the literature on child development, the term "attachment" usually refers to the feelings of a child toward a caretaker. Attachment usually starts to be manifest at about 2 months of age, when infants begin to smile at or reach out for their caretakers. By 6–9 months, these behaviors are displayed for only certain caretakers, and other forms of attachment behavior, such as protest on separation and an increased need for the caretaker in times of stress, begin to appear.

Infants more readily develop attachments to persons who are sensitive to emotional signals. Time spent with an infant simply providing physical care does not seem to increase the chances of being selected as an attachment object. Instead, time spent in stimulating, reciprocal activity plays a bigger role. Attachments can develop with multiple individuals and even to hostile caretakers.

The number of attachments an infant has and their apparent strength are less important markers of healthy relationships than the quality of interaction that takes place with the attachment object. Ainsworth and co-workers have outlined three major types of attachment: secure, anxious-avoidant, and anxious-resistant (discussed in Chapter 13). These patterns appear to persist later in life and to play a role in how children relate to those around them. Children with anxious forms of attachment do not learn well from parents and may do poorly in social situations.

Klaus and Kennell described a type of attachment between mothers and their newborns that they called bonding. Maternal behaviors felt to indicate that bonding is taking place include face-to-face gazing, tender touching, and soothing actions. Experiments with lower primates have suggested that in some species there may be a critical period soon after birth when mothers must bond to their children; otherwise, an abnormally weak relationship will develop, one in which the child may not be sufficiently nurtured.

Because there is no good way to measure bonding itself, research in humans has focused on opportunities for both early and extended interactions between parents and their newborns. These opportunities, it is theorized, should lead to better bonding and subsequently more nurturing relationships.

Early contact between human parents and children (immediately after birth) does not seem to result in long-term changes in the ways that parents and children relate to each other. There appears to be a wide range of culturally and individually determined responses to the birth of a child, and these do not seem to be related to how a parent subsequently feels about the child.

On the other hand, some studies have found that observation of parents and children in the newborn nursery can help identify families at risk for various kinds of maltreatment. Mothers of children who later fail to thrive have been observed to behave differently from mothers who subsequently physically abuse their children. In the study by Altemeir et al. (1985), the latter were more aggressive and overtly rejecting of their children, whereas the former were more likely to simply show a lack of interest.

Extended contact during an infant's first days is thought to produce relatively long-lasting effects on the parents' confidence and skills and thus may reduce the risk of future parenting problems. Although studies have yielded contradictory results regarding bonding and subsequent maltreatment, extended contact does appear to contribute to the parents' enjoyment of a newborn and therefore may well be a good in and of itself.

The Feeding Interaction

PROCESS

Although many other forms of parent-child interaction are important, the feeding interaction has a primary importance in the first year. It takes up a major portion of the infant's waking time, and its success has a great influence on the parent's feelings of competence and satisfaction with child rearing. Some researchers in early child development believe that the parent-child "synchrony" developed during early feeding relationships serves as a model for a strong and flexible relationship later in life.

The feeding interaction has two participants. The child gives cues to start feeding, to alter its pace, to acknowledge the parent's nurturing, and finally to say "enough." It is up to the parent to learn to recognize these cues, to show empathy for the child's needs, and to alter the feeding to fit the child's innate pace and rhythms (Chatoor et al., 1984). Not all babies communicate these needs clearly, and not all parents are capable of recognizing and responding to them. Failure of this communication can result in inadequate feeding and subsequent lack of growth.

Feeding has distinct developmental stages. Motor and behavioral milestones are paralleled by predictable behavioral issues. Problems may arise when parents misinterpret or cannot cope with normal behaviors or limitations; they may also surface when a child is developmentally delayed.

STAGES

Chatoor et al. (1984) divide early feeding development into three stages. Although the boundaries of these stages, like all developmental milestones, may be very blurry, the concepts can help clinicians focus on specific issues that may be contributing to growth failure. Empiric studies have yet to be carried out, however, to show what proportion of failure-to-thrive cases may stem from problems in each of these stages.

Under 2 Months: Homeostasis

The parent's main tasks in this period are to learn the child's cues for hunger and satiety and to learn the environment in which the child will best be able to feed. Parent and child together must work out a mutually agreeable schedule for feeding and a setting that takes account of the child's ability to tolerate stimulation or distraction. Children have varying abilities to remain organized and calm; distractable or intense infants may not be able to resume feeding after an interruption or in a noisy environment. Having decided when and where to feed, the parent must also learn to avoid over- or underfeeding the child.

Oral-motor problems may also be present during this early stage of feeding. Particular problems include difficulties sucking (including the inability to create a good seal around the nipple), gagging, and the persistence of primitive reflexes that make it difficult to remain in the feeding position.

Two to Six Months: Attachment

By age 2–6 months, infants have acquired a number of social skills that make them even more active participants in the feeding interaction. The social smile allows an infant to give selective responses to particular caregivers, helping to reinforce specific relationships. At this point, infants start to become selective about which adults may be their caretakers and start to develop attachments to specific individuals and objects. The development of these relationships may be disrupted by a number of factors. Children with difficult temperaments may continue have problems settling for feeding, or they may not engage in behaviors that promote close relationships, such as smiling at or reaching out for a caregiver. The same problems may occur for children with developmental delays. Parents who remain distant or respond inappropriately to the child's overtures may end up by reducing feeding opportunities or making feeding less efficient.

Six Months to Three Years: Separation/Individuation

The age range of 6 months to 3 years obviously encompasses enormous changes in the child's physical and mental abilities. The parents' main task is to nurture the child while accommodating needs for independence and the mastery of new skills. It is a challenging time during which both parent and child may become easily frustrated over feeding problems.

During this time, the child comes to demand a greater and greater role in feeding. Improving motor skills lead to finger feeding, holding a bottle or cup, and attempts to use utensils. At the same time, increasing intellectual growth makes mealtime (at least from the child's perspective) an opportunity for exploring, for play, and for testing one's ability to control the environment. All of these developments make feeding a lengthy and messy process, a fact that parents must come to accommodate but control. Parents can be helped to see this change in feeding habits as a sign of the child's growth and of their success as parents rather than as an inconvenience and an indication of the child's willfulness or rejection.

This is also a time during which there are great changes in growth patterns and feeding preferences. As weaning takes place a greater variety of foods are offered, along with greater opportunities for pickiness or outright refusal to eat. Parents can be helped to strike a balance between accommodating the child's tastes and setting limits about what foods will be available and at what times. Children can be trusted to regulate their intake appropriately so long as they are offered a range of nutritious foods; the danger of undernutrition arises only when conflicts over control of feeding come to take precedence over the child's hunger or the parents' willingness to offer food at times when the child is receptive to eating.

Problems can also arise when feeding interactions start to take on a disproportionate importance in the parent-child relationship. Whereas feeding time may have been nearly the sole form of parent-child interaction at the time of birth, by the end of the first year there are a variety of other opportunities for play and for nurturing. Failure to interact with the child at other times may result in mealtimes that are a forum more for attention getting than for nutrition.

Endocrine Abnormalities

The endocrine system plays a major role in regulating growth. A small proportion of children who fail to thrive (probably less than 5%) have primary endocrine problems such a hypothyroidism, diabetes mellitus, congenital adrenal hyperplasia, and primary pituitary failure (often secondary to central nervous system malformations or neoplasms). There is increasing evidence that many children who fail to thrive have endocrine abnormalities that arise secondary to a variety of social and sensory stimuli that appear to be be closely linked to the biochemical processes controlling cell metabolism and growth. These stimuli include contingent social interactions (those that are synchronous with the infant's cues and reactions) and stroking or other touch to particular parts of the body. These mechanisms may explain why some infants fail to thrive even though they are taking in food that should be adequate for growth.

Schanberg and Field (1987), for example, conducted experiments in which weanling rats were separated from their mothers and quickly began to eat less and to show alterations in growth metabolism, including decreased release of growth hormone. Normal growth could be restored by providing a specific stimulus: stroking the baby rats with a moist brush that simulated the mother's tongue. Other stimuli, such as sound, motion, or other forms of caressing, did not induce growth. In a similar experiment with preterm human infants, Field and co-workers (1986) randomized feeders and growers (premature infants who were too small to be sent home but who no longer required intravenous fluids or other life support measures) into two groups; one received routine care, and the other received gentle stroking and stimulation for three 15-minute periods each day. The stimulated infants gained nearly 50% more weight per day than those receiving routine care, even though they took in nearly identical amounts of formula. At 12 months of age—well past the time of discharge from the nursery— stimulated infants continued to be heavier and performed better on tests of mental and motor performance.

Human experiments cannot as yet determine whether these long term effects are mediated by persistent endocrine/metabolic changes or by differences in the ways that parents responded to their more stimulated infants. Regardless of the case, these experiments suggest that even if infants receive adequate food, they may still fail to grow, both physically and intellectually, if they are not provided with sufficient and fairly specific sensory stimuli. In older children, the syndrome of psychosocial dwarfism also seems to involve a secondary alteration in endocrine function (see below).

DIAGNOSIS AND EVALUATION

The diagnosis of failure to thrive has two major steps. The first is to separate children who are small but healthy from those who are in fact failing to grow; the second involves identification of specific factors that may be contributing to growth failure.

Case Definitions

Unfortunately, clinicians have used many different ways of deciding when a child is failing to thrive. All are based on the growth parameters height and weight, but they vary in the way these parameters are assessed and whether they consider change in growth over time. Following is a list of several definitions that have been used in clinical work or in research studies. Their best use is perhaps as screening tools: children who fall into one or more of these categories may warrant further attention to see if they are truly failing to thrive.

- Definitions based on growth parameters at a single point in time: height and/or weight less than the 5th percentile for age; weight *for* height less than the 5th percentile; weight less than 80% of the median weight for age.

- Definitions based on pattern of growth over time: growth of normal velocity for age but with weights and/or heights that are below the 3rd percentile for age (even though by definition 3% of "normal" children will be this small); growth at a slower than normal velocity for age (the child fails to gain weight or height as rapidly as expected or actually loses weight).

Growth velocity can be measured in a number of ways. The simplest is to plot serial measurements of weight and height on standard growth charts. Children's growth normally follows a consistent "growth channel" along the chart's percentile bands. Crossing two or more "major" percentile bands (3, 10, 25, 50, 75, 90, and 97) is usually considered to represent a clinically significant change in growth velocity.

In the first 12–18 months of life, however, as many as two-thirds of normal children may cross up or down over one or more major percentile bands, and as many as a quarter may cross over two (Smith et al., 1976). Birth weight and height are strongly related to maternal nutrition and size. Children born to large mothers or who were large for gestational age may have a relative deceleration of growth at 3–6 months and settle in to a new, lower-percentile growth curve at a normal velocity by about 13 months. Thus, in the absence of other problems, it may be necessary to follow growth until it is clear whether the change in velocity is persistent. If the child appears otherwise well and the family's social situation appears stable, small changes in growth velocity may be observed for a month or two before further assessment is undertaken. Dramatic changes in growth, however, should be investigated more promptly.

Assessment of growth velocity with standard charts may not be satisfactory if change must be assessed over relatively short periods of time or if past growth history is unknown. A variety of charts, tables, and formulas are available to assess growth velocity over fixed or variable periods of time (Tanner and Davies, 1985). Care must be taken to get accurate and replicable measurements of weight and height (usually performed by the same person on the same equipment each time) and to take into consideration differences in velocity that may be caused by prematurity.

Comparison of height, weight, and head circumference may also aid in the diagnosis of failure to thrive. The classic failure-to-thrive infant has a weight that is well below normal but a normal or only slightly reduced height and a normal head circumference. More severely affected infants may have markedly reduced weight and height but relative sparing of head growth. When all three parameters are reduced, the possibility of genetic or intrauterine causes of growth problems must be more seriously considered. Failure of height growth more than weight gain strongly suggests a primary endocrine or genetic abnormality rather than failure to thrive. The major exception to this is the syndrome of psychosocial dwarfism, which usually occurs after infancy and is accompanied by marked behavioral as well as growth disorders.

Body proportions are another aid to diagnosis. In infants, the ratio of trunk (top of head to pubic symphysis) to leg length (symphysis to bottom of feet) is about 1.7:1; by maturity, the ratio is about 1:1. Children with some chromosomal abnormalities, skeletal dysplasias, or certain metabolic disorders, such as rickets, may have abnormal proportions, often reduced height accompanied by an increased ratio of trunk to limb size.

It may also be difficult to define "normal" growth for children who were born prematurely, who were small for their gestational age, or who may simply have genetically determined short stature. Premature infants (usually considered to be those born at less than 38 weeks of gestation, with the length of gestation defined as the first day of the mother's last menstrual period to the time of birth) who are of appropriate weight and height for their gestational age (AGA) may not fully catch up with term infants until the beginning of the third year of life (Brandt, 1986). Catching up is defined as having the same growth parameters as a child who is the same age after birth but who was born at term. Until catch-up, correction of the child's postnatal age is required to accurately plot parameters. The corrected age equals the postnatal age (in weeks) minus the number of weeks the child was premature, or corrected age = postnatal age − (40 − gestational age).

Head circumference catches up first. Corrections are necessary up to about 18 months after birth. Weight must be corrected for prematurity until about 24 months, and height until as much as 36 months. AGA premature babies who still appear small after these corrections may be failing to thrive. It is important to use appropriate references of size versus gestational age, however. There is no single accepted standard curve for intrauterine growth, and norms for both relative velocity and absolute weight gain may vary with the population measured.

Assessing growth in premature or term infants who are small for their gestational age (SGA) can be even more complicated. SGA is usually defined as a weight less than the 10th percentile for the chart of intrauterine growth being used. These children are often divided into two broad classes, symmetric and asymmetric (Peterson and Frank, 1987).

Symmetric SGA infants are also called proportional or nonwasted. They have had decreased but proportional growth of both skeletal and soft tissue, and therefore their weights are appropriate for their lengths. These infants, along with AGA but very sick infants, may never catch up but should, once they are well, achieve a normal growth velocity and follow a growth curve that runs parallel to but below the normal curves. Asymmetric SGA infants have decreased masses of soft tissue relative to length and head circumference. Head circumference itself may be appropriate for gestational age. These infants usually do catch up, mostly in the first 3 months, and level off in a new, higher growth percentile by 6–9 months.

In older children, reference to the parents' height may be helpful in deciding whether a child is abnormally small or has been genetically determined to be small. Charts are available that make corrections in expected growth for the correlations observed between parents' and children's measurements (Tanner et al., 1970; Himes et al., 1985). Growth charts are also available for children with Down's syndrome, whose genetic potential for growth differs from that of other children (Cronk et al., 1988).

Medical and Social History

The general approach to medical and social history taking in cases of suspected maltreatment is outlined in Chapter 6. The concern for genetic and gestational influences on growth leads to extra emphasis on the family history and on any complications of conception, pregnancy, labor, or delivery. Additional attention is also given to the child's developmental history, with a heavy emphasis on social and interactive skills and how the child has fit into the structure of the family as he or she has grown. The nutritional history, described below, also receives detailed attention. Identification of the source and type of well-child care received to date may allow collection of other information about growth and health status.

Social and family information can start with three major areas, all of which usually bear further discussion as the evaluation progresses. First, the clinician needs an initial feel for how the family is structured and who provides material and emotional support. One approach is to ask who lives in the home with the child, who takes part in child care, and where funds to run the household come from. Closely related is an exploration of major stresses that may have recently befallen the family. Asking directly often yields a negative answer, so clinicians may have to probe gently by asking about spousal and family relations, problems with jobs or finances, and recent illnesses or deaths in the family. Finally, basic facts about the parents' childhood may help the clinician start to understand the family's behavior and needs. Sketching a family genogram is often a good first step; discussion of feelings and relationships can come later. It may be helpful to know the age and city of residence of each parent's siblings and parents and whether there is ongoing contact among them. Ultimately, details about the parents' own nurturing and their memories from childhood can be elicited.

Physical Examination

After the history, the physical examination is the single most important step in making a diagnosis of failure to thrive. There are three broad goals. The first, which will not be discussed in detail, is to look for evidence of medical problems (heart disease, congenital anomalies) that may be causing growth failure or that may complicate its treatment. The second, which is discussed in Chapters 6-8, is to look for evidence of physical abuse. The third is to aid in the determination of nutritional status.

Most children who fail to thrive have some degree of protein and/or energy malnutrition (PEM). The two prototype symptoms of PEM are marasmus, which results from a balanced deficiency of both protein and total calories, and kwashiorkor, which results from a greater deficit in protein than in calories. Clinically, these two conditions represent the ends of a single spectrum of malnutrition, and aspects of both may often be present in one patient.

Marasmus and kwashiorkor are familiar to clinicians working in underdeveloped countries but are frequently overlooked in industrialized societies. In fact, they are common both among children with socially related failure to thrive and among children with acute and chronic medical problems (Listernick et al., 1985).

Marasmus in developed countries can result from neglect, the use of inadequate or overdiluted infant formulas, unusual diets that do not provide sufficient calories, or simply an inadequate supply of food for the family. Children who lack both protein and overall caloric intake first have a slowed rate of weight gain, then stop gaining weight and height, and finally start to lose weight. Children who are malnourished for a relatively short period of time or have recurring episodes of malnutrition between periods when food is adequate appear thin and wasted. They have decreased amounts of muscle and subcutaneous fat and may have poor skin turgor and a sunken fontanelle. Children who are chronically malnourished usually have deficits of both height and weight: they are stunted. This diagnosis can be difficult to make because marginal nutrition may result in growth just at or below the lower limits of normal. Evaluation of parental height and growth history, as well as anthropometric measures such as skin fold thickness and mid-arm circumference, may help differentiate small children from those who are malnourished.

Marasmus results in profound metabolic changes as the body adapts to decreased intake. Most important to acute therapy is the observation that the proportion of body weight composed of water increases, as does the proportion of total water that is made up of extracellular fluid (MacLean et al., 1980). Total body sodium increases, but laboratory tests usually show hyponatremia because of the even greater increase in body water. These findings are important both because they help confirm the diagnosis of marasmus and because dehydration often enters the differential diagnosis. When marasmus is complicated by acute illnesses that increase fluid losses or decrease intake, dehydration may take place. Because of their sunken fontanelles and decreased skin turgor, however, marasmic infants can look dehydrated when they are not. In these children, inappropriate fluid therapy can exacerbate salt and water overloads and lead to further electrolyte problems or congestive heart failure.

Kwashiorkor results from a greater deficit in protein than of other nutrients. It appears to be less frequent than marasmus among children with psychosocially related failure to thrive, but it may occur in chronically ill children who require dietary manipulations that result in relative protein deficiency. The condition may develop within 2–3 weeks. It often is superimposed on marasmus in marginally nourished children who acutely lose their source of protein intake.

Children with isolated kwashiorkor usually have normal or only slightly decreased weight. As the disease progresses, sodium retention and hypoalbuminemia apparently combine to cause edema, and weight may then even appear elevated. Children with severe kwashiorkor may develop hepatomegaly (from an accumulation of fat), thinning and lightening of the hair, and a desquamating rash. Liver dysfunction can result in hyperbilirubinemia and abnormal coagulation studies. Clues to the type and severity of malnutrition also come from the anthropometric studies described below.

Developmental Assessment

Developmental assessment can help identify causes of failure to thrive and can provide a marker for following the child's progress. Many children with psychosocially related failure to thrive will have normal motor abilities but apparent delays in social and communication skills. The more nutritionally and emotionally deprived a child is, the more important it is that developmental examination results be considered provisional and the assessment be repeated when the child has started to recover. It is especially important that parents who are already ambivalent about caring for a child not be told prematurely that the child is developmentally delayed.

Assessment of Nutritional Status[1]

Once a child has been determined to have growth failure, assessment of diet and nutritional status can be a further aid to diagnosis and planning for therapy. Anthropometric measurements can provide an initial estimate of overall nutrition. The measurement and possible correction for prematurity of height and weight were discussed above. The importance of accurate and replicable measurements cannot be overemphasized.

Table 12.3 shows the classification by Waterlow (1976) of the severity of PEM. Deficits in

Table 12.3 Waterlow (1976) Classification of Protein Calorie Malnutrition[a]

Ratio	Degree of Wasting (weight/height) or Stunting (height/age)(%)[b]			
	Normal	Mild	Moderate	Severe
Weight/height	>90	80–89	70–79	<70
Height/age	>95	90–94	85–89	<85

[a]From Waterlow JC. Classification and definition of protein-energy malnutrition. In: Beaton GH, Bengoa JM, eds. Nutrition in preventive medicine: The major deficiency syndromes, epidemiology, and approaches to control. Geneva: World Health Organization, 1976:23.
[b]Based on the child's measurement compared with the 50th percentile National Center for Health Statistics data.

both height and weight for age can be calculated. Measurements of skin fold thickness (triceps) and mid-arm circumference attempt to determine fat and muscle mass, respectively, as indices of malnutrition. Norms are available in standard publications (Frisancho, 1981). These measurements are not always required in mild to moderate cases of failure to thrive, but they can be helpful in cases where edema or stunting makes it difficult to estimate nutritional status from height and weight alone. Individual measurements are not always useful, but following change over time can help one assess the effects of refeeding. Descriptions of how to perform these tests are available in many standard nutrition texts.

Laboratory Tests

Several authors have noted the relative futility of extensive laboratory investigations in the evaluation of children with failure to thrive (Sills, 1978; Berwick et al., 1982). They point out that, as with most illnesses, the major basis for diagnosis is the history and physical examination. Other than tests or procedures specifically suggested by the history or exam, relatively few routine tests are required. Physical abuse does sometimes occur along with failure to thrive, and skeletal surveys or ophthalmologic exams for hemorrhage may sometimes be appropriate. The decision to perform them can be based on other evidence of physical abuse, a history of past injuries, or observations of the family's behavior during the course of treatment.

Infants with moderate to severe malnu-

---
[1]The author is grateful to Dr. David Tuchman for help with material on nutritional assessment and feeding.

trition, or those who have been given diets known to provoke specific nutritional problems, should be tested for biochemical markers of malnutrition. Although many specific tests are possible, measurement of hemoglobin and serum albumin appear to have the most general clinical utility and are readily available in most settings.

Low hemoglobin may be an indication of a diet deficient in iron. Early feeding with cow's milk, for example, may increase intestinal blood loss and supplant other foods, such as fortified cereals, that are important sources of iron at times of rapid growth. Importantly, however, low hemoglobin is often found in marasmus but is usually not responsive to iron therapy. It is thought that a reduction in oxygen carrying capacity is an adaptation to the body's altered metabolism.

Measurement of serum albumin can help determine the extent to which kwashiorkor has developed. Serum albumin has a half-life of about 16–18 days, which means that it can remain at relatively normal levels in the early stages of malnutrition. Prealbumin, which has a shorter half-life, is a better marker of protein deficiency, but the test is not widely available (Sachs and Bernstein, 1986). Children suspected of having kwashiorkor should also have other liver function tests, including measurement of serum bilirubin and the prothrombin time.

Measurement of serum electrolytes can help evaluate concurrent dehydration and strengthen the diagnosis of PEM. Children with both marasmus and kwashiorkor usually have decreased serum sodium and bicarbonate (see above), children with kwashiorkor may have decreased potassium as well.

Children who are placed on strict vegetarian diets or, because of cultural practices, are kept sheltered from sunlight may develop vitamin D deficiency rickets. Among some cultural groups, children may receive no animal foods except human milk. Human milk has relatively little vitamin D, and the concentration may be further reduced if the mother is a strict vegetarian who also is not regularly exposed to sunlight. Long-bone X rays are the most readily available means of making this diagnosis. When changes consistent with rickets are found, the child's diet can be supplemented with both vitamin D and calcium.

Malnutrition is also known to increase intestinal absorption of lead, a common environmental toxin in many communities. Elevated lead levels have been reported in children with failure to thrive and should be looked for in populations in which lead exposure is a recognized hazard (Bithoney, 1986).

Dietary Assessment

Knowledge of what a child has been eating can be an aid to both medical and psychosocial diagnosis. Many questions about dietary history can be asked informally, but detailed recollection of meals eaten in the past 24 hours or a diet log kept for several days is ideal. It should be said at the outset that the correlation of this history with the child's nutritional status may not be good. Some ill children may not grow well even though they are taking in what would appear to be adequate calories. It may also be difficult for parents to adequately quantify what the child eats, either because there are multiple caretakers or because the child (a toddler, for example) has developmentally normal eating habits and does not eat a good deal of what is offered. Finally, some parents, especially those who are depressed or apathetic, may have such a high degree of denial that the history they give is inaccurate.

Important questions for infants who are bottle fed include the type and caloric strength of the formula used, how the parents are preparing it (including whether any measuring device used is known to be fairly accurate), how much the child takes in during a day, and how much is spit up.

Although it is difficult to quantify intake for breast-fed infants, important clues can be obtained to determine whether the feeding seems to be going successfully. Questions for the parent include:

- How often does the child nurse and for how long each time? Regular intervals between feedings of longer than 3 hours or feedings that last only a few minutes on each breast suggest inadequate intake.
- Is there supplementation with water or formula? If so, how often? Unless the mother is not available to nurse, infants require little or no supplementation in the first months. More than occasional offering of low-nutritional fluids such as water or juices suggests a decreased intake of breast milk.

- Does the baby frequently have a wet diaper? Frequency of urination is related to both fluid intake and the rate of insensible losses, but most infants who are feeding well have several wet diapers a day.
- Can the mother feel the child firmly attach to the breast and generate suction? Do the mother's breasts become engorged between feedings? Does she experience letdown when the child begins to nurse? It may be difficult for mothers who are breast feeding for the first time to know whether the feeding is going well. This is a special problem when no experienced breast feeder is available as a coach or counselor. If the child is attaching well and sucking, the mother's breasts are becoming engorged, and letdown is occurring, it is likely that the mechanics of feeding are going well.

For parents of older infants, questions can be asked about the age at which solids were introduced, whether these are or were of the appropriate texture for the child's age, and to what extent the child self-feeds. Early introduction of solids may prematurely supplant more nutritional breast or bottle feeding. Foods of inappropriate texture, in addition to being choking hazards, may simply not be eaten or lead to active refusal and conflict at feeding times.

Once a dietary history has been established, a rough calculation of daily caloric intake can be made. Most standard infant formulas supply 20 kcal/fluid ounce (or 0.67 kcal/cc). Caloric content of foods can be estimated with the aid of texts that provide lists by both food and portion size (Kraus, 1980; Pennington and Church, 1985). Total daily caloric needs can be estimated from Table 12.4.

Table 12.4 Recommended Energy Intake for Children under 11 Years of Age[a]

Age (yr)	Energy need (kcal/day)	Range (10th–90th percentile)
0 –0.5	kg × 115	95–145
0.5–1	kg × 105	80–135
1 –3	1300	900–1800
4 –6	1700	1300–2300
7 –10	2400	1650–3300

[a]From Committee on Dietary Allowances. Recommended dietary allowances. 9th rev. ed. Washington, DC: National Academy of Sciences, 1980:23, Table 3.

Assessing the Feeding Interaction

Watching parents feed a child can be of great help in making a specific diagnosis for the etiology of failure to thrive. Clues can be obtained about the parent's skills, the child's motor and communication abilities, and the synchrony of the parent-child interaction. Several formal and informal instruments have been developed to help clinicians structure their observations of feeding. One of the most widely used is the Nursing Child Assessment Satellite Training (NCAST) Feeding Scale developed by Barnard and colleagues,[2] a 76-item checklist designed for infants under 1 year of age. Other checklists have been developed by Chatoor et al. (1984). Table 12.2 lists some of the observations recommended by these authors. Ideally, a feeding should be observed in the most relaxed and natural surroundings possible and when there is little chance of interruption. Care must be taken that the feeding take place at a time when the child is interested in food and is alert and awake. Usually this is at a time when the child would regularly be feeding. The observer should try not to talk to or otherwise interrupt the parent until signaled that the feeding has ended. If the feeding has taken place outside the home, it is important to ask the parent whether anything would have been different had the feeding been at home. Fosson and Wilson (1987) have reported cases of failure to thrive in which home feeding was regularly disrupted by a jealous sibling, the mother was interrupted or belittled by a member of the extended family, or the level of chaos in the household precluded quiet feeding.

As noted above, observation of the feeding interaction is useful both for its specific relevance to nutrition and because it is a special case of how the parent and child interact more generally. Observations may also be made during other care-giving tasks such as dressing or bathing, parent-child play, or merely the interaction that takes place in the examining room or hospital ward. In general, one wants to see whether the parent and child are able to match their energy levels and pace to each other's needs

---

[2]Information about the NCAST scales is available from the Nursing Child Assessment Satellite Training Program, CDMRC, Res. 110, WJ-10, University of Washington, Seattle, WA 98195.

and whether they seem to have some degree of attachment. Is the parent distant and poorly interactive or, at the other extreme, overstimulating or overcontrolling? Are the parent's responses consistent, or does he or she sometimes react abruptly but then ignore some of the child's cues? Does the parent seem unable to adapt to the child's temperament or have unreasonable expectations for the child's behavior or responses? Are the child's demands seen as overly burdensome? Which of them are seen as problems and how does the parent react? Can parent and child separate for reasonable periods of time, or does separation appear to cause an unusual amount of stress (Rathbun and Peterson, 1987).

The Child's Temperament

As discussed above, temperamental differences in children may contribute to poor parent-child interactions and thus to failure to thrive. Although identifying a child as having a difficult temperament does not in itself explain growth failure, it may help the clinician better focus explorations of the parent-child relationship. Helping the parent appreciate the child's temperament can also be an important part of treatment. In general, the more parents can be helped to understand why children have certain behaviors, the more they are likely to adapt to them.

Several authors have designed temperament scales based on the NYLS categorization of temperament. Most of these scales involve a relatively long (75–100 items) series of age-specific questions for parents to answer about their children. Buss and Plomin (1984) have devised a shorter scale, the EAS, based on their formulation of temperament (Table 12.5). The scale was designed to be used by parents of children from about 1 year onward. Although it has not been used as widely as the Carey instruments, for example, it can still serve as a useful point of discussion with parents.

It is important to stress to parents that measures of temperament in children less than 1 or 2 years old do not seem to predict what the children will be like during school age or adulthood or whether they will successfully adapt to their social environment. Difficult infants are not necessarily destined to become difficult children, and infants who are easy to care for because they are very quiet may or may not turn out to be overly shy. The main clinical importance of temperament is to help parents understand a child's *present* behavior and to avoid misunderstanding it in ways that could, in fact, have a negative impact on the child's future.

Table 12.5 EAS Temperament Survey for Children: Parental Ratings[a]

Emotionality
1. Child cries easily
2. Child tends to be somewhat emotional
3. Child often fusses and cries
4. Child gets upset easily
5. Child reacts intensely when upset

Activity
1. Child is always on the go
2. When child moves about, he/she usually moves slowly (reversed)
3. Child is off and running as soon as he/she wakes up in the morning
4. Child is very energetic
5. Child prefers quiet, inactive games to more active ones (reversed)

Sociability/shyness
1. Child tends to be shy
2. Child makes friends easily (reversed)
3. Child is very sociable (reversed)
4. Child takes a long time to warm up to strangers
5. Child is very friendly with strangers (reversed)

Instructions: Rate each of the items for your child on a scale of 1 (not like your child) to 5 (very much like your child). For clinical use, items are not presented grouped by categories as shown above.

Scoring: Average the scores for the 5 items in each category (items marked "reversed" should be rescored before averaging so that an initial score of 5 becomes 1, 4 becomes 2, etc.). In preliminary testing, mean scores for 12 and 24 month olds were approximately 2 for emotionality, 2.5 for activity, and 4.2 for sociability/shyness.

[a]From Buss AH, Plomin R. Temperament: early developing personality traits. Hillsdale, New Jersey: Lawrence Erlbaum Associates, 1984:102–103. Used by permission.

Specific Behaviors in Children with Failure to Thrive

Specific behavioral characteristics, including persistence of infantile, flexed posturing, hyperalertness, and self-stimulatory behavior, have frequently been reported to be more prevalent among children with nonorganic failure to thrive (that is, children whose growth failure occurred in a setting of social deprivation) than among children who have identifiable medical reasons for growth failure. Unfortunately, these behaviors do not occur in all children with social deprivation and failure to thrive, and they also occur in many normal children who are suddenly placed in stressful environments such as hospitals. Although no patterns diagnostic of psychosocially induced failure to thrive have yet emerged, several workers have identified behaviors that in controlled studies were more common in this group.

Powell and co-workers (1987) identified three behaviors common in children with nonorganic failure to thrive (found in 60–80% of the children studied) and less common although still fairly prevalent (25–40%) in children with failure to thrive and identifiable illnesses: lack of motor activity or smile when approached socially, general lack of activity when left alone, and abnormality of gaze (including hypervigilance, avoidance of eye contact, and apparent disinterest in social contact). Less common (found only in 30–50% of children in the nonorganic category) but more powerful discriminators because they were rarely found in other children were rumination, excessive thumb sucking, and excessive hand and finger activity.

Rosenn and co-workers (1980) devised a method to look for differences in interactive style that might identify children with psychosocially related failure to thrive. Used formally, the method rates whether the infant has a positive or negative response to nine categories of interaction. The categories are actually part of a single, easily learned, structured encounter with the child.

The method assumes that at the start of the encounter, the child is alone in a crib in his or her room. The examiner notes the infant's positive or negative response to the following:

1. Initial approach: The examiner is in the room but remains quiet and at least a few feet from the crib.
2. Initial socialization: The examiner comes closer and, smiling, speaks to the infant but does not reach out.
3. Presentation of a toy: The examiner offers some age-appropriate toy.
4. Touch: The examiner gently caresses the child on the extremities and trunk.
5. Pick up: The examiner picks up the child and
6. Holds him or her chest against chest for a few minutes, then
7. Repositions the child so that he or she is face to face with the examiner,
8. Returns the child to the crib, and
9. Slowly leaves the room.

Rosenn and colleagues found that children with psychosocially related failure to thrive seemed more comfortable playing with inanimate objects than with people. As they were approached, they became vigilant and distressed. They disliked being touched or held and tried to avoid eye contact. Although they might make some protest when put back in the crib, they quickly returned to a quiet and apparently apathetic state once the examiner started to leave. These findings were markedly different from those for children hospitalized for other reasons. Most important, improvement in the behavior and the beginning of weight gain seemed to be closely related. Therefore, this method may have value both in diagnosis and as a marker for the progress of treatment.

TREATMENT

Inpatient versus Outpatient Treatment

There is no general agreement on whether children with failure to thrive require inpatient diagnosis and treatment or, if so, how long the inpatient stay should last. Likewise, there are no clear guidelines for how long outpatient therapy should be attempted before it is declared unsuccessful and the child is hospitalized. Analysis of published studies that encompass several institutions and approaches suggests that hospitalization increases the chances of sustained weight gain but not necessarily of long-term psychologic recovery (Fryer, 1988).

Some frequently cited specific indications for inpatient treatment include severe malnutrition (grade 2 or 3), severe accompanying illness (especially dehydration), lack of previous medical care (suggesting a more pervasive pattern of neglect), evidence of physical abuse, or serious psychosocial problems already apparent in the family. In particular, chronic stress, evidence of hostility toward the child, and a perception that the child is bad or in some way damaged are related to poor treatment outcomes and a diminished chance that the family will follow through with outpatient care (Evans et al., 1972).

In some communities, alternatives to acute care hospitals may exist. Children may do well in specially trained foster families, although in traditional foster care arrangements it is often difficult for the biologic parent to take as active a role in the child's care as would be possible in a hospital (Karinski et al., 1986). Extended care facilities may be required when children appear to have serious emotional problems and their families are particularly disorganized (Singer, 1987).

Nutritional Treatment

CALCULATING CALORIC NEEDS

Malnourished children require more than maintenance amounts of calories if they are to catch up to their full potential height and weight. These excess needs are highly variable, but they can range up to 50–100% higher than would normally be required. Several formulas have been proposed for calculating catch-up needs (Peterson et al., 1984). All take the form: kilocalories/kilogram/day needed to catch up = kilocalories/kilogram/day for the patient's weight age × ideal weight ÷ present weight.

The calculation starts by determining the patient's present weight. This is usually straightforward except when there is a great deal of edema present. In these cases, actual nonedematous weight may have to be estimated. The patient's weight age is defined as the age for which his or her present weight would be in the 50th percentile. This age is then used with tables of recommended caloric needs (Table 12.4) to determine a maintenance caloric intake.

There are various methods for calculating a child's ideal weight. If the child does not appear to be stunted, ideal weight can be considered as the 50th percentile weight for the child's height. If it is not certain whether the child's height is appropriate, ideal weight can be considered as the 50th percentile weight for the child's age.

The same formula can be used to calculate protein deficits, although in most cases simply calculating caloric deficits and supplying a balanced feeding (about 8–13% of energy as whole protein) is sufficient.

STARTING FEEDS

Mildly malnourished children may simply be offered foods or formula and allowed to eat up to the calculated catch-up requirement. Severely malnourished children or those who have had an acute episode of diarrhea superimposed on chronic undernutrition may have problems absorbing large quantities of food. Both fat and lactose intolerance may be present and complicate refeeding. MacLean et al. (1980) recommend that feeding start at about 25 kcal/kg/day and increase by that amount every other day until the target for catch-up is reached. Stool output can be followed as an index of tolerance; the weight, not the number of stools is important. More than 150–200 g of stool per day is an indication to reduce the number of calories offered until stool output falls. Small, frequent feeds may also be better tolerated than larger meals. Some children, especially those who have marked intolerance or are very weak, may require continuous nasogastric feeding. For all children, a chart should be made to record daily weights and caloric intake. Many intensive care nurseries use similar charts for monitoring feeders and growers. In this way, the occurrence of growth can be matched to a required level of nutrition.

WHAT TO FEED

Oral feeding is always preferred when possible, both because it avoids infection and metabolic problems associated with intravenous nutrition and because it helps stimulate recovery of the gut. If a child's dietary preferences are known, and if these foods appear to be tolerated, it is best to build subsequent diet planning around them. For infants, standard formulas can be made up to whatever concentration provides both the target nutrition and calculated fluid needs. Wide ranges of formula concentrations are acceptable; they become isotonic by the time they are processed in the intestines.

Standard formulas are preferred for infants because they contain balanced amounts of many standard nutrients. Lactose-free varieties are recommended for children at risk for malabsorption. Medium-chain triglycerides can be added if malabsorption of fat becomes a problem. Whole proteins are usually well tolerated.

Children with kwashiorkor may require supplemental potassium.

BEHAVIORAL AND MECHANICAL FEEDING PROBLEMS

Observation of feeding may reveal a variety of mechanical and behavioral problems that contribute to decreased intake. Involvement of physical or behavioral therapists is sometimes required, but preliminary steps are often possible. Developmental delays and abnormal reflexes may require help with positioning of the child in an infant chair or leaning on firm pillows. Tongue thrusting associated with developmental delay or altered sensation in the mouth can sometimes be helped by keeping the head slightly flexed on the neck (Lewis, 1982). Tongue thrusting and other forms of refusal to take food into the mouth may also be encountered with older infants (over 6–7 months) who have never been given solids or who were started on them prematurely and developed an adverse response. For these children, starting with mashed solids or thickened liquids may overcome learned reflexes and serve as a transition to coarser foods. Gentle downward pressure on the tongue with a spoon may also help inhibit thrusting.

Distractable or low-threshold infants may feed better in quiet surroundings and when they are being held securely or swaddled. In general, tension surrounding the eating interaction can be reduced by helping the parent express support of and positive regard for the child and setting liberal but firm guidelines on when and for how long food will be offered (Fraiberg, 1980).

Mealtimes may need careful orchestration for children who are wary of contact with adults or have had negative experiences involving eating.[3] The meal can be preceded by some socially interactive game such as peek-a-boo. This will help the child get used to the caretaker and give the caretaker a sense of how much intimacy the child can tolerate. The caretaker can then try to respect this distance during the meal.

The caretaker should try to make the meal as pleasurable as possible. Negative cues or words should be avoided and opportunities taken to praise and reenforce either good feeding or positive exploring of food. Toddlers need the opportunity to play with their food and become familiar with it, even though this usually is a very messy process. As long as the child is actually eating and seems interested in food, mealtimes should go on as long as is reasonable for the caregiver. The main exception is with children who appear uncertain as to whether they are hungry (frequently requesting food without eating it) or who simply play with the food in a disinterested way. For these children, mealtime must have firm limits.

Parents often need help breaking out of cycles of food refusal and punishment. In severe cases, formal behavioral therapy may be required. One of the most common cycles involves escalating attempts by the parents to feed the child, followed by the child's ultimate refusal and the parents' substitution of some other, less nutritious food (Iwata et al., 1982). This reenforces the refusal because it both gains attention for the child and links the final confrontation to a reward that the child desires. Parents can try instead to associate eating with other positive kinds of interaction with the child, such as play with a favorite toy or simply attention that is not contingent on some particular behavior. They can also give strong positive feedback for small attempts to taste a new food and only gradually attempt to offer greater quantities.

OBSERVING WEIGHT GAIN

Little information is available regarding how long it takes for children with failure to thrive to grow once they are refed. Some children appear to grow quickly once given sufficient calories. Ellerstein and Ostrov (1985), for example, found that about half of infants less than 6 months old at the time of diagnosis began to gain within 3 days of refeeding. Nearly all infants began to grow within 2 weeks. Bell and Woolston (1985) found that more severely malnourished infants with failure to thrive (those whose body weight was less than 80% of ideal) had a more predictable, positive response to refeeding than did those with milder deficits. For many children, emotional and nutritional recovery seem closely linked. Rosenn and co-workers (1980), in work with their interactive assessment tool for failure to thrive, described some infants who suddenly started to grow as

---
[3] Joy Goldberger made suggestions for this section on child's play with food.

they made an affective recovery even though the amount of calories being taken did not change. Some of these children (perhaps those who were more severely malnourished and had excess total body water) actually lost weight before they started to gain.

Most important is that initial growth not be considered satisfactory until it takes place at a clearly greater than normal rate so that catch-up is possible. Although no single formal measure of this rate is generally accepted, children who appeared to have recovered have grown at 1.5 to more than 2 times the average rate expected for children of the same age. One way of calculating this growth quotient is to take the child's average daily weight gain over a few days and divide it by the expected average daily gain for a child of the same age. The expected gain can be estimated from standard growth curves (Ellerstein and Ostrov, 1985).

Checking growth velocity against the expected rate is especially important for older children, who may take longer to establish weight gain and whose growth relative to present weight may not seem as spectacular as that of an infant. Although an older child may not appear to be growing as quickly, the rate of growth compared with that of nonmalnourished children of the same age may be markedly higher.

Social and Emotional Treatment for the Child

The goal of therapy with the child is to teach that it is possible to have consistent, positive interactions with caring adults. If hospitalized, the child should have as few caregivers as possible; it is tempting to use volunteers or students for this seemingly low-technology care, but this approach is acceptable only if these individuals are well supervised and can guarantee to be available for the duration of the child's stay. The child should also spend as much time as possible in a play area or other socially stimulating environment. The child can be offered activities or interaction but should be allowed to choose his or her own pace and distance from others. Toys offered should allow opportunities for expression and fun. Play with water or musical instruments is often easy for children and satisfying. Toddlers may benefit from play that involves food, either pretend play with dishes and pots or mixing and measuring for actual recipes. Older children may also wish to play with dolls. They will often act out the kind of caregiving that they have been receiving, and observers may be able to use this as an opportunity to model other kinds of caregiving and to empathize with the child's experiences.

Caregivers should try to respond to whatever cues to communications the child gives, no matter how ambiguous or inconsistent. Totally maladaptive cues such as tantrums or violence do not need to be reenforced, but it remains important for children to know that communication has taken place and that caregivers are attentive to their needs.

Treatment for Parents

In most cases of failure to thrive, treating the parents is an essential part of treating the child. Only when there are clear indications that the child will not be remaining with the family can the parents' treatment be at all separated.

The single most important principle in treatment of parents is to involve them in treatment of the child. This serves two purposes: it keeps treatment oriented toward the practicalities of child care, and it avoids further diminishing the parents' self-esteem by giving the appearance that the child has been "cured" in their absence, reenforcing their self-image as inadequate parents.

When children are hospitalized for failure to thrive, it is tempting for medical personnel to take charge of their care, start them on the road to recovery, and then return responsibility to the parents. Not only does this approach fit the usual medical model for acute illness, but it also satisfies the clinician's urge to rescue the child from "bad" parents, toward whom the clinician may feel considerable anger. The child's parents may experience this negative response in a number of ways. At the very least, their sense of inadequacy will be validated, and they may further shrink from accepting responsibility for the child's care; at worst, they will become aware of the clinician's anger and incorporate it into their own struggles with parenting and authority, struggles that may have been at the root of the child's failure to thrive. Sometimes they will, temporarily, seem relieved that someone has decided to replace them as parents and simply disappear while the child is hospitalized. These disappearances are often taken as grave signs of the parents' attachment to the child, but they must be interpreted in light of the treatment approach being offered and the messages it may be sending.

It is therefore important to involve the parents in a child's care as much as is medically possible, even if doing so initially seems less efficient or appears to delay the child's rescue. Ideal settings are those special inpatient units in which parents or family members agree to provide the majority of direct care. In regular hospital units, even when rooming in is not possible, the staff can still make an explicit agreement with the family about when they will be present and which feedings, for example, they will routinely give.

As for the child, it is important to have some consistency in who will be helping the parents. A large team may be participating in the child's care, but there needs to be a spokesperson and, preferably, an individual who spends time daily with the parents and child. This person's visits should coincide with times when a parent is feeding or playing with the child. The goal is to learn of the parents' concerns about the child, the parents' opinion of the nature and legitimacy of the child's needs, and conflicts that the parents perceive between their own needs and those of the child (Shapiro et al., 1976). These questions are rarely asked directly. Rather, the clinician tries to listen to what the parents are saying and watch what they do in response to the child's needs. When possible, at least some of these sessions should involve all members of the child's family, including grandparents (if they are active parts of the household) and siblings. Seeing how these individuals interact with the child and how they help or hinder the parents' caregiving can provide other avenues for therapy.

During sessions with parents, it is important to recognize their needs and to try to build self-esteem. Positive aspects of the parent-child interaction can be praised and even small amounts of progress appreciated. When parents discuss major needs and themes in their own lives, it is important to show empathy and interest while encouraging recognition of the child's needs. It is usually not productive or even possible to tackle major parental issues directly except in the most concrete or practical ways. Usually, insight into and resolution of these problems are possible only after the parents have come to trust the clinician and after some successful parenting experiences have reduced their sense of hopelessness.

Sessions with the parents and child can also serve as an informal opportunity to teach child development. The clinician can interpret the child's actions for the parents, explaining, for example, why the child might be crying or why the child clings to the mother's dress. The clinician can also speak for the child, reenforcing positive feedback that the parent could be getting from an interaction. After the child has successfully fed, for example, the clinician can point out how contented or satisfied the child appears or talk about how good it feels to have a full stomach and be cradled in a parent's arms.

It is important, however, that the clinician not take over from the parent or even demonstrate a skill with the parent's own child. It is fine for the clinician to be an expert on children in general, but one goal of therapy is to reenforce the unique nature of the relationship between *this* parent and *this* child. Ideally, demonstrations should be carried out with another child of similar age.

The Decision to Discharge from Hospital

It is often difficult to decide when a child who has failed to thrive is ready for discharge from an acute care hospital. Often there is pressure to end the admission as soon as the child has started to gain weight, and this may be after only 3 or 4 days of care. Obviously, children who are not gaining need to stay until a diagnosis can be made or growth begins. The parents must also have started to recover, however; otherwise children are likely to relapse soon after discharge. Guidelines for discharge are similar to the those for other types of maltreatment. The parents must be willing to acknowledge that their child was not taking in enough food and be willing to take steps to see that feedings are more succcessful. They must be willing to acknowledge the child's needs for nurturing and demonstrate a willingness, at least in the short term, to subordinate their own needs to those of the child. Resolution of acute family crises (loss of housing or of a significant person, financial problems) must at least be underway, and the family must be willing to accept long-term help with chronic problems.

Long-term care facilities or foster care may

be considered when feeding does not go smoothly, when the parents continue to have a predominantly negative or punitive attitude toward the child, or when there has been evidence of physical abuse as well as neglect. Other factors that may warrant delaying the return home include parents who appear too mentally limited (unless appropriate supports can be arranged), parents who have serious psychiatric problems, or families with serious substance abuse problems that are not being treated.

A Plan for Ongoing Therapy

Like inpatient care, treatment of the family of a child who has failed to thrive is a team effort. Great care must be taken, however, to coordinate the team and keep its members from overloading the family or working at cross-purposes. The team should be custom designed for the particular family. As each member or type of intervention is chosen, very specific goals must be outlined, and everyone involved must be convinced that this service is truly essential for this family. It is best to start with the minimum services that seem needed for the child's well-being and to add others as required. Some of those commonly used include:

- Home visitor. Home visiting is the mainstay of treatment in failure to thrive. A visiting nurse, home health aide, or homemaker can provide direct support for the parents and ongoing teaching of practical skills.
- Mental health professional. In some areas, infant mental health programs have therapists who make home visits. In most, however, the parents and child must be seen in an office or clinic. Some parents may need individual psychotherapy, but family therapy or parent-child sessions initially offer the best chance of directly improving family functioning.
- Medical care. Children need frequent follow-up to ensure that they are continuing to gain weight, to continue with nutritional guidance, and to address other medical problems. Parental medical problems need to be addressed as well. It is sometimes hard to strike a balance between monitoring the child's growth and burdening the family with visits. The choice of frequent office or home-based checks by a visiting nurse often depends on who will be the primary therapist for the family. If this is the pediatrician or family practitioner, then office visits will be more frequent (even once or twice a week). If a separate mental health professional is seeing the family regularly, home weight checks plus a monthly office visit may suffice.

When is Failure to Thrive Reportable Child Maltreatment?

As discussed in Chapter 11, cases of possible neglect often pose difficult decisions about the obligation to report to a child protective service agency. In some areas, all cases of failure to thrive that seem clearly nonorganic are reported as suspected neglect; in others, many such cases are not reported. Laws mandating the reporting of neglect are usually vague enough to allow considerable room for clinical judgment.

Definitely reportable cases include those that involve physical abuse or more pervasive patterns of neglect or cruelty and those that involve parents who do not appear capable of caring for the child. The latter might include parents with serious mental illness or substance abuse, severely limited parents, those who are homeless or without resources to provide food and shelter, and those who refuse help for their child's condition. In not all of these situations are the parents at fault, but the state may reasonably be asked to at least temporarily substitute for the parents and provide care for the child.

It is often difficult to think of reporting parents who seem depressed or acutely overwhelmed but who, once engaged in therapy, start to show some positive regard for their child. All of the issues of empathy for and identification with the parents surface, especially if the child proves to have a difficult temperament or a parent's own history is tragic. In the absence of one of the factors mentioned above, not reporting may be an option if this is the first time the child's condition has come to medical attention and if the parents seem receptive to help. As in other cases of potential neglect, however, reporting should never be used as a threat or contingency.

LONG-TERM EFFECTS OF FAILURE TO THRIVE

It is difficult to predict the course of a given child who has been diagnosed as failing to thrive. Older studies of the condition did not make comparisons with control groups, nor did they attempt to look at outcomes within subgroups of children according to sex, initial caloric deficit, parent-child interaction, and other factors. Newer studies have used controls but continue to use different case definitions and draw children from differing populations. In none of the studies is a great deal known about what treatment the children and their families may have received. The following discussion draws on findings from the studies listed in Table 12.6. Reference to specific characteristics of these studies, such as the presence or absence of controls or the type of treatment involved, is helpful in interpreting the results.

Weight and Height

Older, uncontrolled studies such as those by Elmer et al. (1969) and Glaser et al. (1968) found that large proportions of children diagnosed as having nonorganic causes for failure to thrive continued to measure less than the 3rd percentile for weight and/or height several years after diagnosis. Nine of fifteen children in the study by Elmer et al., and fourteen of forty in the study by Glaser et al., continued to weigh less than the third percentile for age. Many of these children were described as being severely ill at the time of diagnosis; some were found to have marked wasting, some ruminated, and some had evidence of physical abuse, including healed long-bone fractures. Two children in the study by Glaser et al. were readmitted between their original hospitalization and the time of follow-up, one reportedly in "moribund" condition. In both studies, referrals were made to social service agencies and for medical follow-up, but details of subsequent treatment were not provided.

Table 12.6 Studies of the Long-Term Effects of Failure-to-Thrive

Study; type	Source of Cases	Number of Subjects; Age at Diagnosis	Case Definition	Age at Follow-up	Treatment Received
Mitchell et al., 1980; case-control	Public primary care clinics	30/12; <24 mo[a]	1. Any weight <80% of normal for age if had previously normal weight or was not premature 2. FTT[b] noted on clinic problem list	3–6 yr	Not stated
Oates, 1985; Oates et al., 1985; Hufton and Oates, 1977; cohort with controls	Hospital	24/14; mean, 1.3 yr	>2 mo old, weight <10th percentile for age, "no discernible cause for poor wt gain," "family factors suggestive of inadequate care"	Mean, 13.8 yr	Nutrition and short-term social support
Elmer, 1977; case series	Hospital (not known how selected)	?/15; 3–30 mo	Final diagnosis of nonorganic failure to thrive (all <3rd percentile for weight)	3–11 yr	Permanent and temporary removal; advice and community support
Glaser et al., 1968; case series	Hospital	50/40; mean, 12 mo	Birth weight >2500 g but admission weight <3rd percentile; no physical cause	Mean, 4.5 yr; range, 8 mo–9 yr	Referrals to medical care and social service agencies

[a]Number at outset/number evaluated at follow-up; age at time of diagnosis.
[b]FTT, Failure to thrive.

More recent studies using control groups have found less striking long-term growth deficits. Oates and co-workers (1985) found that all 14 of the children they could trace an for average of 12 years after diagnosis weighed more than the 3rd percentile, while all but one was taller than the 3rd percentile. However, 6 of the 14 were shorter or lighter than the 50th percentile for their age, compared with only 1 such child in a matched comparison group.

The study by Mitchell et al. (1980) of 30 children drawn from an outpatient population also found smaller deficits in long-term growth but noted striking gender-related differences in the rate and extent of catch-up. By the third year after diagnosis, boys who had failed to thrive were indistinguishable in height and weight from other children. Girls, in contrast, became increasingly different from other children in the years after diagnosis. In infancy, the girls who had failed to thrive weighed, on the average, 83% of what would have been expected for their age; by age 4, they averaged only 77% of the expected weight. Average height also declined relative to what would be expected for age, but to a lesser degree. Mitchell and her co-workers speculated that these gender-related differences might have resulted from a lower social status of women or a lesser value placed on female children in the community under study.

Personality and Behavior

As was the case for weight and height, older studies that did not use control groups or that may have examined more severely ill children found greater long-term changes in the behavior of children who had failed to thrive in infancy. In the study by Elmer et al. (1969), for example, three of eight children followed up when in preschool and four of seven school-age children were reported to have one or more serious behavior problems. Oates and co-workers (1985) also found a high prevalence of reported behavioral problems among the children who had failed to thrive and confirmed that this prevalence was higher than would be expected on the basis of age and socioeconomic status alone. They were able to interview 14 children who had failed to thrive an average of 12 years after diagnosis and compare them with a group of normal children with whom they had been matched according to socioeconomic status. Only 7 of the 14 children were rated by their teachers as having normal behavior, compared with 12 of the 14 comparison children. In general, however, specific psychometric tests found the children who had failed to thrive to be relatively well adjusted. Although they tended to score lower than comparison children on tests of ego strength, self-confidence, and emotional stability, the results were within the ranges considered normal. (This was in contrast to children who had been physically abused in the past, who were different from the both the neglected children and the comparison group.) Mitchell et al. (1980), however, in a study of children from an ambulatory setting, found that parents of children who had failed to thrive were no more likely to report behavior problems than were parents of comparison children.

Intellectual Development

The studies of both Oates et al. and Mitchell et al. used comparison groups and found long-term intellectual deficits in children who had failed to thrive. Using a general intelligence test (the WISC-R), Oates et al. found that at age 13 children who had failed to thrive had lower verbal IQ scores (an average of 90 for the study group versus 102 for comparison children). Performance and full-scale IQ scores were also slightly lower among children who had failed to thrive, but the difference was not statistically significant. Some of these children had previously been tested at age 7, at which time there had been even greater discrepancies between verbal and performance scores. Using a different instrument (the McCarthy Scale of Children's Abilities), Mitchell and co-workers also found differences in cognitive abilities among children who had failed to thrive, but only among girls. Overall, they found no differences in verbal or performance scores between comparison children and those who had failed to thrive.

Physical Abuse Following Failure to Thrive

Many cases have been reported in which children who had failed to thrive were subsequently physically abused. Three of the thirty children studied by Oates et al. were seriously abused in the first years after diagnosis, two fatally. Mitchell et al., in contrast, found no excess of physical abuse among children who failed to thrive in comparison with controls. As discussed above, however, the heterogeneous nature of failure to thrive makes it difficult to generalize from small studies to the general risk of subsequent abuse. Cases in which growth failure has been related to parental rejection or emotional deprivation, for example, may have a higher risk for physical abuse than those in which the difficulty centers on maladaptive feeding patterns.

PSYCHOSOCIAL DWARFISM

Psychosocial or abuse dwarfism are names given to a syndrome of growth failure accompanied by bizarre behaviors and retardation of social, intellectual, and motor development, all of which reverse to a greater or lesser extent when the child is placed in a nurturing environment. The hallmark is a constellation of endocrine abnormalities, including a decreased response of growth hormone and corticosteroids to stimulatory tests (although the adrenals respond to exogenous ACTH) (Powell et al., 1967b). Onset of the syndrome is said to occur before age 2, but the diagnosis is often made much later, sometimes not until the teen years.

Children with psychosocial dwarfism usually come to medical attention because they are short, often only 40-60% of the expected height for age (Powell et al., 1967a). Bone age is delayed, but dentition is appropriate for age. Most children are at or below (in some cases, far below) the appropriate weight for their actual height. This combination of stunting with thinness suggests chronic malnutrition as part of the cause of the syndrome.

The most striking aspect of psychosocial dwarfism is behavioral. Children are described by their parents as having an unusual polyphagia and polydypsia that includes eating from garbage cans, consuming pet food, and gorging that is sometimes followed by vomiting. They are said to drink from toilet bowls or puddles, and parents sometimes report having to put locks on food cabinets or refrigerators to keep the contents from being consumed. Other behavioral problems include encopresis, enuresis, and night awakenings, during which the children are said to wander aimlessly or seek food. Tested intelligence is usually far below normal, and a history of delayed motor and intellectual milestones is usually given. The children may seem isolated and uncommunicative and are said to have few friends or normal social interactions. Checking of the family's accounts may reveal that the child rarely attends school or engages in any other activities outside the home.

For many reasons, the etiology of the syndrome remains obscure. As in cases of other types of maltreatment, much of what is given as medical history may be false or important details may be omitted. Money and Werlas (1976), for example, consider many cases of psychosocial dwarfism to be examples of the Munchausen syndrome by proxy (see Chapter 15), in which the parents collude to create medical symptoms but not reveal their true nature. As some cases of psychosocial dwarfism are evaluated, overt evidence surfaces of severe emotional and physical abuse as well as physical neglect, including deprivation of food and water (Chesney and Brusilow, 1981). This finding suggests that in some cases both the failure to grow and the bizarre food-seeking behaviors may be the direct results of maltreatment; the starving child is forced to take extreme measures to find food or drink (Money, 1977). The endocrine abnormalities seen in the syndrome suggest that some of the growth failure, and possibly the inability to assimilate whatever calories the child is able to consume and retain, are secondary to emotionally mediated neuroendocrine changes similar to those that may occur in infants diagnosed as having nonorganic failure to thrive.

In the original series of cases reported by Powell and co-workers (1967a,b), each child's family was notable for the father's minimal role, either because he was not involved with day-to-day affairs or because marital relations were poor. Sometimes other siblings showed evidence of abuse or neglect, and in two cases siblings also had growth retardation. In many families, however, other siblings or half-siblings may be outwardly normal, while one child has apparently been selected as a victim of maltreatment. In some cases, other family members are threatened with harm if they object to or threaten to disclose the abuse (Money et al., 1985). Money's theory, which is not specific to abuse dwarfism, is that parents may select a certain child to "sacrifice" as atonement for some parental sin, such as an incestuous relationship or a birth out of wedlock. The sacrifice gains potency because the child is not killed but rather is tortured physically and emotionally as an ongoing act of penance. Although such a formulation may seem extreme, Money makes the case that since biblical times children have been used as objects of sacrifice (as exemplified by the binding of Isaac). The details disclosed in present-day fatal cases (McFadden, 1987) suggest that some children continue to be subjected to long-term treatment such as being tied to chairs or in closets, being left in their own excrement, or being given only spoiled food to eat.

The diagnosis and treatment of psychosocial dwarfism usually begins with a hospitalization. The children generally start to grow quickly, even in the relatively deprived hospital environment. Motor and intellectual milestones also improve, although catch-up to expected levels is not felt to be complete. The growth hormone response to stimulatory tests corrects quickly, but steroid response may be delayed for weeks. As with other abused children, adjustment problems are often seen when the child is first placed in a normal environment. Some children seem to invite or provoke abuse, which raises the question of whether they have in some way become conditioned to such treatment, possibly because it is the only way they have learned to interact with adults or because they still do not trust those around them to love them on any other basis. This behavior requires intense support for the staff or foster family caring for the child and sometimes short-term psychiatric hospitalization for the child.

Psychosocial dwarfism is a syndrome that resists classification: it has parallels with failure to thrive and in some cases probably has components of physical and emotional abuse. Although its incidence is not known, the occasional fatal cases reported in the press suggest that it is unfortunately not as rare would be hoped.

References

Altemeier WA, O'Connor SM, Sherrod KB, Vietze PM. Prospective study of antecedents for nonorganic failure to thrive. J Pediatr 1985;106:360–365.

Bell LS, Woolston JL. The relationship of weight gain and caloric intake in infants with organic and nonorganic failure to thrive syndrome. J Am Acad Child Adolesc Psychiatry 1985;24:447–452.

Berwick DM, Levy JC, Kleinerman R. Failure to thrive: diagnostic yield of hospitalization. Arch Dis Child 1982;57:347–351.

Bithoney WG. Elevated lead levels in children with non-organic failure to thrive. Pediatrics 1986;78:891–895.

Bithoney WG, Newberger EH. Child and family attributes of failure-to-thrive. J Dev Behav Pediatr 1987;8:32–36.

Brandt I. Growth dynamics of low-birth-weight infants with emphasis on the perinatal period. In: Falkner F, Tanner JM, eds. Human growth: a comprehensive treatise. Vol. 1. New York: Plenum Press, 1986:415.

Buss AH, Plomin R. A temperament theory of personality development. New York: John Wiley & Sons, 1975.

Buss AH, Plomin R. Temperament: early developing personality traits. Hillsdale, New Jersey: Lawrence Erlbaum Associates, 1984.

Chatoor I, Schaefer S, Egan J. Non-organic failure to thrive: a developmental perspective. Pediatr Ann 1984;13:829–843.

Chesney RW, Brusilow S. Extreme hypernatremia as a presenting sign of child abuse and psychosocial dwarfism. Johns Hopkins Med J 1981;148:11–13.

Cronk C, Crocker AC, Pueschel SM, et al. Growth charts for children with Down syndrome: 1 month to 18 years of age. Pediatrics 1988;81:102–110.

Ellerstein NS, Ostrov BE. Growth patterns in children hospitalized because of caloric-deprivation failure to thrive. Am J Dis Child 1985;139:164–166.

Elmer E, Gregg GS, Ellison P. Late results of the 'failure to thrive' syndrome. Clin Pediatr 1969;8:584–589.

Evans SL, Reinhart JB, Succop RA. Failure to thrive. A study of 45 children and their families. J Am Acad Child Psychiatry 1972;2:440–457.

Field T, Schanberg SM, Scafidi F, et al. Effects of tactile/kinesthetic stimulation on preterm neonates. Pediatrics 1986;77:181–185.

Fosson A, Wilson F. Family interactions surrounding feedings of infants with nonorganic failure to thrive. Clin Pediatr 1987;26:518–523.

Fraiberg S. Clinical assessment of the infant and his family. In: Fraiberg S, ed. Clinical studies in infant mental health: the first year of life. New York: Basic Books, Inc, 1980:28.

Frisancho A. New norms of upper limb fat and muscle areas for assessment of nutritional status. Am J Clin Nutr 1981; 34:2041.

Fryer GE Jr. The efficacy of hospitalization of nonorganic failure-to-thrive children: a meta-analysis. Child Abuse Negl 1988;12:375–381.

Gibbs MV, Reeves D, Cunningham CC. The application of temperament questionnaires to a British sample: issues of reliability and validity. J Child Psychol Psychiatry 1987;28:61–77.

Glaser HH, Heagarty MC, Bullard DM Jr, Pivchik EC. Physical and psychological development of children with early failure to thrive. J Pediatr 1968;73:690–698.

Himes JH, Roche AF, Thissen D, Moore WM. Parent-specific adjustments for evaluation of recumbent length and stature of children. Pediatrics 1985;75:304–313.

Hufton RW, Oates RK. Non-organic failure to thrive: a long-term follow-up. Pediatrics 1977;57:73–77.

Iwata BA, Riordan MM, Wohl MK, Finney JW. Pediatric feeding disorders: behavioral analysis and treatment. In: Accardo PJ, ed. Failure to thrive in infancy and early childhood: a multidisciplinary team approach. Baltimore: University Park Press, 1982:297–330.

Karinski W, Van Buren L, Cupoli JM. A treatment program for failure to thrive: a cost/effectiveness analysis. Child Abuse Negl 1986;10:471–478.

Kotelchuck M, Newberger E. Failure-to-thrive: a controlled study of familial characteristics. J Am Acad Child Adolesc Psychiatry 1983;4:322–328.

Kraus B. Caloric guide to brand names and basic foods. New York: Signet, 1980.

Lewis JA. Oral motor assessment and treatment of feeding difficulties. In: Accardo PJ, ed. Failure to thrive in infancy and early childhood: a multidisciplinary team approach. Baltimore: University Park Press, 1982:265–295.

Listernick R, Christoffel K, Pace J, Chiaramonte J. Severe primary malnutrition in US children. Am J Dis Child 1985;139:1157–60.

MacLean WC Jr, Lopez de Romana G, Massa E, Graham GG. Nutritional management of chronic diarrhea and malnutrition: primary reliance on oral feeding. J Pediatr 1980;97:316–323.

McFadden RD. Parents of girl, 6, charged with murder after she dies. New York Times 6 Nov 1987:B3.

Mitchell WG, Gorrell RW, Greenberg RA. Failure-to-thrive: a study in a primary care setting: epidemiology and follow-up. Pediatrics 1980;65:971–977.

Money J. The syndrome of abuse dwarfisms (psychosocial dwarfism or reversible hyposomatotropinism): behavioral data and case report. Am J Dis Child 1977;131:508–513.

Money J, Werlwas J. *Folie à deux* in the parents of psychosocial dwarfs: two cases. Bull Am Acad Psychiatr Law 1976;4:351–362.

Money J, Annecillo C, Hutchinson JW. Forensic and family psychiatry in abuse dwarfism: Munchausen's Syndrome by Proxy, atonement, and addiction to abuse. J Sex Marital Ther 1985;11:30–40.

Oates K. Child abuse and neglect, what happens eventually. Sydney: Butterworths, 1985.

Oates RK, Peacock A, Forrest D. Long-term effects of nonorganic failure to thrive. Pediatrics 1985;75:36–40.

Pennington J, Church HN. Food values of portions commonly used. New York: Harper and Row, 1985.

Peterson KE, Washington JW, Rathbun JM. Team management of failure to thrive. J Am Diet Assoc 1984;84:810–815.

Peterson KE, Frank DA. Feeding and growth of premature and small-for-gestational-age infants. In: Taeusch HW, Yogman MW. Follow-up management of the high risk infant. Boston: Little, Brown and Co, 1987:135–148.

Powell GF, Brasel JA, Blizzard RM. Emotional deprivation and growth retardation simulating idiopathic hypopituitarism. I. Clinical evaluation of the syndrome. N Engl J Med 1967a;276:1271–1278.

Powell GF, Brasel JA, Raiti S, Blizzard RM. Emotional deprivation and growth retardation simulating idiopathic hypopituitarism. II. Endocrinologic evaluation of the syndrome. N Engl J Med 1967b;276:1279–1283.

Powell GF, Low JF, Speers MA. Behavior as a diagnostic aid in failure-to-thrive. J Dev Behav Pediatr 1987;8:18–24.

Rathbun JM, Peterson KE. Nutrition in failure to thrive. In: Grand RJ, Suthpen JL, Dietz WH Jr, eds. Pediatric nutrition in theory and practice. Boston: Butterworths, 1987:163–184.

Rosenn DW, Loeb LS, Jura MB. Differentiation of organic from non-organic failure to thrive syndrome in infancy. Pediatrics 1980;66:698–704.

Sachs E, Bernstein LH. Protein markers of nutrition status as related to sex and age. Clin Chem 1986;32:339.

Schanberg SM, Field TM. Sensory deprivation and supplemental stimulation in the rat pup and preterm human. Child Dev 1987;58:1431–1447.

Shapiro V, Fraiberg S, Adelson E. Infant-parent psychotherapy on behalf of a child in a critical nutritional state. Psychoanal Study Child 1976;31:461–491.

Sills RH. Failure to thrive: the role of clinical and laboratory evaluation. Am J Dis Child 1978;132:967–969.

Singer L. Long-term hospitalization of nonorganic failure-to-thrive infants: patient characteristics and hospital course. J Dev Behav Pediatr 1987;8:25–31.

Smith DW, Truog W, Rogers JE, Greitzer LJ, Skinner AL, McCann JJ, Harvey MAS. Shifting linear growth during infancy: illustration of genetic factors in growth from fetal life through infancy. J Pediatr 1976;89:225–230.

Tanner JM, Davies PSW. Clinical longitudinal standards for height and height velocity for North American children. J Pediatr 1985;107:317–329.

Tanner JM, Goldstein H, Whitehouse RH. Standards for children's height at ages 2–9 years allowing for height of parents. Arch Dis Child 1970;45:755–762.

Thomas A, Chess S, Birch H, Hertzig M, Korn S. Behavioral individuality in early childhood. New York: New York University Press, 1963.

Waterlow JC. Classification and definition of protein-energy malnutrition. In: Beaton GH, Bengoa JM, eds. Nutrition in preventive medicine: the major deficiency syndromes, epidemiology, and approaches to control. Geneva: World Health Organization, 1976:23.

13 Emotional Abuse

RELUCTANCE TO RECOGNIZE EMOTIONAL MALTREATMENT

Society's response to emotional abuse and neglect has lagged behind the response to other forms of child maltreatment. Whereas cases of physical and sexual abuse are being detected with increasing frequency, recognition and reporting of emotional maltreatment have shown little change in the last decade (US Department of Health and Human Services, 1988). From a historical perspective, it is only within the last two or three centuries that parents have been generally seen as playing a role in a child's healthy psychologic and emotional development (Kagan et al., 1978). Prior to that time, faith, fate, or communal values were seen as more important forces determining what a child would be like as an adult. Children did not necessarily spend a great deal of time with their parents, and their nurturing and education was often delegated to others. Although parents are now considered important to a child's development, how they should relate to their children remains a matter of controversy. While a warm and loving parent-child relationship is widely advocated as essential, significant minorities still feel that strict discipline and a certain detachment (especially from fathers) are important elements of child rearing.

The last 100–200 years have also seen a parallel evolution in the status of children in society. Children have ceased to be seen as the property of their parents and have gained the status of individuals who possess rights and are due protection, if necessary, by authorities outside the family. Ironically, this justice or rights-based perspective on parent-child relationships, although seemingly vital to protecting children's physical safety, may be one of the roadblocks to defining and treating emotional abuse. It has placed the emphasis on balancing a parent's rights and duties rather than trying to encourage parents to communicate with and understand their children.

Rights-based ethical systems emphasize adherence to basic rules (such as respect for autonomy, the duty to do good, and the need for fairness) as a foundation for interpersonal relationships. In a society based on rights, feelings and motivations have little importance except to the extent that they reinforce or subvert adherence to rules. Applying a rights perspective to interpersonal conflicts transforms the conflicts into discussions of rules rather than of emotional needs (Gilligan, 1982). Such a system may be appropriate for relationships among adults, but it creates a framework within which parents may provide only minimal, mechanistic care for their children and have society accept the situation as unfortunate but not unfair.

Philosophers have proposed an alternative ethical model that places a higher value on human, affective relationships than on rights. Called the care perspective, it is based on the need for communication, understanding, and the recognition of mutual dependencies. Within the care perspective, dilemmas are approached not as potential hierarchies of rules but rather as situations in need of discussion. The ultimate goal is that those who have immediate needs are understood and helped by the other individuals involved. One view of the care perspective is that its objective is to resolve conflicts rather than to determine who is right.

GOALS OF EMOTIONAL DEVELOPMENT

The general goal of emotional development is to attain a certain psychologic and social competence that complements other aspects of intellectual growth. The desired nature of this competence varies from society to society. Kagan et al. (1978) see Western society as valuing emotional development in three major areas, each of which involves a balancing of opposite tendencies. The first area encompasses autonomy and sociability. On the one hand, the ideal adult is seen as solving most problems alone, "respected by peers whose help he does not need." On the other hand, adults are also expected to respect human mutual dependence and the need for social interaction. They are expected to balance personal needs with the constraints involved in respecting the needs of others.

In the second area, the goal is to modulate sensual and emotional feelings so as to achieve some inner peace and equilibrium when faced with either very exciting or very unpleasant stimuli. Closely related is the third area, which is to balance the urge to act with the ability to contemplate and plan. Western society, say Kagan and colleagues, seems to prefer that its adults be more autonomous than sociable, somewhat more sensual and emotional than serene, and more active than contemplative. Other cultures have quite different preferences and therefore might view emotional maltreatment in a different light.

Garbarino and Garbarino (1980) see emotional competence as the ability to love others and to love one's self, to be free of extreme self-destructive or antisocial impulses, and to effectively receive, process, and send complicated emotional messages to other people. All of these qualities are basic to adults' ability to get along with others, live with themselves, and withstand the stresses of day-to-day existence. They are not qualities that develop overnight; like other mental capacities, they grow and evolve from early childhood through adulthood. Evidence of how they grow, and how their growth may be disrupted, forms the basis for defining emotional maltreatment.

FORCES BEHIND EMOTIONAL DEVELOPMENT

Early efforts to demonstrate the existence of emotional maltreatment yielded inconsistent results (Kavanagh, 1982). It was postulated that emotional harm, if it could be found anywhere, would be seen among children of so-called deviant parents (defined as those with schizophrenia, psychoses, and substance abuse problems). These children, however, did not appear uniformly to develop psychologic problems. Recent studies that looked more closely at specific aspects of emotional development have cast light on why some children are harmed by less than optimal parenting while others develop normally. For example, in the view of Kagan and colleagues (1978), one of the most powerful forces in psychologic development involves encounters with information about the self. In the same way that encounters with new facts change a child's understanding of the outside world, information from parents, other adults, and peers shapes children's views of themselves and their abilities. According to Kagan and co-workers, a child's belief that he or she is valued or disliked is a "guess" based on a variety of interactions. If this guess does not fit the child's present vision of self, he or she is more apt to change and adapt behavior to fit the guess than to gather additional information. These changes in self-perception can happen quickly and even in apparently stable, well-adjusted children. Krugman and Krugman (1984) described a group of 17 third- and fourth-grade children who suddenly came into contact with an unpredictable, verbally abusive teacher. Within a matter of weeks, 13 of the 17 started telling their parents that they felt "dumb" and that school was bad, even though they had previously been good students.

This mechanism of emotional growth has several important consequences for a conceptualization of emotional maltreatment. First, it suggests that there is not a one-to-one correlation of parent behaviors and child reactions. Each child processes the information coming from the parent differently and develops different guesses about what he or she is like. The less information available (because of more restricted social experiences or younger age), the less predictable may be the outcome. On the other hand, the idea that more opportunities to get information lead to better guesses about the self predicts what has been observed about children who survive extremely dysfunctional environments (Rutter, 1987). Many children seem to have successfully adapted because a "normal" individual, often a teacher or adult friend, was able to give them a truer reflection of their worth. A greater variety of social experiences, and thus exposure to more social information, also probably contributes to later competence by helping individuals make better inferences when they encounter unusual, discordant information about themselves.

One way in which the long-term consequences of early childhood relationships have been studied is by relating parent-child attachment patterns observed in infancy with later behavior in childhood. Troy and Sroufe (1987), for example, looked at the behaviors of kindergarten-aged children whose attachment with their mothers had previously been studied when the children were 12–18 months old. Attachment patterns are felt to represent a relatively stable picture of how children see their competency to handle stressful events and their relationships with potentially helpful and powerful figures in their life (Minde, 1986). Distinct attachment patterns are felt to evolve from fairly specific styles of parenting, with secure attachment coming from responsive and consistent care and anxious attachment coming from either active rejection of the child's needs or ambivalent and inconsistent responses (Egeland and Farber, 1984).

In Troy and Sroufe's 1987 study, pairs of children were observed during play. Children who had been anxiously attached in infancy, when paired with each other, almost always fell into victim-bully roles, becoming physically aggressive, displaying verbal hostility, and in some cases appearing to seek out punishment from the other child. In the 14 pairs of children studied, bullying or victim behavior never occurred as long as one of the children in the pair had been observed to be securely attached in infancy. Thus, there seemed to be good evidence that parent behaviors could lead to maladaptive social behavior on the part of the children. These behaviors had the potential for severely harming the children's ability to function in school and other group settings.

OBSTACLES TO A WORKING DEFINITION OF EMOTIONAL MALTREATMENT

Most practical, clinical definitions of emotional maltreatment have actually consisted of catalogs of actions or inactions (discussed in Chapter 1) rather than a unifying statement from which the catalog could be deduced. One working group sponsored by the National Institute of Mental Health and the National Center for Child Abuse and Neglect proposed the following definition, but considered it too broad and difficult to interpret for legal use. They defined emotional maltreatment as

> . . . an injury to the intellectual or psychological capacity of the child, as evidenced by an observable and substantial impairment in his or her ability to function within his or her normal range of performance and behavior with due regard to his or her culture. (Lourie and Stefano, 1978)

In requiring that the child be visibly impaired to be considered emotionally abused, the definition reflected the controversy within the broader child maltreatment field concerning whether harm was required to justify any allegation of abuse. In the case of emotional abuse or neglect, however, the harm dichotomy seemed even more important because whether harm occurred seemed to depend on characteristics of both the child and the parents. The parents of a psychologically very vulnerable child could readily be accused of emotionally abusive behaviors, while the parents of a very resilient child might get away with fairly extreme and unusual treatment. What the work group finally suggested was that clinicians adopt a two-level system for approaching emotional maltreatment. In the absence of specific local law,[1] they felt that clinicians should first try to treat potentially emotionally abusive families without reporting them to protective service systems and without waiting until harm had occurred. This would allow clinicians to recognize and treat situations that seem to fall short of those currently justifying legal intervention. These might include consistent penalizing of a child for normal, developmentally appropriate activities, failing to reinforce or encourage self-esteem, and limiting normal social contacts within and outside the family (Garbarino and Garbarino, 1980). If the treatment was unsuccessful, if the family refused help, or if more serious concerns for maltreatment surfaced, then a report could be made and social service intervention sought.

DIAGNOSING EMOTIONAL MALTREATMENT

The possible manifestations of emotional abuse run the gamut of childhood behavioral disorders. Chronic symptoms in older children may include hostility or aggression, extreme dependency, and a pervasive negative self-esteem and world view (Junewicz, 1983). Older children may develop suicidal or apparently psychotic behavior, while younger children may develop failure to thrive or psychosocial dwarfism. More acute symptoms include nightmares, regression in social functioning, somatic com-

---

[1] State laws have enormous variation, ranging from specific mention of "mental injury" to only general references within broader definitions of abuse and neglect.

plaints, and unusual fearfulness or anxiety. Sometimes children may act normally in an emotionally abusive environment but then display aggressive or dependent behaviors when they are in a safer setting.

Emotional maltreatment can take place any time there is close, prolonged contact between an authority figure and children who depend on that individual for recognition and nurturing. Teachers and athletic coaches can inflict emotional injury as effectively as parents, since many educational systems still stress discipline and the threat or use of degradation as a way of toughening students. Emotional maltreatment is also almost always a part of other forms of child abuse.

Junewicz (1983), in a study of children referred to a county welfare agency, identified five general types of family situations in which emotional maltreatment had occurred. The most common situation (17 of 66 families) involved victimization of children because of the parents' preoccupation with their own interpersonal conflicts. In these families, the children were often unwanted and rejected as either inferior to planned children or as symbols of relationships the parents had sought to avoid or terminate. Some children appeared to have been rejected because they had handicaps or limitations that jeopardized the parents' self-esteem. Other children in this group appeared to have developed maladaptive behaviors as attention-getting strategies because their parents were so preoccupied with job or social interests that the children felt left out. Finally, some of the parents were so emotionally needy that they had turned their own children into parents (role reversal).

A second large group (15 of the 66 families) consisted of children of parents with mental illnesses. In some of these families, the parents had refused to seek treatment for themselves and had no other family members who could help care for the children. Some of the parents were severely depressed, while others had delusions and considered their children to be defective or possessed. Some mentally retarded parents may also become emotionally abusive or neglectful, especially if they are unable to understand the normal developmental changes and needs of their children.

The third group (14 families) was characterized by parents who were diagnosed as having "borderline" or "inadequate" personalities. These parents led tumultuous and intense but seemingly aimless lives to which their children were largely peripheral. In some ways they were similar to the 11 families in the fourth group who had drug and alcohol problems. Children of these families were often physically as well as emotionally neglected. Their parents were frequently absent, preoccupied, or incapacitated, and family resources were used to buy drugs or alcohol.

The fifth and smallest group (nine families) in Junewicz's series may actually represent the most common setting of emotional maltreatment, that of stressful conflict within the family. Because on the surface they are more normal, these families are much less likely to be reported to social service agencies. In most cases, Junewicz found serious conflict between the parent figures. Children were harmed emotionally in two ways: they developed extreme anxiety from witnessing physical or sexual violence, and they faced double binds from being recruited to take sides in the adults' emotional combat or being blamed for what had happened. Other authors (Preston, 1986) have observed that in many cases even divorce or separation do not end maltreatment caused by parent conflict. Ongoing litigation over property and custody rights keep the children at the center of the parents' struggles while the parents' emotional needs perpetuate infantilization or role reversal.

CONSEQUENCES AND TREATMENT

All forms of child maltreatment involve some emotional component, and thus the consequences of emotional abuse are similar to effects of other trauma that takes place continually and from an early age. One longitudinal study of high-risk families, however, suggests that emotional maltreatment may have the most serious consequences for a child's intellectual and social development (Egeland et al., 1983). A group of parents and children were followed from the late stages of pregnancy through preschool. Some of the children were abused or neglected; others who were not served as controls. All forms of maltreatment (physical abuse, neglect, verbal abuse, and psychologic unavailability) led to anxious rather than secure attachment and to increased anger, frustration, and hostility. In addition, in the two groups of emotionally maltreated children (verbal abuse and unavailability), developmental quotients also declined over time. The children were easily frustrated with new tasks, approaching them with anxiety and a negative mood. Emotional maltreatment caused alterations in children's performance equal to or more serious than those caused by physical abuse or neglect. The researchers, in fact, postulated that emotional maltreatment might have been a more serious psychologic threat than physical maltreatment, since the physical abuse was often sporadic whereas the verbal abuse or parental detachment was usually constant.

The first step in treating emotional abuse is, when possible, to stop the abuse from taking place. This intervention may require removing a child from a classroom with an abusive teacher or trying to recruit a family into therapy to alleviate the conflicts. Some families may accept a home aid or "big brother" who can provide some emotional stability while other treatment begins. Longer-term help for older children may require individual or group psychotherapy; younger children may respond to group or individual play sessions in which they can experience a safe and nurturing environment (for example, a preschool program such as Head Start). Groups for children whose parents are or were alcoholics or drug abusers, or who are from separated families, are available in many communities. Specific treatment for the parents' psychologic or substance abuse problems is important but may be difficult to achieve.

Emotional maltreatment may be the most difficult form of abuse to prove in court. Yates (1982) suggests three types of cases that seem more likely to succeed than others:

- Those in which specific symptoms appear causally linked (usually because of time sequence) to a particular adult. Such cases involve, for example, children who have marked behavioral changes when they start with a new teacher or show a sudden improvement or relief when they are moved to a new home or when a particular individual leaves the home.
- Cases involving single acts that appear particularly bizarre or cruel, such as severe public humiliation or close confinement.
- Cases characterized by documented unwillingness to seek treatment for a child's emotional problems. These situations may also be approached as cases of medical neglect, but adding concern for the long-term emotional consequences, as well as the acute behavioral problem, may strengthen the argument for intervention.

References

Egeland B, Farber EA. Infant-mother attachment: factors related to its development and changes over time. Child Dev 1984;55:753–771.

Egeland B, Sroufe A, Erickson M. The developmental consequences of different patterns of maltreatment. Child Abuse Negl 1983;7:459–469.

Garbarino J, Garbarino AC. Emotional maltreatment of children. Chicago: National Committee for the Prevention of Child Abuse, 1980.

Gilligan C. In a different voice: psychological theory and women's development. Cambridge: Harvard University Press, 1982.

Junewicz WJ. A protective posture toward emotional neglect and abuse. Child Welfare 1983;62:243–252.

Kagan J, Kearsley RB, Zelazo PR. Infancy: its place in human development. Cambridge: Harvard University Press, 1978.

Kavanagh C. Emotional abuse and mental injury: a critique of the concepts and a recommendation for practice. J Am Acad Child Adolesc Psychiatry 1982;21:171–177.

Krugman RD, Krugman MK. Emotional abuse in the classroom: the pediatrician's role in diagnosis and treatment. Am J Dis Child 1984;138:284–286.

Lourie IS, Stefano L. On defining emotional abuse: results of an NIMH/NCCAN workshop. In: Lauderdale M, Anderson R, Cramer S, eds. Child abuse and neglect: issues in innovation and implementation. Vol. 1. US Department of Health, Education, and Welfare Publ. (OHDS) 78-30147. Washington, DC: US Government Printing Office, 1978:201–208.

Minde K. Bonding and attachment: its relevance for the present-day clinician. Dev Med Child Neurol 1986;28:803–806.

Preston G. The post-separation family and the emotional abuse of children: an ecological approach. Aust J Sex Marriage Fam 1986;7:40–49.

Rutter M. Psychosocial resilience and protective mechanisms. Am J Orthopsychiatry 1987;57:316–331.

Troy M, Sroufe LA. Victimization among preschoolers: role of attachment relationship history. J Am Acad Child Adolesc Psychiatry 1987;26:166–172.

US Department of Health and Human Services. Study findings: study of national incidence and prevalence of child abuse and neglect: 1988. Washington, DC: US Government Printing Office, 1988.

Yates A. Legal issues in psychological abuse of children. Clin Pediatr 1982;21:587–590.

14 Corporal Punishment

Corporal punishment, the inflicting of physical pain for the purpose of discipline, is a practice that dates to the beginnings of Western civilization. The Proverbs attributed to King Solomon suggest:

> If folly settles in the heart of a lad,
> The rod of discipline will remove it. (22:15)

Lest he who wields the rod become faint hearted, the Proverbs counsel further:

> Do not withhold discipline from a child;
> If you beat him with a rod he will not die.
> Beat him with a rod
> And you will save him from the grave.
> (23:13–14)[1]

The King James translation of Prov. 23:14 goes even further, suggesting that a beating will serve not only the cause of discipline but the cause of salvation as well: "Thou shalt beat him with the rod, and shalt deliver his soul from hell." These admonitions have been incorporated into both children's literature (the old woman who lived in a shoe, for example) and into Anglo-Saxon common law. As of 1987, only nine American states had acted to ban or limit corporal punishment in the home or school. In the remaining 41, the practice either was not prohibited or was specifically excluded from criminal codes, although it may have been banned locally in some school districts. Europe is somewhat ahead of the United States in this regard: Norway and Sweden have enacted legislation that specifically outlaws corporal punishment by parents or teachers, and the practice is banned in schools throughout most of western Europe.

The tolerance for physical punishment of children stands out against a general prohibition of the practice in nearly any other authoritarian setting. Corporal punishment is outlawed in the military (10 USCA Sec. 855, Article 55) and for adults and juveniles in correctional facilities (Jackson v. Bishop, 404 F. 2d 571, 1968; Nelson v. Heyne, 491 F. 2d 352, 1974; 417 US 976, 1974 [certiorari denied]). Although lower federal courts have found "excessive" physical punishment in schools to violate the Bill of Rights' prohibition against cruel and unusual punishment (Bramlet v. Wilson, 495 F. 2d 714, 1974), the Supreme Court's landmark corporal punishment case did not find it to be constitutionally objectionable. That case, Ingraham v. Wright (430 US 651, 1977), involved junior high school students in Florida who alleged that their punishment not only was cruel and unusual but also deprived them of their 14th Amendment right to due process. One of the boys in the case had received more than 20 blows with a wooden paddle while being held over a table in the principal's office for having been "slow to respond to a teacher's instructions." Another child had been hit on the arms. Both were said to have been incapacitated for several days as a result of their injuries. The boys' allegations were not disputed. The court, however, ruled that the "cruel and unusual" prohibition applied only to those convicted of crimes and that "due process" protections were not required in the "open" school environment. Since that time, lower federal courts have in some cases found that school paddling violated student rights (Schmidt, 1987), but no ruling has had a broad impact on the practice.

Although corporal punishment is formally opposed by many professional groups, including the American Academy of Pediatrics (Committee on School Health, 1984), it is widely supported by a majority of parents and educators. In the 1975 National Family Violence Survey (Straus et al., 1981), over 70% of parents said that spanking or slapping were necessary and good parts of child rearing. Adults who did not have children were even more supportive of these practices. About 60% of parents said that they had slapped or spanked one of their children in the past year, and about 70% said

---

[1] These versions of the Proverbs are from a modern translation (The Torah, Philadelphia: The Jewish Publication Society, 1962).

they had done so at some time in their children's lives. These figures appear to have remained fairly stable over time; there was only a slight decrease in the proportion of parents reporting slapping or spanking when the study was repeated in 1985 (see Table 1.2).

One factor that has helped perpetuate the acceptance of corporal punishment among professionals is the belief that the practice is more prevalent among lower socioeconomic groups. The supposition that the use of force is in some way a manifestation of poor breeding or ignorance has led many observers to believe that corporal punishment will simply go away. However, an analysis of data from a survey taken by the 1968 National Commission on the Causes and Prevention of Violence (Erlanger, 1979) found relatively little difference in social class among individuals who reported having experienced corporal punishment or who said they condoned its use. The incidence did decrease somewhat with increasing levels of education but rose with increasing levels of income. Among both middle- and working-class families and among both whites and blacks, over 90% of the adults questioned said that they had been spanked as children.

These trends in corporal punishment in the home are reflected in the schools. Rose, in a study published in 1984, surveyed 232 school principals sampled from around the United States. Of those surveyed, 74% (84% in elementary schools and 55% in high schools) said they used corporal punishment in their schools. In some ways, physical punishment in schools parallels its use in homes: younger children and boys are more frequently targets than older children or girls (Straus et al., 1981). On the other hand, while there seem to be little differences among racial groups in the use of corporal punishment in the home, minority students appear to be more likely than whites to be physically punished in school (Schmidt, 1987).

The school principals in Rose's study overwhelmingly felt that corporal punishment was necessary both for keeping discipline and for maintaining teacher morale. It was meted out mostly for fighting, but also for truancy, "horseplay," and other forms of classroom disruption. Wooden paddles were used in most cases, but 5% of the principals reported that they sometimes used pinches or hair pulling. The full extent of physical punishment in schools is not known. In Florida, where central records of paddlings are kept, just over 10% of the schools' 1.5 million students were said to have been paddled at least once during the 1983–84 school year (Maeroff, 1985).

Although some parents have taken exception to these practices and even gone to jail for retaliating against a teacher (Smothers, 1987), most appear to agree with educators that physical punishment belongs in schools. One survey of parents at a United States military installation found that about 50% supported the practice in schools, with 20–30% believing that it helped both school performance and behavior (Kelly et al., 1985). Similar findings were reported from a 1985 survey of British parents (Thomas, 1985). Proponents in the educational field generally claim that some children, especially those with conduct disorders, respond only to threats of force, which are therefore necessary to maintain order in the classroom. Some adults feel that physical punishment is character building, especially for boys, and that boys, who are seen as more difficult to raise, benefit from its "toughening" effects (Straus, 1971).

Proponents of physical punishment also have traditionally cited studies of laboratory animals or severely handicapped individuals that find aversive, negative stimuli to be effective tools for modifying behavior. Opponents counter that it is not reasonable to extend such findings to normal children, who, in fact, react quite differently (Maurer, 1974). Perhaps the most compelling criticism is that those who advocate corporal punishment as a means of discipline seriously confuse both their own motivations and the definitions of "punishment" and "discipline." Bettelheim (1985), for example, points out that while punishment involves concepts of suffering, pain, and retribution, the roots of the word "discipline" stem from learning, molding, and perfecting one's skills or character. Bettelheim argues that if an adult truly wants to instill a child with discipline, an internally and not externally derived quality, the most effective way to do so is to build on the child's desire to be like and to please the adult. Punishment, with its attendant degradation, is more likely to cause resentment and a desire to hurt or defy the parent in return.

Clinical observations (Maurer, 1974) strongly support the contention that corporal punishment has negative consequences. Punishment decreases a child's self-esteem and can lead to symptoms of depression or anxiety (Krugman and Krugman, 1984). It can also backfire, making the victim into a hero or martyr who subsequently gets even more peer attention for unacceptable behavior.

Perhaps the most serious consequence of physical punishment is the risk that it will lead to more violence. Generally unable to strike back at adults, children who are physically punished may transfer their anger to objects around them or to other children. In the National Family Violence Survey (Straus et al., 1981), children who were physically punished were more likely to be violent to their siblings and more likely to have tried to hit their parents. The punishers themselves are also likely to become carried away. Although the true incidence is not known, examples of school punishments that become "excessive" and result in relatively severe injury are widely reported (Maurer, 1979). Evidence from the National Family Violence Survey (Straus et al., 1981) suggests that physical violence in the family tends to repeat and advance in severity over time and that adults who were physically punished as children are more likely to physically punish their own children. The researchers concluded that physical punishment teaches three unfortunate lessons that serve to perpetuate multigenerational patterns of family violence: (1) those who love you most are the ones most likely to hit you; (2) physical punishment is justified if it is for a good purpose, such as discipline or character building; and (3) violence is an acceptable last resort if other attempts at communication fail.

There are few guidelines for the clinician seeking to draw a line between what might be considered acceptable corporal punishment and that which is excessive and therefore constitutes abuse. Even in areas where corporal punishment is permitted, punishments that are excessively degrading or disfiguring or that risk or cause serious internal injury are generally considered abusive, as are injuries that appear to indicate fixated or sadistic thinking. These terms are subjective, however, and they may be harder to assert in cases of school punishments than those occurring at home. One possible policy is to systematically report any situation in which it appears that the punisher was losing control. Support for this opinion might include evidence of anything more than the most superficial and transiently visible injury or injuries that extend beyond the buttocks. Lesions on both the front and back of the body, that extend up the trunk and down the legs, or that are on the underside of the upper arms (possibly incurred when the victim was trying to protect his or her face) suggest an adult who was not able to control the blows. Likewise, evidence that any more than a few blows were delivered also suggests either a loss of control or deliberately excessive punishment. Even schools that condone physical punishment generally allow only a few blows per punishment, although such policies seem to be poorly enforced.

Clinicians can also try to advocate and teach alternative methods of discipline (Bettelheim, 1985; Committee on Psychosocial Aspects of Child and Family Health, 1983; Dubanoski et al., 1983). These include:

- Trying to model controlled, nonviolent behavior.
- Using the child's desire to be with or please the adult—paying attention to good behaviors and rewarding them with the adult's presence or praise.
- Decreasing rewards for negative behavior (such as having the adult pay attention to the child when he or she misbehaves or allowing punishment to retrieve the child from an anxiety-producing situation such as taking a test).
- Trying to be a better listener and a clearer speaker; taking time to hear what the child is saying and feeling; taking time to let the child know what you are feeling.
- Warning children when changes of activity will be imminent ("we will have to stop playing in a few minutes") so as to avoid sudden confrontations.
- Trying to reduce the chances of confrontations (removing objects the child cannot play with before the child sees them; trying to plan at least some time and place where the child can set the agenda or pace of activities).

References

Bettelheim B. Punishment versus discipline. Atlantic Monthly 1985;Nov:52–59.

Committee on Psychosocial Aspects of Child and Family Health. The pediatrician's role in discipline. Pediatrics 1983;72:373–374.

Committee on School Health. Corporal punishment in schools. Pediatrics 1984;73:258.

Dubanoski RA, Inaba M, Gerkewicz K. Corporal punishment in the schools: myths, problems, and alternatives. Child Abuse Negl 1983;7:271–278.

Erlanger HS. Social class and corporal punishment: a reassessment. In: Gil DG, ed. Child abuse and violence. New York: AMS Press Inc, 1979:484–515.

Kelly PC, Weir MR, Fearnow RG. A survey of parental opinions on corporal punishment in schools. J Dev Behav Pediatr 1985;6:143–145.

Krugman RD, Krugman MK. Emotional abuse in the classroom. The pediatrician's role in diagnosis and treatment. Am J Dis Child 1984;138:284–286.

Maeroff GI. Spare the rod and spoil the school? New York Times 24 Nov 1985:IV7.

Maurer A. Corporal punishment. Am Psychol 1974;29:614–626.

Maurer A. It does happen here. In: Hyman IA, Wise JH, ed. Corporal punishment in American education. Philadelphia: Temple University Press, 1979:219–236.

Rose TL. Current uses of corporal punishment in American public schools. J Ed Psychol 1984;76:427–441.

Schmidt WE. Paddling in school: a tradition is under fire. New York Times 9 July 1987:A1.

Smothers R. Jailed for paddling the paddler. New York Times 13 Nov 1987:A1.

Straus MA. Some social antecedents of physical punishment: a linkage theory interpretation. J Marriage Fam 1971;33:658–663.

Straus MA, Gelles RJ, Steinmetz SK. Behind closed doors: violence in the American family. Garden City: Anchor Books, 1981.

Thomas J. British school issue: spare the rod and . . .? New York Times 18 Aug 1985:A6.

15 Munchausen Syndrome by Proxy

Munchausen syndrome by proxy (MSBP) is the name given to a broad group of situations in which parents simulate, falsely report, or actually create symptoms of medical illness in their children. At one end of the spectrum, MSBP shares many of the characteristics of fatal child abuse and includes deliberate suffocation (Geelhoed and Pemberton, 1985) or poisoning (Dine and McGovern, 1982). At the other extreme, it shares the dynamics of parent-child separation problems seen in school avoidance (Guandolo, 1985) and results in extensive, sometimes harmful, and generally unnecessary medical care. At either extreme, it is a serious condition. Death or serious physical morbidity is described as the outcome in some 20% of cases reported in the medical literature (Rosenberg, 1987), and psychologic sequelae are probably much more common. Since its initial description in the 1970s (Money and Werlas, 1976; Meadow, 1977), MSBP has been increasingly recognized as a cause of diagnostic dilemmas and unexplained life-threatening illnesses.

The term "Munchausen syndrome" was originally coined to describe adults who gave exaggerated or fanciful reports of their own illnesses (Asher, 1951). When parents seek medical attention by proxy, via their children, typical presentations include:

- Long but vague histories of difficult-to-document medical complaints (hyperactivity, somnolence, seizures, or abdominal, chest, or head pains) accompanied by doctor shopping, erratic compliance with suggested treatment, or lack of satisfaction with negative findings on work-up.
- Bleeding, hematuria, or hematemesis. Parents have been known to put their own blood in a child's urine or stool samples during the course of an evaluation or to purposely induce bleeding. There have been reported cases of blood removal from indwelling central venous catheters (Table 15.1).
- Central nervous system problems (drowsiness, coma, seizures, apnea). When these are actual presenting problems (as opposed to events observed only by the parent), they may be symptoms of poisoning, head trauma (including the shaken baby syndrome), or suffocation.
- Biochemical chaos; that is, laboratory values that do not make sense, either because the findings suggest too many simultaneously occurring illnesses or because the values lack internal consistency. When real, such findings may be the result of salt or fluid poisoning or administration of drugs that alter metabolism (Table 15.1); when factitious, they may be the result of deliberately altered lab specimens.
- Sudden change in the status of a hospitalized child when discharge is planned, especially if a work-up has been negative and the child is likely to receive a clean bill of health.

CHARACTERISTICS

In the overwhelming majority of cases of MSBP, the child's mother is found to be the perpetrator (Meadow, 1984). Often she will be perceived by clinicians as a model parent during the time that the child is hospitalized, always being very helpful on the ward and solicitous of the staff. It is not clear whether this behavior represents a conscious effort to deceive the staff or whether it is a reflection of the mother's abnormally great need for affection and belonging. In some cases, exacerbations of the syndrome (new complaints presented to physicians or new episodes of poisoning or suffocation) occur during stressful points in the mother's life or at times when other family members observe her behavior to be more erratic. This observation supports the hypothesis that at some level the mother may be seeking recognition and security within the medical system. Alternatively, these may also be times when the mother's anger or ambivalence toward the child, or need to atone for some wrong the child represents, are surfacing more strongly (see Chapters 12 and 16).

The deceptions involved in MSBP are often quite complex and may be carried out for long periods of time. Some workers have suggested that the mother, child, or entire family

Table 15.1. Substances and Maneuvers Creating or Simulating Illness in Victims of Munchausen Syndrome by Proxy[a]

Psychoactive drugs
    Phenothiazines
    Imipramine
    Amitriptylene
    Codeine
    Chloral hydrate
    Methaqualone
    Amphetamines
    Barbiturates

Drugs/substances altering fluid and electrolye balance
    Excessive table salt
    Excessive water
    Insulin (Mayefsky et al., 1982)
    Furosemide
    Chlorthalidone
    Phenformin
    Salicylates
    Theophylline

Miscellaneous toxins
    Pepper
    Laxatives
    Naphtha
    Lye (Friedman, 1987)
    Warfarin (White et al., 1985)

Other mechanisms
    Starvation
    Suffocation (Rosen et al., 1986)
    Fabricated history of previous diagnosis of serious illness
        Operable cardiac disease (Small, 1988)
        Various conditions (Woolcott et al., 1982)
        Epilepsy (Meadow, 1984)
    Inflicted vaginal/rectal injury to produce bleeding
    Altered laboratory studies
        Simulation of cystic fibrosis by obtaining contaminated sputum samples, putting salt in collection for sweat test, adding fat to stool collection (Orenstein and Wasserman, 1986)
        Injection of contaminated material into intravenous lines (Halsey et al., 1983)
        Putting parent's blood on child (Kurlandsky et al., 1979)
        Putting parent's blood in urine (Waller, 1983)
        Removal of blood from child's central venous line (Malatack et al., 1985)

[a]References refer to case reports describing abuse involving the indicated maneuver or substance. Citations for many of the unreferenced items can be found in Dine and McGovern (1982) and Rosenberg (1987).

may be participants in a delusional state and truly believe that the child is ill (Money and Werlas, 1976; Richtsmeier and Waters, 1984). On the other hand, some cases involve deliberate harmful or deceitful acts that, when discovered, contrast sharply with the mother's often ostentatious demonstrations of care for her child. Such parents may fit a syndrome of "sick but slick" behavior that has been observed in other forms of child abuse (Wright, 1976). Sick but slick parents can demonstrate near-psychopathic ideation but succeed in projecting an image of normality that withstands all but the most skilled psychiatric assessment. For example, the first sign that one is involved with a case of MSBP is often an uncomfortable feeling evoked by a mother who appears friendly and solicitous but simultaneously guarded and unreachable on anything more than a superficial level (Zitelli et al., 1987). Many MSBP parents are supremely shrewd observers of human behavior. When their facade is challenged, they have an uncanny ability strike back with challenges that divide and cripple the medical staff. Attempts to learn more about the parent may meet with the formation of secret alliances between the parent and selected staff members and simultaneous accusations of professional misconduct against others. Sometimes a mother develops somatic complaints herself and uses these as a way to temporarily leave the child's bedside or to appeal to sympathetic staff members in the role of a victim. The parent often wins in this situation because the turmoil among staff members prevent them from organizing a methodical investigation.

The ability to deceive clinicians in MSBP is often enhanced by the fact that the mother has a history of medical illness or complaints similar to that of the child. She may have been prescribed the drugs that have been used to poison the child. Alternatively, she may have a history of medical training or extensive contact with medical care settings; she knows what kinds of symptoms will elicit attention from the staff and is able to give fairly convincing descriptions of these symptoms. As in school avoidance problems, the child may sometimes have had an illness, usually minor, that serves both as a model for elaboration of other symptoms (or provides a drug useful for poisoning) and as the initial opportunity to avoid separation of mother and child.

The father in MSBP cases classically takes a distant or passive role in all of the child's illnesses and in the life of the family. He may leave medical decisions regarding the child to the mother and may seem to have little regard for the child's apparently serious illness. Again, his lack of participation and the way in which this facilitates an overly involved relationship between the mother and the child are similar to the dynamics of school avoidance (see Chapters 5 and 11).

DETECTION

Meadow (1982) has proposed a list of "warning signs" that may raise the clinician's suspicion of MSBP:

- Persistent or recurrent illnesses for which no medical explanation can be found, which suggest new syndromes not previously seen even by experienced clinicians, or which suggest only very rare disorders.
- Discrepancies between the child's apparent condition (good) and the results of laboratory tests or the history of recent symptoms (grave).
- In the context of the above, mothers who are overly attentive to their children in the hospital or who will not leave even for brief periods. This devoted concern is often in contrast to the mother's affect toward the clinical staff, which may be inappropriately cheerful and helping, given the supposed severity of the child's illness.
- Symptoms or signs that do not occur when the child is away from the mother.
- Routine treatments (e.g., casts, bandages, or intravenous lines) or medications (e.g., anticonvulsants) that are curiously and consistently not tolerated or fail to work for the particular patient.

Several factors often make it difficult to diagnose MSBP. There are usually no other signs of physical or sexual abuse (Rosenberg, 1987), although failure to thrive (Money and Werlas, 1976) and emotional abuse may be inherent parts of the syndrome. Physicians often play into the parents' agenda by giving into pressure to vigorously investigate vague symptoms or unexpected laboratory results for an otherwise healthy-appearing child. These investigations are difficult to avoid when parents have actually caused problems such as sepsis or apnea; even then, however, taking a comprehensive, multisystem view of the child's condition and carefully checking past medical history may provide early clues to the true nature of the problem (Guandolo, 1985). Unless there is a primary care clinician who takes responsibility for integrating findings, subspecialty consultation frequently serves only to compound difficulties. Rather than illuminating the child's condition, it serves instead to create confusion as the parent, who seems informed and reliable, conveys partial or misleading data among the subspecialists and recruits new allies who are willing to pressure their colleagues into performing additional tests.

Initial steps in the diagnosis of MSBP include obtaining and verifying details about the child's or siblings' past illnesses and health status. It is common for parents to report that records have been lost or that names of hospitals or physicians have been forgotten, but attempts to obtain this information must be pursued tactfully and in a nonaccusatory fashion. Clinicians sometimes worry that the mother will detect their suspicions and withdraw the child from care or, perhaps even more seriously, will see any hesitancy as a sign that the child needs to be even sicker to gain medical attention. These risks suggest that any inquiries into past findings should be accompanied by demonstrated attention to the parent's present concerns.

Once MSBP is suspected, deliberate steps must be taken to obtain proof. Law enforcement and social service agencies have historically been reluctant to believe that MSBP can exist as a clinical entity, and their disbelief is aided by the parents' outwardly normal appearance and striking ability to deny what they have done. Premature reporting of abuse or unprepared confrontation with the parent that fails to lead to adequate treatment can be fatal for the child. Several cases have been reported in which children died after ineffective intervention resulted in their return to untreated families (Rosenberg, 1987). At present, MSBP may represent the only exception to the rule (though not the law) that clinicians should report suspected rather than certain abuse. In some jurisdictions, good working relationships with social service agencies may allow confidential reporting and an agreement to delay any intervention until more information is gathered. In all cases, close consultation among members of the care team, including legal counsel, is necessary to coordinate an evaluation while simultaneously ensuring the child's short-term safety.

Hospitalization is often a final step in the evaluation of MSBP, although it functions differently than in other cases of maltreatment. Whereas hospitalization is usually thought of as providing a safe environment within which the family can be evaluated, in MSBP hospitalization often appears to be a trigger for accelerated abuse. In reported cases, anywhere from one-third to two-thirds of children admitted suffer ongoing abuse in the hospital. Thus, hospitalization offers some of the traditional opportunities to observe the child's symptoms firsthand and to interview the child alone, but it also offers an opportunity to observe the parent carrying out the abuse. Surveillance must be carefully planned to protect the child while allowing the parent a sufficient sense of privacy to act. Measures taken have included hidden video cameras (Epstein et al., 1987; Rosen et al., 1983; Meadow, 1987), radioisotope labeling of transfused blood to establish a source of bleeding (Kurlandsky et al., 1979), administration of ascorbic acid to verify the source of urine (Nading and Duval-Arnould, 1984), and measurement of serum C-peptide levels to detect insulin-induced hypoglycemia (Mayefsky et al., 1982). Complete toxicology screens can be obtained for patients with altered mental status or inexplicable metabolic problems. Because many screening systems available in hospitals may not be sufficiently sensitive, extra urine and serum samples can be frozen for further testing if required. The laboratory can be asked to test for specific drugs or toxins known to be in the home. Standard hospital epidemiology techniques may also be used to demonstrate that the parent was the only person with the patient each time an untoward event occurred (Halsey et al., 1983).

TREATMENT

The treatment phase in MSBP cases begins when the offending parent is confronted with evidence of intentional injury to the child or deliberate deception of medical staff. Careful preparations for this meeting must be made. Emergency psychiatric services must be available for either mother or child. Notification of the local child protective service agency before the confrontation can ensure that an emergency order for shelter care of the child can be obtained if the mother's reaction is to remove the child from the hospital. Social service intervention will be required in nearly all cases until the mother and other family members can have full psychiatric evaluations. The medical staff should not agree to any plan for such evaluations, however, unless the assessment will be carried out in depth, over several visits, and possibly use psychological testing to penetrate the parents' ability to project a normal appearance. Short-term assessments by inexperienced mental health professionals are notorious for their ability to exonerate parents involved in MSBP.

Until treatment is well underway, return to the home with the perpetrator poses undue risks for the child. While a temporary home for the child is being arranged, supervised contact with the parents can take place in the hospital.

Treatment plans must include all members of the family. The child may have evolved into a role in which he or she has become a participant in the abuse, adopting sick behaviors and becoming dependent on the overly close relationship with the mother. Some mothers have become suicidal upon being discovered; all require psychiatric care of various types and length (Nicol and Eccles, 1985).

References

Asher R. Munchausen's syndrome. Lancet 1951;i:339–341.

Dine MS, McGovern ME. Intentional poisoning of children—an overlooked category of child abuse: report of seven cases and review of the literature. Pediatrics 1982;70:32–35.

Epstein MA, Markowitz RL, Gallo DM, Holms JW, Gryboski JD. Munchausen syndrome by proxy: considerations in diagnosis and confirmation by video surveillance. Pediatrics 1987;80:220–224.

Friedman EM. Caustic ingestions and foreign body aspirations: an overlooked form of child abuse. Ann Otol Rhinol Laryngol 1987;96:709–712.

Geelhoed GC, Pemberton PJ. SIDS, seizures or 'sophageal reflux'? Another manifestation of Munchausen syndrome by proxy. Med J Aust 1985;143:357–358.

Guandolo VL. Munchausen syndrome by proxy: an outpatient challenge. Pediatrics 1985;75:526–530.

Halsey NA, Frentz JM, Tucker TW, Sproles T, Redding J, Daum RS. Recurrent nosocomial polymicrobial sepsis secondary to child abuse. Lancet 1983;ii:558–560.

Kurlandsky L, Lukoff JY, Zinkham WH, Brody JP, Kessler RW. Munchausen syndrome by proxy: definition of factitious bleeding in an infant by ^{51}Cr labelling of erythrocytes. Pediatrics 1979;63:228–231.

Malatack JJ, Wiener ES, Gartner JC, Zitelli BJ, Brunetti D. Munchausen syndrome by proxy: a new complication of central venous catheterization. Pediatrics 1985;75:523–525.

Mayefsky JH, Sarnaik AP, Postellon DC. Factitious hypoglycemia. Pediatrics 1982;69:804–805.

Meadow R. Munchausen syndrome by proxy: the hinterland of child abuse. Lancet 1977;ii:343–345.

Meadow R. Munchausen syndrome by proxy. Arch Dis Child 1982;57:92–98.

Meadow R. Factitious illness—the hinterland of child abuse. In: Meadow R, ed. Recent advances in paediatrics. Edinburgh: Churchill & Livingstone, 1984:217–232.

Meadow R. Fictitious epilepsy. Lancet 1984;ii:25–28.

Meadow R. Video recording and child abuse. Br Med J 1987;294:1629–1630.

Money J, Werlas J. *Folie à deux* in the parents of psychosocial dwarfs: two cases. Bull Am Acad Psychiatry Law 1976;4:351–62.

Nading JH, Duval-Arnould B. Factitious diabetes mellitus confirmed by ascorbic acid. Arch Dis Child 1984;59:166–169.

Nicol AR, Eccles M. Psychotherapy for Munchausen syndrome by proxy. Arch Dis Child 1985;60:344–348.

Orenstein DM, Wasserman AL. Munchausen syndrome by proxy simulating cystic fibrosis. Pediatrics 1986;78:621–624.

Richtsmeier AJ Jr, Waters DB. Somatic symptoms as family myth. Am J Dis Child 1984;138:855–857.

Rosen CL, Frost JD Jr, Bricker T, Tranow JD, Gillette PC, Dunlavy S. Two siblings with recurrent cardiorespiratory arrest: Munchausen syndrome by proxy or child abuse. Pediatrics 1983;71:715–720.

Rosen CL, Frost JD Jr, Glaze DG. Child abuse and recurrent infant apnea. J Pediatr 1986;109:1065–1067.

Rosenberg DA. Web of deceit: a literature review of Munchausen syndrome by proxy. Child Abuse Negl 1987;11:547–563.

Small G. Boy's heart surgery plight called phony. The Evening Sun [Baltimore] 22 Jan 1988:A1, A20.

Waller DA. Obstacles to treatment of Munchausen syndrome by proxy. J Am Acad Child Adolesc Psychiatry 1983;22:80–85.

White ST, Voter K, Perry J. Surreptitious Warfarin ingestion. Child Abuse Negl 1985;9:349–352.

Woolcott P Jr, Aceto T, Rutt C, Bloom M, Glick R. Doctor shopping with the child as proxy patient: a variant of child abuse. J Pediatr 1982;101:297–301.

Wright L. The "sick but slick" syndrome as a personality component of parents of battered children. J Clin Psychol 1976;332:41–45.

Zitelli BJ, Seltman MF, Shannon RM. Munchausen's syndrome by proxy and its professional participants. Am J Dis Child 1987;141:1099–1102.

16 Fatal Maltreatment

Death in childhood is always disturbing to clinicians. Deaths that involve obvious neglect or intentional injury evoke reactions ranging from rage to depression. These feelings often get in the way of effectively pursuing a possible perpetrator or protecting siblings. Deaths that are simply sudden or unexplained can also pose emotional problems for professionals (Mandell et al., 1987). Feelings of guilt and helplessness may make it difficult to pursue a thoughtful evaluation of why the death occurred and whether the consideration of intentional injury is appropriate.

Clinicians faced with an unexpected death must strike a difficult balance between competing professional tasks. A first priority is always to support and counsel the child's family. On the other hand, finding out why the child died is of utmost importance, whether the death ultimately is found to have been caused by an illness or by an inflicted injury. In either case, the well-being of the parents, siblings, and potential future children all depend on coming as close as possible to making a correct diagnosis. Developing the diagnosis in the most nonaccusatory, supportive way possible, however, requires an understanding of the epidemiology and possible etiologies of sudden death in childhood.

EPIDEMIOLOGY OF HOMICIDE AND FATAL ABUSE IN CHILDHOOD

Homicide is among the leading causes of death for American children ages 1–14 (Table 16.1). Beyond the first year of life, death rates from homicide among children are of the same order of magnitude as death rates from other major pediatric medical problems such as cancer, heart disease, and congenital malformations. Homicide takes a relatively greater toll among children than among adults. It accounts for about 5% of deaths among those 1–17, compared with only about 1% of deaths among those 18 and over (Anonymous, 1982).

Child homicide is a "syndrome" whose characteristics vary by the age of the victim (Table 16.2). Its incidence has a bimodal distribu-

Table 16.1. Ten Leading Causes of Death, United States, 1985[a]

Age (yr)	Cause	n	Rate/ 100,000
1–4	All causes	7339	51.4
	1. "Accidents"	2856	20.0
	2. Congenital anomalies	840	5.9
	3. Cancer/leukemia	543	3.8
	4. Homicide	348	2.4
	5. Heart disease	305	2.1
	6. Pneumonia/influenza	219	1.5
	7. Meningitis	159	1.1
	8. Perinatal complications	139	1.0
	9. Septicemia	92	0.6
	10. Other neoplasms	68	0.5
5–14	All causes	8933	26.3
	1. "Accidents"	4252	12.5
	2. Cancer/leukemia	1183	3.5
	3. Congenital anomalies	469	1.4
	4. Homicide	417	1.2
	5. Heart disease	322	0.9
	6. Suicide	278	0.8
	7. Pneumonia/influenza	130	0.4
	8. Asthma/obstructive lung disease	115	0.3
	9. Other neoplasms	87	0.3
	10. Cerebrovascular disease	82	0.2

[a]Source: National Center for Health Statistics. Advance report of final mortality statistics, 1985. Monthly Vital Stat Rep 1987;36:20, Table 7. Publ. (PHS) 87-1120.

tion: mortality rates are highest in the first year of life and then fall rapidly, not to rise again until the teen years. Most of the deaths among children under age 3 represent fatal child abuse. Two-thirds or more of the children killed in the first year of life are killed by a parent, compared with only a quarter to a half of all child homicide victims (Jason et al., 1983). Homicide deaths among older children, especially those over 12, fit more closely the adult pattern of violence at the hands of acquaintances or unknown assailants.

Homicide figures alone probably underestimate the extent of fatal maltreatment, however, at least in part because FBI statistics

Table 16.2. Homicide of Children by Age of Victim, United States, 1987[a]

Age (yr)	All Children		Whites		Blacks	
	n	Rate/100,000	n	Rate/100,000	n	Rate/100,000
<1	232	6.15	141	4.62	79	11.02
1–4	303	2.09	170	1.45	125	4.50
5–9	119	0.67	67	0.47	48	1.40
10–14	205	1.24	108	0.82	92	2.84
15–19	1539	8.32	654	4.35	854	24.72

[a]Sources: Federal Bureau of Investigation. Crime in the United States. Uniform crime reports, 1987. Washington, DC: US Department of Justice, 10 July 1988:9; Bureau of the Census. United States population estimates, by age, sex, and race: 1980 to 1987. Series P, No. 1022. Washington, DC: US Department of Commerce, 1988:11, Table 1.

purposely exclude deaths attributable to negligence. The 1986 Study of National Incidence and Prevalence of Child Abuse and Neglect (NIS) estimated that in that year there were 1100 fatalities that could be attributed to some form of abuse or neglect, or about 2/100,000 children. Although the NIS noted that the incidence of maltreatment in general increased with age, all of the fatalities found in the study involved children under 6 (National Center on Child Abuse and Neglect, 1988).

FATAL ABUSE IN INFANCY

Characteristics

Various terms are used to signify the deaths of children at the hands of parents. "Infanticide" is sometimes used as a general term for any death of a child under age 1 caused by either parent (Jason et al., 1983) and sometimes specifically to indicate that the assailant was the mother (Emery, 1985). "Neonaticide" is often used to refer to the death of a child in the first day of life, and "filicide" denotes the death of a child of any age at the hands of a parent. Regardless of the terms used, fatal child abuse in early infancy is itself a heterogeneous group of problems.

Deaths in the first year of life include both homicides and fatal abandonment or other forms of neglect. The intentional killing or abandoning of unwanted newborns has been practiced since antiquity (Bloch, 1988). It continues to be practiced in many cultures where strong traditions attach more value to a child of a particular sex or where premarital pregnancy can make it difficult to find a mate (Rule, 1987). In Western cultures, episodes of abandoned newborns are still frequently reported in the popular press, although their true incidence is not known.

Deaths in the first year of life that are identified as homicides are more readily quantified. About 20% occur in the first month of life, at a rate of about 1.4/100,000 live births (National Center for Health Statistics, 1986). Although the available data are incomplete, statistics collected by the FBI suggest that women are much more likely to kill children in the first weeks of life, while as children get older, male and female perpetrators are found in relatively equal proportions (Jason et al., 1983). The methods used to kill infants differ from those involved in homicides of older children. In cases tabulated by the FBI, over 80% of deaths of children under 1 year were known or suspected to involve the use of personal force (strangulation, asphyxiation, blows), with only 10% involving a deadly weapon or blunt object (Table 16.3). By age 5, 50% of child homicides involve a gun or knife, a figure that rises to over 80% among victims 15–19. Even after adjustment for age of the victim, however, the data show that parents used a higher proportion of firearms than did other perpetrators. Fathers are more likely than mothers to use guns, while mothers are more likely than fathers to strangle or drown a child (Jason et al., 1983).

Young children are more likely than older children to be killed at home. In a study of child homicides in Atlanta, Georgia, over a 10-year period, Blaser (1983–85) found that 11 of 12 victims under age 2 died at home, compared with 14 of 20 who were 2–7 years old and only 12 of 47 who were 8–15. Again, the deaths of

Table 16.3. Murder Victims: Weapons Used by Age of Victim, United States, 1987[a]

Age (yr)	No. of Victims	% of Victims Murdered by Given Weapon Type			
		Gun or knife	Blunt object	Personal force[b]	Other or not known
<1	232	6	4	58	32
1–4	303	17	9	54	20
5–9	119	50	6	24	20
10–14	205	74	3	14	12
15–19	1539	88	3	6	3

[a]Source: Federal Bureau of Investigation. Crime in the United States. Uniform crime reports, 1987. Washington, DC: US Department of Justice, 10 July 1988:10.
[b]Includes strangulation, asphyxiation, and blows with hands, fists, and feet.

older children fit a pattern more consistent with adult homicide, whereas the younger children were more likely to be victims of fatal abuse by caretakers. As will be discussed in more detail below, young children, at least those beyond the first few weeks of life, appear more likely to be the victims of prolonged, progressively intensifying violence, while older children are more likely to die in sudden confrontations that involve lethal force.

Both published homicide statistics and special studies of fatal child abuse suggest that children in lower socioeconomic groups are at a higher risk of death. In urban Atlanta, child homicide rates in the lower two socioeconomic quartiles were nearly twice those in the upper two quartiles (Blaser, 1983–85). In a statewide study of fatal abuse in Georgia, Jason and Andereck (1983) also found an increased risk among poor children. Racial patterns have been less consistent. Although reported child homicide rates at all ages are higher among blacks than whites (Table 16.2), Jason and Andereck found an interaction of urban residence with race. Fatal physical abuse in Georgia had its highest incidence among low-income rural white families (a rate of 3.3/100,000 children) and was next highest among low-income urban black families (2.4/100,000 children).

Studies of fatal abuse in the general population may underestimate the risk among more impaired families. Oliver (1983) reviewed case files of all families in a single health district in England who were known to social service agencies and in which at least two children had been neglected or abused. In addition, in all of the families at least one parent had been abused in childhood and had been the subject of social service intervention. Of 560 children in 147 families, 41 (just over 7%) died over a 20-year follow-up period. All of the children died before their eighth birthday, with the majority dying in the first year of life. All but 12 of the deaths were felt to be related to abuse or neglect. Importantly, only three of the cases resulted in convictions for manslaughter or infanticide.

Failure to prevent these deaths or recognize their intentional nature was often related to an inaccurate impression of the family's past history. Parents consistently failed to reveal that other children in the family had either died or been removed. Officials also consistently failed to recognize the suspicious nature of previous deaths or injuries of which they were aware. This problem is hardly limited to Great Britain. In a 1986 United States case that received wide publicity, a mother was charged with the suffocation death of a 3-month-old daughter and suspected of having killed eight other of her children over a 14-year period (Wallace, 1986). Six of the nine children died before they were a year old; one child, who was 2, died while adoption proceedings were being finalized. It was not known whether officials supervising the adoption knew that seven of the mother's children had died previously, some from undetermined causes. This type of case emphasizes the importance of reviewing and verifying family and medical histories, especially in situations of unexplained or multiple injuries or deaths (see Chapter 15).

Causes of Neonaticide and Infanticide

As mentioned above, in some cultures neonaticide is considered a more or less acceptable method for disposing of unwanted children. It is more comfortable to believe that in Western culture neonaticide is more likely to be caused by some form of mental illness. Indeed, although it has not been universally accepted, temporary insanity based on postpartum depression has been invoked as a reason for the killing of infants (Anonymous, 1988; Sullivan, 1988).

There is a long-standing debate in the psychiatric literature over the nature of postpartum mental illness. Some clinicians view the postpartum period as causing unique forms of illness, while others view it as simply another stressful time of life capable of evoking symptoms in susceptible individuals. The general symptoms of depression or anxiety that develop in women in the postpartum period are similar to symptoms developed by women at other life stages, but the themes appear to be different. Women in the postpartum period are more likely to have guilt feelings, obsessions, or paranoias that relate to their newborn children or to their ability to care for them. There is therefore an increased risk that these distortions of perception could have adverse consequences for the children's care.

Depression appears to be the most common postpartum psychiatric disorder, although this finding comes from series of hospitalized patients among whom psychoses and more serious thought disorders are also found in high numbers (Dean and Kendell, 1981). Hopkins and co-workers (1984) identify three types of postpartum depression. The most common is the so-called maternity blues, a condition that may affect 50–60% of women in the first few days after they give birth. The blues may be more common in women having their first child and is often characterized by tearfulness, crying, and more tension or anger than sadness. Although it appears to be a self-limited condition lasting only 24–48 hours, it may be more common among those who later develop more serious psychiatric problems.

The second type, the form of postpartum depression that usually comes to medical attention, has symptoms that are similar to those of other depressions but are marked less by self-destructive ideation than by feelings of inadequacy, inability to cope with the task of parenting, and medical concerns for the child or for the parent. This type of postpartum illness may effect 10–30% of women giving birth. Its onset is variable, as is its course; symptoms may persist for several months. Despite the degree of dysfunction involved, relatively few women seek treatment.

The least common but perhaps most serious of the postpartum mental conditions is psychosis, reported to follow 1–2 live births per 10,000. Major depressions and thought disorders such as schizophrenia are the most common manifestations (Dean and Kendell, 1981), but as with other postpartum conditions, the themes appear to vary (Herzog and Detre, 1976). Among depressed women, preoccupations may include a perceived inability to care for the child, feeling unable to give enough love, and infanticidal thoughts. All of these feelings may be accompanied by intense guilt. Women who develop symptoms of schizophrenia in the postpartum period may develop delusions that include supernatural connotations of the child's birth or origin. It is felt that some of these women kill their infants while in a delusional state, perhaps believing that the child is possessed or in some way evil. It is not known what proportion of infanticides is attributable to this mechanism.

DEATHS OF OLDER CHILDREN

More complex mechanisms may underlie the killing of an older child, in theory because that child now has a role in the family; whatever value the family places on having that role filled competes with what motivation the parent has to kill. Resnick (1969), in a review of published cases, identified several patterns that seemed to offer differing explanations for deaths among older children.

One pattern was labeled "accidental." Children who died in this manner were killed as the endpoint of a long period of recurring abuse (Korbin, 1987). The death was accidental in the sense that the parent did not set out to cause fatal injury but did repeatedly cause severe harm. Money (Chapter 15) has suggested that such parents have a need to keep the child alive as a "living sacrifice" that in some way atones for a parental transgression such as giving birth out of wedlock. Steele (1980) observed that some severely abusive parents may want to keep a child alive because they obtain gratification from the child's continued fear and obedience.

About half of the child deaths in Resnick's series fit a second pattern of apparently altruistic motives, although the basis for this altruism was often delusional. In several cases the mother, depressed, planned her own suicide and felt that the child would be better off dead than without her. In other cases the mother, possibly projecting feelings about herself onto the child, saw the child as irrevocably ruined or in some way defective. Thus, killing the child was seen as a humane act. One hallmark of altruistic killings was that parents were much less likely to hide what they had done, in contrast to "accidental" killings, which tended to be denied.

Some of these children may have been victims of what Green and Solnit (1964) called a vulnerable child syndrome, although the existence of such a syndrome continues to be debated (Scheiner et al., 1985). It is postulated that some small proportion of parents never emotionally recover from the fact that a child has had a life-threatening illness. Their perception of the child as weak or fragile may seem to be supported by the child's quiet temperament or some minor handicap that diminishes the child's ability to elicit nurturing. The illness may also evoke in the parent fears of his or her own death or memories of someone who has died or is ill. As a result, the parent comes to feel hopeless and defective. Consequences may include a preoccupation with the child's health, infantilization of the child as he or she grows older, and problems with separation. Less commonly, parents become resentful that the child makes them feel depressed or see the child's quiet nature or expressive limitations as a sign of rejection. It is perhaps these conscious ambivalent feelings about the child and a bleak view of the child's future that lead to intentional injury or fatal neglect.

Other causes of fatal abuse found in Resnick's review included acute delusional episodes in which parents saw their children as possessed or evil and more paranoid states in which the parent felt that the child was a rival for a mate's affection or a cause of the family's misfortunes. Recently, the concern has been raised that the use of cocaine, especially in its smokable form crack, has been associated with violent outbursts and with an increased incidence of fatal physical abuse and violent sexual abuse (see Chapter 17).

PHYSICAL EXAMINATION OF CRITICALLY INJURED VICTIMS OF SUSPECTED ABUSE

The physical examination has special importance in cases of very severe or fatal injury. Because the victim cannot speak, physical findings may be the only clues to the injury mechanism and possibly to the identity of the perpetrator. As outlined in Chapter 6, special attention must be paid to marks that may represent inflicted injuries, especially knife or gunshot wounds. To the extent possible, these should be examined and documented before they are altered by life-saving efforts or by death (Smialek, 1983). When the cause of illness is unknown or when toxins are suspected, it is important to obtain samples of body fluids (blood, stomach contents, urine) as soon as possible, preferably before intravenous therapy is administered. Administration of large quantities of saline or blood products, as is frequently necessary in life-threatening conditions, may dilute the toxins or hasten their excretion. The time the body fluid samples were obtained should be recorded, as the pharmacokinetics of known toxins may be used to estimate the timing and amount of exposure. Procedures in the urgent care setting should be documented so that iatrogenic trauma can be differentiated from previously inflicted injuries. Clothing should be carefully saved, preferably with the patient laying on a clean sheet that can then be wrapped up to enclose the clothing and any small objects that may have fallen from it. As in cases of sexual assault, areas of skin that appear to have fresh bite marks or residues of body fluids such as semen should be swabbed with a saline-moistened applicator that is then allowed to air dry and placed in a clean envelope (see Chapter 10).

Physicians treating a patient who is critically ill or dead on arrival in an emergency room must be careful in interpreting physical findings. Several phenomena that happen near or at the time of death may produce signs that can be confused with intentional injury. Jumping to conclusions about their meaning may result in inappropriate accusations or misleading notes in the medical record. Findings should be described as completely as possible, with interpretations clearly labeled as such. For example, livor mortis (the pooling of blood in dependent parts of the body soon after death) may produce blotches or marks suggestive of bruises. Similarly, administration of vasopressor drugs to support blood pressure can result in changes in the peripheral circulation and produce both blotching and extreme friability of the skin. Frequent instrumentation, such as taking rectal temperatures, can then cause the skin to break down and resemble findings seen in intentional injury. With death, body orifices may gape; the female genitalia, for example, may assume dimensions suggestive of abuse. Foamy white or bloody discharge from the nose and mouth, caused by hemorrhagic pulmonary edema and rupture of mucosal capillaries, may occur after shock or death unrelated to a history of trauma. Agonal or postmortem relaxation of the esophageal sphincter can result in reflux of stomach contents and the presence of food in the mouth or nose, giving the impression that death was caused by aspiration. When a child dies at home and is not found for some time, insects or rodents may inflict damage to the body that can resemble burns or blunt trauma (Smialek and Lambros, 1988).

DECISION MAKING FOR CRITICALLY INJURED CHILDREN

Medical decision making in cases of suspected near-fatal abuse, especially with respect to termination of life support, is often complicated by apparently competing ethical and legal considerations. Usually, the first concern that arises is that the parents, if they are suspected of being abusers, have a conflict of interest when making decisions about the child's treatment. The medical staff's fear is that in order to escape murder or manslaughter charges, the parents will insist on heroic measures that could save the child's life but at a cost in quality of life that the staff feels is unreasonable. Alternatively, one parent may seem to want the child to die in order to see the other parent punished. Just how often parents actually behave in this manner is not known, but concern on the part of the medical staff often creates a great deal of anxiety. Although there are no clear legal guidelines available, some thoughts for managing this sort of situation are as follows.

First, the medical staff should remember that they are the ones who basically determine which treatments are medically indicated and which are essentially futile. In any critical care situation, this determination defines the limits within which treatment decisions can be made. Patients and their proxy decision makers should always have access to an ethics committee or other form of second opinion if they disagree with the definitions of "indicated" or "futile," but many ethicists argue that patients generally, and proxy decision makers in particular, do not have an unqualified right to insist on futile treatment.

Second, even parents who have been charged and incarcerated do not lose decision-making authority for their children unless authority has been formally reassigned. In fact, the biggest problem in such severe cases is trying to gain the parents access to the hospital where the child is being treated. Likewise, a parent who has been living outside the home may arrive and assert decision-making authority when the child is ill. This individual would seem to have little standing in comparison with the parent with whom the child has been living, but both share decision-making authority unless there has been some formal arrangement assigning guardianship. A prudent course is to (1) promptly ask the hospital attorney to help clarify any questions about decision-making authority and (2) seek to involve both parents in all decisions, especially those that involve heroic measures or termination of life support. If the parents cannot agree, or if they insist on a course of treatment that the treating physicians feel is either futile or, at the other extreme, insufficient given the child's prognosis, the juvenile or family court should be petitioned to appoint a medical guardian for the child.

Finally, it may be true that if a seriously injured child survives, even in a severely impaired state, the criminal charges levied against an abuser may be of lesser magnitude than if the child had died. This outcome may be disappointing to clinicians who are angry and wish to see the abuser punished as severely as possible, but it should not alter the finding that abuse had taken place and other children in the home require protection. Once a child has been declared brain dead, however, or when it is determined that further treatment would be futile (Freeman and Ferry, 1988), termination of life support, rather than treatment until cardiorespiratory arrest takes place, does not detract from a murder or manslaughter charge. Such charges are based on the degree of premeditation or negligence involved in the lethal act, not in its proximity to the time of death. In writing death notes and filling out death certificates, physicians can specify that injury was the cause of death and that brain swelling and cardiorespiratory arrest, for example, were not causes but only predictable sequelae of the injury.

THE AUTOPSY

Official responsibility for investigating suspicious or unexplained deaths varies with jurisdiction (Anonymous, 1989). In the United States, responsibility may rest with a coroner (generally an elected official without medical or forensic training) or a medical examiner, who is a physician with training in pathology. Medical examiners may serve only a local area such as a city or county, or there may be a single statewide office responsible for all death investigations.

Two important aspects of a medical examiner's role are the mandatory nature of the duties and the fact that these duties are not limited to an autopsy but include a comprehensive investigation into the cause of death. Statutes vary from area to area but, in general, the coroner or medical examiner has the authority to investigate any death that is sudden and unexpected, not caused by a readily recognizable disease, or for which there is a suspicion of violence or foul play. In these situations, next of kin should not be asked permission for an autopsy to be performed. Rather, they must be informed that one is required by law and that questions as to its necessity and extent must be addressed to the medical examiner. Likewise, next of kin should not be asked for permission to donate the patient's organs or other tissues unless the medical examiner agrees that doing so will not interfere with the investigation of the cause of death.

The autopsy itself can be disappointingly unrevealing in cases of suspected abuse, especially in young children. FBI homicide statistics (Table 16.3) show that no mechanism of injury is determined in a substantial proportion of cases of legally proven murder, and another large proportion involve mechanisms such as hyperthermia or asphyxiation that may produce few physical signs (Zumwalt and Hirsch, 1980; Norman et al., 1984). Head trauma may be difficult to diagnose because large concussive forces can cause death without causing skull fractures or even microscopically visible injury to the brain. Contre-coup injuries frequently found in adults who suffer head trauma are reportedly found less frequently in children (Lindenberg and Freytag, 1969). There may be few signs of asphyxia, especially in children who have no teeth. So-called gentle smothering may not result in the telltale injuries to the nose, lips, or buccal mucosa often found in older victims. Even drowning may be wet or dry (without or with spasm of the larynx); therefore, the absence of water in the lungs may not rule out drowning as the cause of death. Toxicology and electrolyte studies are important to discover poisonings or forced ingestions of water or salt (see Chapter 15). The vitreous humor of the eye can be sampled for electrolyte studies, and samples of blood, urine, bile, stomach contents, liver, kidney, brain, and lung can be saved in separate containers for toxin analysis. Clues from a death scene investigation are important in deciding when toxiocologic studies should be performed and which toxins should be suspected (Smialek and Lambros, 1988).

These difficulties with the autopsy itself emphasize the importance of other aspects of the medical examiner's investigation. The child's medical and social history may play a central role in the interpretation of autopsy findings. In cases of suspected suicide, for example, so-called psychological autopsies (Litman et al., 1963) have been used to augment pathologic data and improve accuracy in determination of the cause of death (Jobes et al., 1986). Importantly, they also may help compensate for biases in medical examiner judgments, such as a tendency to over- or underdetermine suicide as a cause of death. Krugman's review of a group of fatal abuse cases (1983–85) suggested the following list of points to look for in a child or family's history as clues to occult trauma:

- Inconsistent or vague accounts of how the child was injured or the sequence of events leading to the critical illness.
- A delay in seeking care, measured either from the time an injury took place or from the time that it would have been reasonable to recognize that the child was seriously ill. Krugman hypothesized that some abusive parents reacted promptly to their child's symptoms, but that those symptoms had occurred some-

time after a severe shaking or beating that itself should have triggered a call for help.
- A recent crisis in the family, including financial, legal, or interpersonal problems. As discussed in Chapter 17, a family history of drug or alcohol abuse, especially abuse of cocaine, may also be related to the violent death of a child.
- Some triggering act of the child, such as a problem toileting, a spell of inconsolable crying, a refusal to eat, or an act of physical aggression against the parent.

It is equally important to obtain as much information as possible about previous deaths, injuries, or illnesses of the injured child or of siblings. As noted above, parents may neglect to mention other children or the fact that siblings have been placed out of the home, and patterns of illness or injury potentially linking the deaths may consequently be missed.

Another important step in any abuse investigation, but especially in fatal cases, is a visit to the site where the child was either injured or discovered to be ill. Although the diagnostic power of such visits has at times been overstated (Bass et al., 1986), information vital to the investigation may often be found (Wagner, 1986). Neighbors can be questioned about aspects of a child's behavior, general care, health, or relations with parents. They may be able to describe injuries that were never brought to medical attention or that were purposely cared for at a site different from the one where the child usually received care. Exact descriptions or photographs can be obtained of beds, floors, or objects said to be involved in the injury. Critical issues include the composition of floors (wood versus concrete), whether they are covered with a rug, and, if so, the thickness of the rug. The height of furniture involved in falls, or of bathtub sides that a child is alleged to have climbed over, can also be measured. If the visit can take place promptly, families should be asked not to disturb anything at the site where the child's body was found. Impressions or stains in bedclothes may suggest the position in which the child died. The laundry and garbage can be checked for articles of clothing that are bloodstained or soiled with bodily fluids. When tapwater scalds are being investigated, measuring the accessibility of the water spigots and the temperature of the hot water (including how fast it gets hot) may reveal discrepancies in the history that has been provided. When the cause of death is completely unknown, the scene can be examined for evidence that the ambient temperature was extremely hot or cold or that fumes from a heater or flue pipe were present.

In some areas, very comprehensive evaluations of sudden deaths in childhood are available. In the area surrounding Sheffield, England, for example, information from police and autopsy reports, from a home visit by a physician, and from primary care providers for the entire family can be integrated into a single file and discussed confidentially with a child's parents (Taylor and Emery, 1982). This type of approach can greatly reduce the number of deaths that remain unexplained and offers the family a greater opportunity for counseling and necessary treatment. Unfortunately, this degree of coordination and thoroughness is not available in the majority of cases.

SIDS AND THE DIFFERENTIAL DIAGNOSIS OF SUDDEN, UNEXPLAINED DEATH OF CHILDREN

In developed countries, sudden infant death syndrome (SIDS) is the leading cause of infant death beyond the first month of life, accounting for about half of all mortality among children from 8 days to 1 year of age. Because it is so common and has no specific markers for diagnosis, it is frequently mentioned as a possible explanation when infants die unexpectedly. As its name implies, it is a cluster of phenomena without a known cause. A variety of causes have been postulated, most thought to relate to abnormal regulation of respiration and an impaired response to asphyxia during sleep.

SIDS is formally a diagnosis of exclusion, specifically, "the sudden death of any infant or young child that is unexpected by history and in which a thorough postmortem examination fails to demonstrate an adequate cause" (Hunt and Brouillette, 1987). A number of autopsy findings, such as pulmonary congestion or edema, thyroid petechiae, retained periadrenal brown fat, hepatic erythropoiesis, and brainstem scarring may be found with increased frequency in SIDS deaths but are not specific markers for the condition. Thus, an autopsy diagnosis of SIDS depends on the combination of negative findings and a suggestive premortem history.

Given the lack of a standard for diagnosis, the epidemiology of SIDS remains somewhat problematic. In general, however, the peak incidence of SIDS is felt to occur between age 9 and 12 weeks, with cases being rare in children under 1 month or older than 12 months. Only about 10% of SIDS deaths occur among children 6 months of age or older (Peterson, 1988). Death usually occurs at night, during sleep, and somewhat more commonly in winter. There is usually no previous illness or warning, although in many cases, possibly related to the winter predominance, there is mild upper respiratory infection at the time of death. Only a small proportion of children who die from SIDS are reported to have had a previous episode of apnea or an apparent life-threatening event, although when closely monitored in large-scale prospective studies, some have been found to have more frequent episodes of apnea or airway obstruction during feeding.

Some groups of infants, including black and Native American infants, those born at low birth weight, and those born to families of low socioeconomic status, do seem to be at higher risk of SIDS (Kelly and Shannon, 1982; Black et al., 1986). Children of intravenous drug abusers (see Chapter 17) also appear to be at increased risk, although this remains a matter of controversy. Unfortunately, some of these characteristics are risk factors for many other causes of morbidity, including child abuse.

Given the observed clustering of infanticide in families and the fact that previous deaths may have been ascribed to SIDS, is important to consider how often SIDS recurs within sibships. Infants are felt to be at an increased risk of SIDS if a sibling has previously died of the syndrome. In a self-reporting study of about 1100 mostly Caucasian families, Peterson and co-workers (1980) found 18 in which there had been a repetition of SIDS. The risk for each successive child born after the child who had died of SIDS was about 2%, about 10 times the United States national rate of about 2–5/1000. The risk of repetition was similar for successive siblings and for heterozygous and homozygous twins. In contrast, some case reports of simultaneous sudden death in twins have been closely investigated and felt to represent SIDS (Smialek, 1986). Some of these cases, however, had epidemiologic characteristics less often seen in SIDS, such as death in the daytime, or were marked by extreme economic deprivation.

The difficulty with this sort of analysis, of course, is that one is dealing with what is ultimately a subjective diagnosis. There is always the question of whether further investigation would have found other clues, perhaps psychosocial, that could have led to a different determination of the cause of death. In the study by Peterson and co-workers (1980), for example, the mothers of families in which there had been a repeat SIDS death were much more likely to have had a half- or step-sibling than were mothers of families in which there had been only one SIDS death. Perhaps this was a marker for a more disrupted early childhood, which might be a risk factor for later infanticide. Emery and Taylor (1986), from the Sheffield area of England, reported on a series of 12 families in which two or more "cot deaths" were reported to have occurred. By their analysis, the deaths were truly unexplained in only two of the families. In five infanticide was probably involved, and in the rest familial diseases, neglect, or extreme poverty played a role. These findings came from detailed autopsies and from interviews with the families and their health care providers, although the conclusions were still to a large degree subjective.

The Sheffield data give what is perhaps the best estimate of the extent to which infanticide is misdiagnosed as SIDS. From 1975 through 1984, there were 106 unexpected postneonatal deaths in the Sheffield area (Emery, 1986). Of these, five deaths were known to have resulted from nonaccidental injury. After investigation, another 10 (about 10% of all of the unexpected deaths) were felt most likely, but not unequivocally, to have been caused by abuse.

Numerous case reports have discussed children who were said to have suffered apnea, seizures, pallor, or cyanosis at home and who were later found to have been smothered or poisoned by their parents. These cases are taken to be examples of the Munchausen syndrome by proxy (Chapter 15) and raise the question of "near-miss" SIDS (or an "apparent life-threatening event" [ALTE]) in the differential diagnosis of intentional injury. An ALTE is generally defined as an episode in which an infant is found "apparently dead" and requires vigorous stimulation or mouth-to-mouth resuscitation before normal breathing resumes. Afterwards, the infant appears normal, and no obvious cause for the episode is found (Dunne and Matthews, 1987). The large majority of these episodes respond to stimulation alone. About 90% of children with ALTEs have a first episode before the age of 4 months, and about half have one or more subsequent episodes.

One difficulty involved in interpreting ALTEs comes from the problem of establishing when they have actually occurred. Krongrad and O'Neill (1986) monitored 20 infants thought to be at high risk for apnea. The children were monitored at home with either recording devices or telephone telemetry to preserve electrocardiographic data. Parents reported 93 episodes that they considered to be real on the basis of changes in breathing, decreased muscle tone, or color; for 11 episodes the parents gave the child tactile stimulation, but none were felt to require cardiopulmonary resuscitation (CPR). None of the children were found to have electrocardiographic changes suggestive of cardiorespiratory distress during the episodes, and on follow-up all were alive at more than 1 year of age.

One reason that this study may have had negative findings is that other studies have found that the subgroup of children who apparently require CPR to end an ALTE are those at higher risk of death rather than those who end the episode spontaneously or require only stimulation. In a group of 166 infants followed after 1 or more ALTEs, Kelly and Shannon (1982) reported 7 deaths among 69 children (10%) who had required CPR but none among 97 who had required only stimulation. Among the group who required CPR, the mortality rate was further increased (up to rates of 25–50%) among children who had multiple episodes, who were siblings of SIDS victims, or who developed seizures (Oren et al., 1986).

These risk factors, however, overlap considerably with the presentation of children who are intentionally injured by their parents. Rosen and co-workers (1986) were able to retrospectively identify factors that were related both to death and to a high likelihood that the episodes were the result of intentional injury. In a group of 17 infants who were all said to have required CPR to terminate prolonged episodes of apnea, they determined which of the children's caretakers had been present when an episode began and who else had subsequently witnessed the episode before it was terminated. In 11 of the 17 cases, the episode was witnessed and treated by the parent alone, or others were present when the episode began and witnessed the entire resuscitation. There were no deaths in this group and no siblings with similar conditions. Only two of the infants, when hospitalized for observation, had a subsequent event requiring resuscitation in the hospital. This was in contrast to the six cases in which the parent was alone at the time the episode started but others were summoned and witnessed the resuscitation. Importantly, some of the parents in this group initially claimed that others had witnessed the onset of the episode, but this was later found not to be the case. There were three deaths in this group; in the other three cases no further episodes occurred after the children were removed from their parents. Four of the five children had siblings with similar histories, and all of the children had repeat episodes requiring resuscitation in the hospital. In two of these episodes, viewed with a hidden camera, the parent was seen to provoke the spells. All of the other in-hospital episodes began when the parent and child were alone. None of the children had any demonstrable cardiorespiratory abnormality between episodes. The two parents observed harming their children fit the described characteristics of mothers in the Munchausen syndrome by proxy: they were seemingly model parents, cheerfully cooperative with the medical staff in the hospital and agreeable to all diagnostic procedures, even the most invasive.

The frequency of abuse as a cause of ALTEs is not known. Kahn and co-workers (1988), in a review of 2779 infants admitted to a Belgian hospital for evaluation of ALTEs, found four cases in which the children had apparently been smothered and one in which an infant had been given insulin injections by his emotionally disturbed mother. Overall, however, they felt that only about 40% of the cases met the diagnosis of ALTE given above in that no apparent cause for the events could be found. For the remaining 60% of the cases, they identified a specific medical condition that appeared to have caused the episode.

Overlying, the accidental smothering of a child who is sleeping in bed with an adult, is frequently raised as a possible explanation for unexplained infant deaths. The possibility that such tragedies can occur is part of the Western cultural heritage (see, for example, William Butler Yeats's "The Ballad of Moll Magee"). Bass and co-workers (1986), in their study of death scene investigations, felt that 6 of 26 cases of unexpected infant deaths originally diagnosed as SIDS had, in fact, been caused by overlying. In two cases, obese mothers were said to have fallen asleep while nursing their children; the children presumably were smothered under the mother's breast. In three cases the mothers were said to have been in an altered sensory state (one "exhausted," one suspected of drug use, and another with a history of syncopal attacks), and in one the child may have become entrapped in a makeshift bed composed of plywood and pieces of foam rubber. Although all of these explanations seem plausible, they were supported by only circumstantial evidence.

Cosleeping of parents and children is quite common in many societies. Lozoff and colleagues (1984) interviewed families with children under 4 who were coming for well-child care in Cleveland. They found that 43% of white families and 86% of black families said that a child had slept at least part of the night in the parents' bed one or more times in the past month. Nearly half of the black families reported that a child slept with the parents all night on a regular basis (three or more times a week). Given that cosleeping is this common, it seems unlikely that it is particularly hazardous except, perhaps, when the parents are impaired in some way, such as by drug or alcohol use. Unfortunately, the sample studied by Lozoff et al. was not large enough to address issues of physical morbidity stemming from the practice.

A related explanation often offered for deaths of undetermined cause is that the children smothered in the bedclothes or between a mattress and the sides of a crib. Strangulations on hanging crib toys, between crib slats, and under loose-fitting mattresses have been well documented, although they should be much less likely if parents have the means to purchase infant toys and furniture that conform to present-day safety standards (Baker and Fisher, 1980). In contrast, a healthy term infant placed prone should be capable of clearing the nose, and the risk of asphyxia should be present only if the bedclothes include plastic sheeting or other materials that do not allow the diffusion of air.

PREVENTION OF FATALITIES

Preventing child abuse fatalities has proved to be a difficult task. As many as a third of known victims are already involved with a local child protective service system, and an additional proportion have been previously reported for suspected abuse, although at the time the suspicion could not be substantiated (Mitchell, 1987). A lack of previous reports or system involvement is not necessarily comforting, however. In their study of child abuse fatalities in Georgia, Jason and Andereck (1983) found no difference between fatal and nonfatal abuse cases in the incidence of previous reports.

Although many protective service agencies have elaborate processes for reviewing fatalities among active cases, little information has been gained to help predict lethal abuse. In addition, the heterogeneity of apparent causes of fatalities makes it difficult to make a simple list of warning signs that might prompt preventive efforts. Some factors that appear to be markers of increased risk can be described, although their predictive value for any one case is not known:

- Parents' excessive, vocalized fear of hurting a child or that the child's health (when the child is doing well) is somehow in danger. Probes for these fears, when they are suspected by the clinician but not vocalized, include: "I think you are very worried about your child's health. Has he/she ever been seriously ill?"; "Have you ever been afraid that you might lose your child?"; "When you were pregnant, did you ever worry that you or your baby might die?"; "Has anyone else you know ever been seriously ill?"; "Have you ever lost a child or a pregnancy?" (Green, 1988).
- A mother's own suicidal thoughts.
- A prompt replacement (with another pregnancy) of a child who has died under unclear circumstances.
- An infant who is gaining weight slowly or has a difficult or overly passive temperament coupled with a parent who is isolated, stressed in other ways, and may have been emotionally deprived as a child.
- Children who are brought repeatedly for vague or mysterious medical problems, for minor injuries that are inappropriate for their ages (especially unusual bruises or broken bones in infants), or for behavioral or feeding

problems that seem minor in comparison to the parents' level of concern.
- Families in which one parent (usually the father) appears to have little involvement in child rearing.

Reviews of reported cases of fatalities (Greenland, 1980) and discussions with fatally abusive parents (Korbin, 1987) have also suggested some guidelines for professional intervention in cases where severe abuse has already occurred and the risk of fatalities appears to be high:

- It is important not to rely on medical judgments about an infant's health status that are made by nonmedical personnel making home visits. Frequent office visits or in-home assessments by health professionals are required to monitor growth and to look for evidence of injury.
- Parental concerns for minor medical problems should never be taken lightly. They may be calls for emotional help or represent concern for the sequelae of an intentional injury and should be seen urgently.
- The person offering support or therapy for the family should not be the same person who is taking responsibility for the child's interests. The latter individual needs to communicate closely with the family but needs to avoid becoming overly sympathetic with or aligned with the parents. In addition, the parents need their own support system. Many have poor self-esteem and see concern for the child as evidence that no one cares about them.
- The period immediately following the reunification of a parent and child who have been separated (for foster placement or because the parent was incarcerated, for example) may have an extremely high risk of fatal abuse. The parent's idealized vision of again having custody of the child may be dashed, and an older child may display ambivalence or even hostility about being moved back to the parent's home.

References

Anonymous. Child homicide—United States. MMWR 1982;31:292–294.
Anonymous. Jury rejects rare defense, convicts woman. The Evening Sun [Baltimore], 13 Nov 1988:A3.
Anonymous. Death investigation—United States, 1987. MMWR 1989;38:1–4.
Baker SP, Fisher RS. Childhood asphyxiation by choking or suffocation. JAMA 1980;244:1343–1346.
Bass M, Kravath RE, Glass L. Death-scene investigation in sudden infant death. N Engl J Med 1986;315:100–105.
Black L, David RJ, Brouillette RT, Hunt CE. Effects of birth weight and ethnicity on incidence of sudden infant death syndrome. J Pediatr 1986;108:209–214.
Blaser MJ. Epidemiologic characteristics of child homicides in Atlanta, 1970–1980. Pediatrician 1983–85;12:63–67.
Bloch H. Abandonment, infanticide, and filicide: an overview of inhumanity to children. Am J Dis Child 1988;142:1058–1060.
Dean C, Kendell RE. The symptomatology of puerperal illnesses. Br J Psychiatry 1981;139:128–133.
Dunne K, Matthews T. Near-miss sudden infant death syndrome: clinical findings and management. Pediatrics 1987;79:889–893.
Emery JL. Infanticide, filicide, and cot death. Arch Dis Child 1985;60:505–507.
Emery JL. Families in which two or more cot deaths have occurred. Lancet 1986;313–315.
Emery JL, Taylor EM. Investigation of SIDS [Letter]. N Engl J Med 1986;315:1676.
Freeman JM, Ferry PC. New brain death guidelines for children: further confusion. Pediatrics 1988;81:301–303.
Green M. Vulnerable children, vulnerable mothers. Contemp Pediatr 1988;Nov:102–116.
Green M, Solnit M. Reactions to the threatened loss of a child: a vulnerable child syndrome. Pediatrics 1964;34:58–66.
Greenland C. Lethal family situations: an international comparison of deaths from child abuse. In: Anthony EJ, Chiland CC, eds. The child in his family. Vol. 6. New York: John Wiley & Sons, 1980:389–408.
Herzog A, Detre T. Psychotic reactions associated with childbirth. Dis Nerv Syst 1976;37:229–235.
Hopkins J, Marcus M, Campbell SB. Postpartum depression: a critical review. Psychol Bull 1984;95:498–515.
Hunt CE, Brouillette RT. Sudden infant death syndrome: 1987 perspective. J Pediatr 1987;110:669–678.
Jason J, Andereck ND. Fatal child abuse in Georgia: the epidemiology of severe physical child abuse. Child Abuse Negl 1983;7:1–9.
Jason J, Gilliland JC, Tyler CW Jr. Homicide as a cause of pediatric mortality in the United States. Pediatrics 1983;72:191–197.
Jobes DA, Berman AL, Josselson AR. The impact of psychological autopsies on medical examiners' determination of manner of death. J Forensic Sci 1986;31:177–189.
Kahn A, Rebuffat E, Sottiaux M, Blum D. Management of an infant with an apparent life-threatening event. Pediatrician 1988;15:204–211.

Kelly DH, Shannon DC. Sudden infant death syndrome and near sudden infant death syndrome: a review of the literature, 1964 to 1982. Pediatr Clin North Am 1982;29:1241–1261.

Korbin JE. Incarcerated mothers' perceptions and interpretations of their fatally maltreated children. Child Abuse Negl 1987;11:397–407.

Krongrad E, O'Neill L. Near miss sudden infant death syndrome episodes? A clinical and electocardiographic correlation. Pediatrics 1986;77:811–815.

Krugman RD. Fatal child abuse: analysis of 24 cases. Pediatrician 1983–85;12:68–72.

Lindenberg R, Freytag E. Morphology of brain lesion from blunt trauma in early infancy. Arch Pathol 1969;87:298–305.

Litman RE, Curphey T, Shneidman ES, Farberrow NL, Tabachnick N. Investigations of equivocal suicides. JAMA 1963;184:924–929.

Lozoff B, Wolf AW, Davis NS. Cosleeping in urban families with young children in the United States. Pediatrics 1984;74:171–182.

Mandell F, McClain M, Reece RM. Sudden and unexpected death: the pediatrician's response. Am J Dis Child 1987;141:748–750.

Mitchell L. Child abuse and neglect fatalities: a review of the problem and strategies for reform (working paper 838). Chicago: National Center for Child Abuse Prevention Research, National Committee for Prevention of Child Abuse, 1987.

National Center on Child Abuse and Neglect. Study findings: study of national incidence and prevalence of child abuse and neglect: 1988. Washington, DC: US Government Printing Office, 1988.

National Center for Health Statistics. Vital statistics of the United States, 1982. Vol. II. Mortality, part A. Department of Health and Human Services Publ. (PHS) 86-1122. Washington, DC: US Government Printing Office, 1986:Table 2–6.

Norman MG, Newman DE, Smialek JE, Horembala EJ. The postmortem examination on the abused child. Perspect Pediatr Pathol 1984;8:313–343.

Oliver JE. Dead children from problem families in NE Wiltshire. Br Med J 1983;286:115–117.

Oren J, Kelly D, Shannon DC. Identification of a high-risk group for sudden infant death syndrome among infants who were resuscitated for sleep apnea. Pediatrics 1986;77:495–499.

Peterson DR. Clinical implications of sudden infant death syndrome epidemiology. Pediatrician 1988;15:198–203.

Peterson DR, Chinn NM, Fisher LD. The sudden infant death syndrome: repetition in families. J Pediatr 1980;97:265–267.

Resnick PJ. Child murder by parents: a psychiatric review of filicide. Am J Psychiatry 1969;126:325–334.

Rosen CL, Frost JD, Glaze DG. Child abuse and recurrent infant apnea. J Pediatr 1986;109:1065–1067.

Rule S. A Zimbabwe issue: killing of babies. New York Times 17 May 1987:11.

Scheiner AP, Sexton ME, Rockwood J, Sullivan D, Davis H. The vulnerable child syndrome: fact and theory. J Dev Behav Pediatr 1985;6:298–301.

Smialek JE. Forensic medicine in the emergency department. Emerg Med Clin North Am 1983;1:693–704.

Smialek JE. Simultaneous sudden infant death syndrome in twins. Pediatrics 1986;77:816–821.

Smialek JE, Lambros Z. Investigation of sudden infant deaths. Pediatrician 1988;15:191–197.

Steele B. Psychodynamic factors in child abuse. In: Kempe CH, Helfer RE, eds. The battered child. 3rd ed. Chicago: University of Chicago Press, 1980:49–85.

Sullivan R. Jury, citing mother's condition, clears her in deaths of 2 babies. New York Times 1 Oct 1988:B1.

Taylor EM, Emery JL. Two-year study of the causes of post-perinatal deaths classified in terms of preventability. Arch Dis Child 1982;57:668–673.

Wagner GN. Crime scene investigation in child-abuse cases. Am J Forensic Med Pathol 1986;7:94–99.

Wallace A. After 9 deaths in 14 years, mother arrested. New York Times 8 Feb 1986:1.

Zumwalt RE, Hirsch CS. Subtle fatal child abuse. Hum Pathol 1980;11:167–174.

17 Suspected Abuse or Neglect in the Prenatal and Perinatal Periods

INTRODUCTION

The growing fetus is vulnerable to physical assault, exposure to teratogens, and general medical or nutritional neglect. Difficulty deciding when the fetus should be regarded as a separate individual and the obvious conflict between maternal and fetal rights have made this an area to which the label "child abuse" has only gingerly been applied. Although injury to the fetus probably constitutes the single largest avoidable form of harm to children, it clearly illustrates how the definition of maltreatment is shaped by cultural and political constraints.

Condon (1986), for example, separates the issue of elective abortion from the problem of fetal abuse. Although many see no difference between these two acts, Condon and others (Robertson, 1983) take the position that elective abortion is an act justified by a balancing of fetal and maternal rights and directed against the state of pregnancy per se. In their view, fetal abuse, in contrast, is an act triggered by the perception of the fetus as a specific, separate being, often at a point in pregnancy when the parents have presumably made a choice not to have an abortion and thus signaled their intent to produce a healthy child. On the other hand, supporters of women's rights strongly defend the right to abortion but are wary of the fetal rights movement as a further attempt to control women and to reduce their status vis à vis men and children. They contend that a balancing of fetal and maternal rights overlooks the strong tradition of respect for an individual's rights to self-determination and bodily integrity as well as the fact that society generally does not assign individuals a duty to rescue persons in distress, however laudable such actions might be (Gallagher, 1987). The fetus's needs are hardly to be neglected, but they should be approached from the direction of changes in societal and clinical policies that improve the environment for pregnancy rather than by developing new methods to coerce a woman to alter her behavior.

Although fetal abuse is usually thought of as involving women, men may be either active or passive participants. The male role is most explicit when it involves direct blows to the mother, particularly to the abdomen, but it may also involve facilitating maternal behaviors such as drug or alcohol abuse or participation in denial of the pregnancy and subsequent lack of material support or prenatal care. Lack of emotional support from the father or other family members may encourage maternal ambivalence toward a pregnancy and slow or stop the woman's process of assuming a mothering role. Maternal attachment to the developing child does not come instantaneously and requires validation from the mother's partner and extended family.

Gelles and co-workers, in their research on family violence, found evidence that spouse abuse, and thus physical attacks on the fetus as well, occurs with increased frequency and intensity during pregnancy (Gelles, 1975). Fathers may see the fetus as a rival for the mother's attention, or they may see pregnancy as the sign of a commitment they are unwilling to make. Even in more mature relationships, a father may react adversely to the changes in his partner's appearance and behavior that normally accompany pregnancy.

Condon suggests that the traditional dichotomy between wanted and unwanted pregnancies can be misleading. A pregnancy may be wanted initially but only because at that time it represents an idealized fantasy through which a partner will be retained or the mother will gain someone (the baby) who can give her unconditional love. Later, when the realities of pregnancy become clear, the same fetus can come to be seen as attacking the mother or as diverting love and attention from the mother rather than providing them for her.

Passivity is a frequently found characteristic of mothers who kill their newborns (Resnick, 1970) and may play a role in fetal neglect. The failure to use contraceptives or to terminate an unwanted pregnancy may be part of a more pervasive pattern of victimization and inability to seek help or take action.

SUBSTANCE ABUSE DURING PREGNANCY

The fetal alcohol syndrome (FAS) is the leading known cause of mental retardation and birth defects and it is, by far, the leading preventable cause. Overall, the full syndrome is found in 1–2/1000 live births, although the risk is 10–20 times as great among women who drink heavily (about six "hard" drinks a day) (Anonymous, 1984). The three major manifestations of FAS include microcephaly with mild to moderate mental retardation, intrauterine and postnatal growth deficiency, and characteristic facial abnormalities such as short palpebral fissures, a diminished or absent philtrum, and a hypoplastic upper lip (Clarren and Smith, 1978).

Studies suggest that there is a dose-response relationship between the extent to which the syndrome is expressed and the amount of alcohol consumed. Unfortunately, these studies do not suggest a threshold below which alcohol consumption is safe or establish whether it is chronic ingestion, peak levels, or both that are teratogenic. Distinct alcohol effects have been found in children whose mothers reported only moderate drinking. Drinking little or no alcohol during a pregnancy is the most prudent course. Although, women generally report drinking less than men, in one recent survey about 5% of all women over age 18 said that they had five or more drinks in one sitting at least once a week (Maryland Center for Health Statistics, 1985).

Cigarette smoke is one of the few avoidable teratogens that is even more prevalent than alcohol. About 30–40% of women over 18 report that they smoke. The average smoker among both men and women consumes 15–20 cigarettes a day (Maryland Center for Health Statistics, 1985). Smoking more than five cigarettes a day (about a quarter of a pack) has been linked to symmetrical growth retardation of the developing fetus (Nieburg et al., 1985). Estimates are that 20–40% of the prevalence of below-normal birth weight is attributable to smoking (Rush and Kass, 1972; Meyer et al., 1976).

Drugs of abuse present some of the most difficult questions of fetal maltreatment because they are strongly associated with other health and social risks. Distinct syndromes of fetal drug exposure have been difficult to describe, both because drug users may not give accurate histories of what they have taken and because many use more than one drug. In addition, street drugs may be adulterated with phencyclidine, diazepam, quinine, procaine, chalk, sugar, talc, or other substances that may themselves have effects on the developing child.

Until recently, the best defined syndromes of fetal-maternal drug dependency involved use of opiates such as heroin. The introduction of methadone, a long-acting, orally administered opiate, created the possibility of shifting users away from some of the social and medical complications of intravenous drug use, although it does not necessarily control the desire for simultaneous use of other, nonopiate drugs (Newman, 1987). Methadone, at least in high doses, appears to result in more severe neonatal withdrawal and perinatal complications, but it offers an opportunity for an addicted woman to improve her nutritional and social status and thus to generally improve the outcome of her pregnancy (Keith et al., 1986).

The rapidly increasing use of cocaine, especially in its smokable form known as crack, has posed new problems in the detection and control of fetal exposure. Crack is less expensive and more available than opiates, and it appears to be much more powerfully and rapidly addictive. Because it is a stimulant and is often used communally, crack has been associated with a greatly increased frequency of sexual activity among its users and thus a greatly increased risk of pregnancy and the acquisition of sexually transmitted diseases. Sudden increases in the prevalence of syphilis have been linked to crack use, as has concern that sex in "crack houses" is a major means of heterosexual transmission of the human immunodeficiency virus (HIV) (Kerr, 1988a,b).

Perhaps most alarming, crack appears to be responsible for recently observed increases in the proportion of drug addicts who are women (Kerr, 1988a,b). Women who would not use intravenous drugs such as heroin apparently are willing to smoke crack. Some observers fear that crack use will seriously jeopardize the stability of female-headed households, which predominate among poor minority families. Crack use has been reported to be so compelling that women may quit their jobs, sell their possessions in order to buy drugs, or abandon their children for extended periods. Crack also appears to be associated with an increased level of interpersonal violence, linked either to the effects of the drug itself or to conflicts among drug traffickers. Increases in the proportion of fatal child abuse and neglect cases that are associated with drug use have been attributed to crack.

Cocaine use in pregnancy can have particularly serious consequences. In addition to nutritional and infectious risks posed by the drug-associated life style, pregnant women who use cocaine have an increased incidence of spontaneous abortion, placental abruption, and premature labor (Chasnoff et al., 1985). Children exposed to cocaine during gestation appear to have an increased rate of genitourinary malformations (Chasnoff and Chisum, 1987), abnormal behavior in the neonatal period, and possibly an increased risk of sleep disorders (Chasnoff, 1986). It is also thought that infants exposed to cocaine in utero have an increased risk dying from sudden infant death syndrome, although the extent of this risk is not known and may not be higher than would be expected from risk factors associated with maternal drug use (Zuckerman et al., 1988). Table 17.1 summarizes the consequences of in utero exposure to commonly encountered drugs of abuse.

Unlike heroin, for which methadone maintenance offers a path to control, there is no substitute for cocaine that can be used in detoxification programs. Cocaine addiction appears to be much harder to control than heroin or alcohol addiction, with much higher rates of recidivism and dropout from treatment programs (Kolata, 1988).

CLINICAL INTERVENTIONS

Case Findings during Pregnancy

Some families in which a pregnancy is being neglected may appear normal, although for many the first sign of a problem is in the use of prenatal services. Some mothers come for care later in gestation, denying that they knew they were going to have a baby; others never come for medical care but instead give birth at home and subsequently attempt to hide or kill the child. In most of these cases, it is not the mother alone who is placing the fetus at risk, but also those around her who deny or fail to support the pregnancy (Ratner, 1985).

Standard prenatal care includes warnings that various substances or activities may be harmful to the growing fetus. Although such warnings may produce some behavioral change in low-risk groups, they are unlikely to help individuals with serious addictions or poor support for their pregnancies. In these situations, education when offered alone may stimulate guilt and denial rather than healthful change (Chisum, 1986). Instead, education should be linked to identification of specific substance abuse or emotional problems and coupled with supportive, empathetic care.

As mentioned previously, asking whether a given pregnancy was planned or is now desired may have limited use in understanding a family's feelings toward the unborn child. It is important to ask specifically how the parents think other family members feel about the pregnancy and whether they perceive support, antagonism, or ambivalence. The parents should be asked, separately if necessary, how they feel the pregnancy is affecting them and whether they perceive it as depriving them of social or sexual interactions or posing a threat to their family economics or life style. These questions can be asked in an empathetic, permissive way. For example, an expectant father could be asked, "Most men feel, at least some time, that their wives pay more attention to the baby in their belly than they do to them. Do you ever feel that way?" Positive answers can be used as a lead-in for further discussion, and emphatic negative responses can gently be tested for denial. If the clinician suspects that a woman may, in fact, have focused a great deal of anger or resentment on the fetus, Condon (1986) suggests the following question: "Some pregnant women find that they (or their partner) get so frustrated and irritated with the pregnancy that they want to take it out on the baby. Have you ever felt that way?"

Constructing a simple family genogram and asking about the social and emotional relationships among its members may also help elicit feelings toward the pregnancy. Simple genograms are usually a routine part of prenatal care as a means of identifying heritable risks to the fetus. This discussion can be extended to questions such as the circumstances of the parents' own birth and their perceptions of their own childhood nurturing. It can also be a chance to find out which relatives live nearby

Table 17.1. Observed Sequelae of Fetal Drug Exposure According to Type of Drug Predominantly Used[a]

Drug	Congenital Malformations	Decreased Intrauterine Growth	Abortion, Abruption, or Premature Labor	Neonatal Withdrawal or Symptoms	Risk of SIDS	Mental Retardation or Developmental Delay
Opiates		Yes, independent of nutritional status		Yes, can be prolonged for months	Appears to be increased	Probably none directly attributable
Cocaine	Probably yes, genitourinary	Uncertain	Yes	Yes, shorter duration than opiates	Increased rate of sleep problems	May be persistent motor problems
Psychotropics (PCP)	Uncertain			Yes, shorter duration than opiates		Probable decreased fine motor, language, and adaptive skills
Alcohol	Yes, FAS	Yes		Yes		Mental retardation part of FAS; less affected children may have behavior or learning problems
Cigarette smoking		Yes, but possible confounding with highly related use of alcohol	Yes			
Marijuana	Possible	Probably yes		Yes		?Ophthalmologic/visual abnormalities

[a] Data from references cited in text and Braude MC, Szeto HH, Kuhn CM, et al. Perinatal effects of drugs of abuse. Fed Proc 1987;46:2446-2453; Cregler LI, Mark H. Medical complications of cocaine abuse. N Engl J Med 1986;1495-1500. FAS, Fetal alcohol syndrome; PCP, phencyclidine; SIDS, sudden infant death syndrome.

and with whom there may be some long-standing disputes that could have a bearing on support for the pregnancy.

Self-reports of alcohol or substance abuse usually lead clinicians to underestimate the extent of an individual's problems. Several techniques may make it easier for parents to disclose current or past activities. Starting with a general conversation about medical and social problems may both elicit clues about dysfunctional behavior and help establish rapport between the physician and the parent. In some settings, particularly those in which clinicians are also probing for risk factors associated with HIV infection, anonymous questionnaires can be used. The questionnaires can be filled out in private and then destroyed after the contents have been discussed.

Standardized screening questionnaires have been successfully used in the diagnosis of alcoholism and other drug dependencies. One instrument that has gained wide acceptance is the Michigan Alcoholism Screening Test (MAST) (Selzer, 1971). The MAST has 24 questions that require yes-no answers. It usually takes about 5 minutes to administer and does not ask how much an individual drinks, a question that is generally felt to yield unreliable answers. Rather, it asks how often the individual has symptoms or life style changes that are related to alcohol use. MAST questions include "Has drinking ever created problems between you and your wife, husband, and parent, or other relative?" and "Do you drink before noon fairly often?" The MAST can be used to probe for other substance abuse problems by replacing "alcohol" in each of the questions by "drugs" or some specific substance. It can also be given to a proxy respondent who knows the patient well.

Another instrument, which is shorter than the MAST and can be used as a screening device, is the CAGE, a series of four questions that also focus on life-style alterations that may be engendered by substance abuse (Mayfield et al., 1974; Ewing, 1984). The name of the instrument comes from key words in each of its four questions:

- Have you ever felt that you should *cut* down on your drinking?
- Have people *annoyed* you by criticizing your drinking?
- Have you ever felt bad or *guilty* about your drinking?
- Have you ever had a drink first thing in the morning to steady your nerves or to get rid of a hangover (an *eyeopener*)?

Positive answers to two or more of these questions are felt to be relatively specific for problems with alcohol abuse (Halliday et al., 1986). Glibness, avoidance, anger, and defensiveness when discussing substance abuse issues are felt to be particular indicators of problems. Patients who say that they could stop anytime or do not need the drugs or alcohol they are using are very likely to be addicted (Whitfield et al., 1986).

Clinicians can also probe for medical problems that may be clues to drug abuse. These include a history of hospitalizations for hepatitis, cellulitis, pneumonia, and other complications of drug use or an obstetrical history suggestive of drug effects.

Screening of blood and urine for traces of drugs and alcohol can help confirm concerns about substance abuse, but testing must be done in an ethically acceptable manner. If a patient appears to be acutely intoxicated, especially at the time of delivery, testing without consent may be justifiable, since treatment decisions must be based on accurate knowledge of the patient's condition (Colquitt et al., 1987). Other patients should be asked for consent to screening, as they would be asked for consent to any other laboratory test. Talking with the patient about what has led the clinician to be concerned for drug use and why exact knowledge of present drug levels will help best manage the pregnancy may be effective in gaining consent.

In performing toxicology tests, it is important to know the characteristics of the tests being used and the metabolism of the drugs involved. Blood tests for alcohol may detect only very recent use, for example, while metabolites of marijuana, because this drug is stored in body fat, may be excreted in the urine of heavy users for several days after the last use. The very sensitive screening tests used to detect trace amounts of drug metabolites in urine must be confirmed with more specific tests (Council on Scientific Affairs, 1987). Many clinicians believe that a carefully conducted interview is a more sensitive tool for detecting drug use than are toxicology screens.

Goals for Treatment during Pregnancy

Many treatment goals for at-risk pregnancies are similar to those for lower-risk groups. Mothers can be helped to obtain proper nutrition and health care, sometimes with specific counseling and assistance with enrollment in programs such as WIC (Women, Infants, and Children, the federally sponsored nutrition supplementation program) or Medicaid.

Parenting and preparation for childbirth education may be especially critical for high-risk parents. Drug-using parents especially may seek escape from the discomforts of labor and delivery, and childbirth classes (with training in Lamaze or other techniques) can help reduce fear and offer an alternative to drugs as a means of feeling in control. Parenting classes can build confidence by supplying practical information about child care but can also give special attention to questions of infant temperament and how behavior may be altered by drug or alcohol withdrawal. Again, helping the parents anticipate these problems may help alleviate guilt and increase tolerance for what could be an especially irritable and difficult infant. These activities are important on another level because they involve the parents in a community of care that can provide nurturing for themselves and support for the pregnancy.

Drug and alcohol detoxification are often seen as desirable goals for the parents, but, at least for opiates, even slow detoxification during pregnancy may have risks for the fetus. Withdrawal from opiates in the first and third trimesters may be particularly dangerous, increasing the risk of spontaneous abortion and premature labor (Rementeria and Nunag, 1973). Pregnant opiate addicts can be converted to methadone maintenance with beneficial effects on nutrition and other medical and social problems. There is some evidence that the methadone dose can be safely decreased in the second trimester; for patients using moderate or low doses, however, detoxification may best be reserved until after delivery.

Some high-risk mothers, especially if they are homeless, malnourished, or appear to have other medical problems, may benefit from a short, acute care hospitalization early in pregnancy or at the time the pregnancy is discovered (Iennarella et al., 1986). If appropriate resources are available in the hospital, a complete social, nutritional, and medical evaluation can take place, with an opportunity to coordinate services that will be needed during the remainder of the pregnancy. Such hospitalizations must be handled carefully, however, lest they serve only as opportunities for confrontation between the patient and the hospital staff. The patient should be helped to see the hospitalization as supportive and not punitive. If there is a drug or alcohol problem, plans should be made for adequate maintenance and open discussion of the patient's fear of withdrawal. Hospital staff members must meet frequently to coordinate their efforts and to ensure that the patient is not able to generate antagonisms among them regarding the treatment plan or the reason for admission. Drug-addicted patients, like parents who abuse children, evoke strong emotions among health care workers, often recruiting both strong allies and hostile adversaries.

There must also be prior discussion of how the staff will react to hostile or abusive behavior on the part of the patient, since such reactions may be provoked by drug withdrawal, staff-patient problems, or the low self-esteem and ambivalence often associated with drug dependency. Immediate responses may include reasonable limit setting for behavior within the hospital, perhaps coupled with an unusually lenient policy of allowing the patient to leave the hospital "against medical advice" but with an invitation to return. Most important, the staff should meet immediately to determine why the outburst occurred and how that information can be used to better understand the patient and her needs.

LEGAL CONSIDERATIONS

In some cases, clinicians may believe that a mother is either deliberately harming her unborn child or disregarding advice that could result in minimizing risks. Legal intervention is often considered, but its success is highly dependent on local legal precedent and attitudes.

It is only within the past few decades that the fetus has gained some consideration as a potential individual separate from the mother. Some legal scholars have seen in the United States Supreme Court's historic abortion decision, Roe v. Wade, a recognition of fetal interests that might be balanced against maternal rights (Robertson, 1983). Not every scholar has seen the opinion in this light, however (Gallagher, 1987). Most courts, in fact, have not granted rights to the unborn, although a few cases suggest settings in which some rights might be recognized. Although a hardly universal approach, some courts have used cases involving neonatal drug withdrawal to recognize some "right to begin life with a sound body and mind" (In the matter concerning Baby X, a minor, 293 N.W. 2d 736, 1980). Some courts also recognize the right of a child, once born, to take legal action against a third party (such as a mother's physician or employer) for "wrongful life," i.e., the responsibility for some prenatal event that prevented the child from being born without as sound a mind and body as would otherwise have been possible (Fleisher, 1987; Anonymous, 1988). In some jurisdictions, the child must be born alive in order for action to be taken; in others, the allegedly harmful event must have happened at a point in gestation when the fetus would have been viable. Other courts, however, have allowed claims of harm earlier in pregnancy and even claims of harm to the mother that occurred prior to conception that subsequently resulted in fetal injury (such as negligent Rh sensitization).

Responsibility for prenatal injury has been extended, although to a much more limited extent, to the fetus's mother. Potential cases of in utero abuse or neglect can be broadly divided into two categories: one in which the child is still in utero and the other in which the child has been born but injury in utero is alleged to have occurred. The thrust of the first type is generally the prevention of immediate risk to the developing fetus. The child's mother is felt to be engaging in some activity (or neglecting others, such as nutrition or prenatal care) that could potentially harm the fetus. The second type generally asks a court to find in the mother's behavior during pregnancy sufficient cause for seeking protection from further or potential harm for the now born child.

There is little firm legal precedent or explicit law regarding fetal abuse. Information about many potentially applicable cases is available only in the form of accounts in the popular press. While some cases have reached the level of appeals courts and thus received thoughtful deliberation, many have apparently been hastily decided almost literally at the bedside, without adequate legal representation for all parties (Kolder et al., 1987).

Allegations of abuse or neglect while a child is still in utero are obviously problematic because they directly weigh benefit to the fetus against potential risk or loss of liberty for the mother. Some state courts have addressed this issue by including fetuses as children who are protected under abuse and neglect statutes (Hoener v. Bertinato, 67 N.J. Super 517, 171 A. 2d 140, 1961; Jefferson v. Griffin Spaulding Cty. Hospital 274 S.E. 2d 457 [Ga. 1981]). Alternatively, mandatory maternal transfusions during pregnancy have been rationalized on the grounds that benefits would accrue to both the mother and the fetus (Memorial Hospital v. Anderson, 201 A. 2d 537, 1964). Most difficult are cases in which intervention on behalf of the fetus may be of no benefit or even pose a risk to the mother. Reasoning in these cases has been that demonstrable conditions threatening the life of the fetus may be grounds for overriding maternal rights. Even the one major case that pioneered application of this principle, however, demonstrated the difficulty of proving risk in utero. In that case (Jefferson v. Griffin), a court ordered a caesarean section for a woman diagnosed as having a placenta previa but who had insisted on a vaginal delivery. The woman reportedly had an uneventful vaginal delivery before the order could be enforced. In spite of this problem, a scattering of courts in both the United States and Canada have been willing to order caesarean sections for women whose fetuses were threatened with Rh disease, or mandatory hospitalization for poor compliance with control of diabetes or general disregard of maternal health status (Kolder et al., 1987; Brahams, 1988). Whether this willingness continues may depend on the outcome of legal action surrounding the case of a forced caesarean section for the 25-week fetus of a terminally ill woman (Greenhouse, 1987). Although both the fetus and the mother died soon after the procedure, the decision is being appealed on the grounds that it was contrary both to the mother's right to make decisions regarding her pregnancy and to the right of individuals to refuse medical treatment. The court originally defended its ruling on the disputed understanding that the fetus was viable; an appeals panel refused to alter the ruling, although it recognized that the fetus's chance of survival was slim. Both decisions would appear to differ from the ethical position that patients have a right to decide on a course of treatment either when medical experts cannot offer a unified opinion or when the chances of successful treatment are small. Successful appeal may help to better define both procedures and standards for fetal intervention.

Courts have sometimes intervened when physicians allege that maternal behaviors such as smoking and use of alcohol or illegal drugs could endanger a fetus. In one case, evidence that the unborn child was growing poorly and thus might already have been harmed was part of the evidence leading a Maryland court to order a 20-year-old woman, who was 7 months pregnant and alleged to be a multiple-drug abuser, to enroll in a treatment program and submit to weekly drug testing (Bainbridge, 1983). According to newspaper accounts, the mother had already violated a court order to seek drug treatment stemming from concerns for maltreatment of an older child.

Legal authorities have shown more willingess to act once a potentially affected child is born. In some states (Utah and New York, for example), laws explicitly include the fetal alcohol syndrome or signs of neonatal drug withdrawal as reasons for mandated reporting to a child protective service agency. In other states, case law has established evidence of neonatal withdrawal either as prima facie evidence of maltreatment or as evidence that a child is in need of protection (Michigan: In re Baby X; New York: In re Vanessa 351 N.Y.S. 2d 337,340). Physicians who are concerned about maternal substance abuse can help press their cases by carefully documenting any symptoms of maternal or neonatal withdrawal (Tables 17.2 and 17.3) and by emphasizing to social service agencies the long-term consequences of the drug exposure involved, including the effects of withdrawal on infant behavior and its implications for difficult parenting. Use of structured observational tools can help clinicians have more confidence in their observations and lend more emphasis to a report. General behavioral instruments, such as the Brazelton Neonatal Behavioral Assessment Scale, or scales designed specifically to rate the severity of neonatal withdrawal (Finnegan et al., 1975) can be used.

Close cooperation between pediatricians and obstetricians is required so that an acceptable treatment plan can be developed for both mother and child. Ideal arrangements include

Table 17.2. Signs of Neonatal Substance Withdrawal[a]

Drug	Signs
Opiates	Diarrhea, vomiting
	Frantic sucking but poor feeds with decreased suck rate and pressure
	Tremors
	Sweating
	Increased activity, irritability, skin abrasions from increased movement
	Sneezing
	Yawning
	Tachypnea
	Altered sleep cycles: decreased periods of quiet sleep
	Seizures (probably more with methadone)
	Onset usually within 24–48 hr for heroin but can be delayed or recur several weeks later with methadone
Phencyclidine	Tremulousness
	Sensitivity to touch and environmental stimuli
	Increased tone
Cocaine	Early lethargy
	Quiet staring spells
	Rigid muscle tone
	Writhing of upper extremities
Marijuana	Tremors
	Increased spontaneous and provoked startles (but easily consolable, in contrast to opiate-withdrawing infants)
	Decreased response to light
Alcohol	Increased activity, tremulousness, and irritability
	Decreased tone
	Decreased arousal and poor habituation to stimuli
	Altered sleep patterns

[a] Sources: Braude MC, Szeto HH, Kuhn CM, et al. Perinatal effects of drugs of abuse. Fed Proc 1987;46:2446–2453; Neumann LL, Cohen SN. The neonatal narcotic withdrawal syndrome: a theraputic challenge. Clin Perinatol 1975;2:99–109; Rothstein P, Gould JB. Born with a habit: infants of drug-addicted mothers. Pediatr Clin North Am 1974;21:307–321; Fried PA. Marijuana and human pregnancy. In: Chasnoff IJ, ed. Drug use in pregnancy: mother and child. Lancaster: MTP Press Ltd, 1986:64–74.

Table 17.3. Signs of Maternal Withdrawal[a]

Time of onset	Signs
Early	Craving for drugs
	Thirst
	Anxiety and restlessness
	Lacrimation
	Tremors
	Hot and cold flashes
	Sweating
	Nausea
	Yawning
	Mydriosis
	Early postpartum discharge against medical advice
Late	Bone pain
	Vomiting
	Diarrhea
	Hypertension
	Hyperpyrexia
	Tachypnea
	Seizures

[a]Adapted from: Keith L, Donald W, Rosner M, Mitchell M, Bianchi J. Obstetric aspects of perinatal addiction. In: Chasnoff IJ, ed. Drug use in pregnancy: mother and child. Lancaster: MTP Press Ltd, 1986:35, Table 3.8.

immediate involvement of the mother in a drug or alcohol treatment program, with intensively supported or shared parenting responsibilities for the child. The longer-term medical consequences of fetal opiate and cocaine exposure, including prolonged withdrawal syndromes and the possible increased risk of sudden infant death syndrome, may make it necessary for another adult to formally take responsibility for the newborn while the mother's social and medical situation is stabilized. Early intervention with the mother must minimize feelings of hostility and guilt. These feelings may increase maternal ambivalence toward the child and make it more difficult for the mother to accept help with the child's care.

References

Anonymous. Fetal alcohol syndrome: public awareness week. MMWR 1984;33:1–2.
Anonymous. Wrongful life. Hospital Law Man 1988;115:(March)82–84.
Bainbridge JS Jr. Doctor asks court to force pregnant woman off drugs. The Sun [Baltimore] 26 April 1983:1.
Brahams D. Fetus as ward of court? Lancet 1988;i:369–370.
Chasnoff I, Chisum G. Genitourinary tract dysmorphology and maternal cocaine use. Pediatr Res 1987;22:225A.
Chasnoff IJ. Perinatal addiction: consequences of intrauterine exposure to opiate and nonopiate drugs. In: Chasnoff IJ, ed. Drug use in pregnancy: mother and child. Lancaster: MTP Press Ltd, 1986:52–63.
Chasnoff IJ, Burns WJ, Schnoll SH, Burns KA. Cocaine use in pregnancy. N Engl J Med 1985;313:666–669.
Chisum GM. Recognition and initial management of the pregnant substance-abusing woman. In: Chasnoff IJ, ed. Drug use in pregnancy: mother and child. Lancaster: MTP Press Ltd, 1986:17–22.
Clarren SK, Smith DW. The fetal alcohol syndrome. N Engl J Med 1978;298:1063–1067.
Colquitt M, Fielding P, Cronan JR. Drunk drivers and medical and social injury. N Engl J Med 1987;317:1262–1266.
Condon JT. The spectrum of fetal abuse in pregnant women. J Nerv Ment Dis 1986;174:509–516.
Council on Scientific Affairs. Scientific issues in drug testing. JAMA 1987;257:3110–3114.
Ewing JA. Detecting alcoholism: the CAGE questionnaire. JAMA 1984;252:1905–1907.
Finnegan LP, Connaughton JF Jr, Kron RE, Emich JP. Neonatal abstinence syndrome: assessment and management. Addict Dis 1975;2:141–158.
Fleisher LD. Wrongful births: when is there liability for prenatal injury? Am J Dis Child 1987;141:1260–1265.
Gallagher J. Prenatal invasions & interventions: what's wrong with fetal rights. 10 Harvard Women's Law J 9, 1987.
Gelles RJ. Violence and pregnancy: a note on the extent of the problem and needed services. Fam Coord 1975;24:81–86. (Reprinted in: Gelles RJ. Family violence. 2nd ed. Newbury Park: Sage Publications, 1987.)
Greenhouse L. Wide appeal filed on forced caeserean delivery. New York Times 25 Nov 1987:A15.
Halliday A, Bush B, Cleary P, Aronson M, Delbanco T. Alcohol abuse in women seeking gynecologic care. Obstet Gynecol 1986;68:322–326.
Iennarella RS, Chisum GM, Bianchi J. A comprehensive treatment model for pregnant chemical users, infants, and families. In: Chasnoff IJ, ed. Drug use in pregnancy: mother and child. Lancaster: MTP Press Ltd, 1986:42–51.
Keith L, Donald W, Rosner M, Mitchell M, Bianchi J. Obstetric aspects of perinatal addiction. In: Chasnoff IJ, ed. Drug use in pregnancy: mother and child. Lancaster: MTP Press Ltd, 1986:23–41.
Kerr P. Addiction's hidden toll: poor families in turmoil. New York Times 23 June 1988a:A1,B4.
Kerr P. Syphilis surge and crack use raising fears on spread of AIDS. New York Times 29 June 1988b:B1.
Kolata G. Drug researchers try to break a nearly unbreakable habit. New York Times 25 June 1988:1, 30.

Kolder VEB, Gallagher J, Parsons MT. Court-ordered obstetrical interventions. N Engl J Med 1987;316:1192–1196.

Maryland Center for Health Statistics. Health Maryland, 1985. Baltimore: Department of Health and Mental Hygiene, 1985.

Mayfield D, McLeod G, Hall P. The CAGE questionniare: validation of a new alcoholism screening instrument. Am J Psychiatry 1974;131:1121–1123.

Meyer MB, Jonas BS, Tonascia JA. Perinatal events associated with maternal smoking. Am J Epidemiol 1976;103:464–476.

Newman RG. Methadone treatment: defining and evaluating success. N Engl J Med 1987;317:447–450.

Nieburg P, Marks JS, McLaren NM, Remington PL. The fetal tobacco syndrome. JAMA 1985;253:2998–2999.

Ratner RA. A case of child abandonment—reflections on criminal responsibility in adolescence. Bull Am Acad Psychiatry Law 1985;13:291–301.

Rementeria JL, Nunag NN. Narcotic withdrawal in pregnancy: stillbirth incidence with a case report. Am J Obstet Gynecol 1973;116:1152–1156.

Resnick P. Murder of the newborn. Am J Psychiatry 1970;126:1414–1420.

Robertson JA. Procreative liberty and the control of conception, pregnancy, and childbirth. 69 Virginia Law Rev 405, 1983.

Rush D, Kass EH. Maternal smoking: a reassessment of the association with perinatal mortality. Am J Epidemiol 1972;96:183–196.

Selzer ML. The Michigan Alcoholism Screening Test: the quest for a new diagnostic instrument. Am J Psychiatry 1971;127:1653–1658.

Whitfield CL, Davis JE, Barker LR. Alcoholism. In: Barker LR, Burton JR, Zieve PD, eds. Principles of ambulatory medicine. 2nd ed. Baltimore: Williams & Wilkins, 1986.

Zuckerman B, McClain M, Frank D, Fried LE, Kayne H. Risk of sudden infant death syndrome among infants with in utero exposure to cocaine. J Pediatr 1988;113:831–834.

18 Children as Child Abusers

CHILD PERPETRATORS OF PHYSICAL ABUSE

The question of whether one child might intentionally harm another sometimes arises as part of an an explanation offered by an adult for an otherwise inexplicable injury. Small children are frequently alleged to have been injured by older siblings who shut doors on them, drop them on the floor, or hit them with toys. Some of these stories are likely to be fabrications intended to displace blame from an adult abuser, but evidence suggests that violence among children, especially siblings, is quite prevalent and perhaps likely to increase as more single and working parents are forced to leave small children in the care of older ones. The following two cases illustrate situations that the clinician may encounter:

> Case 1: A single mother brought her 4-month-old child to the emergency room because he had been fussy since she had returned home from work that afternoon. She had also noticed that his leg was swollen. An X-ray examination found a spiral fracture of the femur, but the child was otherwise well and developmentally normal. At first the mother said that the child had been well in the morning and fussy only since she had picked him up from the babysitter. Later, another account was obtained: Not wanting to be late for work at her new job, she had left the infant that morning in the care of her 12-year-old son. The two boys were to wait at home for a delivery of supplemental nutritional supplies (from the WIC program), and then the older child was to take the infant across town on a bus to the babysitter's home, which was near the older child's school. The older boy reported that at one point in the morning, when the supplies had still not arrived, the infant became fussy and he had picked up the baby to comfort him. The Infant, however, started to fall from his brother's arms, apparently injuring his leg. Confused about what to do and somewhat angry that he had had to miss school, the older boy proceeded with the day's plans and took the infant to the baby sitter (who presumably did not notice anything unusual about the child's leg).
>
> Case 2. A 3-year-old developmentally disabled girl was brought to the emergency room by ambulance. She had shallow respirations and was unresponsive except to deep pain. Radiologic studies found subarachnoid bleeding but no bone lesions. Her weight was less than the 5th percentile for her height. She had retinal hemorrhages, a torn frenulum, marks on the neck and at the corners of her mouth suggestive of a gag, and multiple bruises on the trunk and legs, some of which were in the shape of looped cords. Her 14-year-old twin brothers, who were not attending school regularly, told police that they frequently had to care for her during the day when their mother was "out on business." They disclosed that they sometimes shook her and put things in her mouth to keep her quiet. A 4-year-old sibling told police that the twins sometimes burned the younger girl with matches, kicked her, pushed her down the stairs, and locked her in the basement.

While in neither of these cases can a sibling's "confession" be taken at face value, in both there were circumstances that might increase the risk of an older child harming a younger one. In the first case, the 12 year old was part of an overly close mother-child relationship that involved frequent role reversal: the mother considered her older son to be her best friend and to be much more mature than the average adult. As a consequence, the child's activities came to be quite restricted. He had few friends and was given major responsibilities for care of his younger brother, who was, in turn, a "special" child for whom the mother had long waited. These responsibilities, plus the periodic burden of his mother's needs, created emotional demands that the 12 year old was unable to fulfill.

In the second case, the twins were left with the care of their disabled sister, a situation that would have been a challenge for an adult. The general environment was one of neglect. The boys' education was a low priority, and the girl had not been enrolled in early intervention programs that would at least have helped her nutritional status and provided some respite for her caretakers at home. There had been previous episodes of violence in the home, and the boys' conduct, although hardly forgivable, was apparently modeled on behaviors they had seen enacted by both adults and peers.

Even in less troubled families, violence among siblings is alarmingly common. The 1975 National Family Violence Survey (Straus et al., 1981) found sibling "abuse" to be 10 times more prevalent than spouse or child abuse. Forty percent of children were said to have kicked, bitten, punched, or hit a sibling with an object within the past year. Twenty percent were said to have at some time in the past "beaten up" a sibling, and 5% were said to have at one time threatened or injured a sibling with a gun or a knife. Boys were only slightly more likely than girls to engage in this type of behavior, although violence was greatest in all-male sibships. The prevalence of sibling violence declined as children got older, but even among 15–17 year olds, more than half reported some form of violent interaction within the past year.

The use of firearms by children in both intra- and extrafamilial violence is a rapidly growing problem. Deaths from firearms have increased sharply in the past two decades, especially among males 15–34 (Wintermute, 1987). Children increasingly have access to guns, either because one is kept in the home or because inexpensive weapons are readily available on the street, often from individuals involved in the sale of illicit drugs (Hilson, 1985). In the 2-year period 1983–84, 226 children age 17 and under were arrested for carrying a deadly weapon in Baltimore. Nearly all were boys, and 60% were under 15.

Unintentional injuries frequently occur in the home when children discover and attempt to play with weapons, whereas intentional injuries are reported from schools and other public areas. Obviously, the determination of intentional versus unintentional injury is one that is difficult to make. If the use of guns by children in any way parallels that of adults, intentional injuries (either suicides or homicides) are likely to be far more common than accidents (Kellerman and Reay, 1986).

CHILDREN AS SEX OFFENDERS

The fact that children are sometimes sexually abusive with each other has not always been taken as a serious problem. Potentially traumatic incidents have often been dismissed by blaming the victim for being seductive or curious, observing that "boys will be boys," or confusing assaults with sexual experimentation. Examination of the issue has also become caught up in a larger debate over child sexuality. One extreme feels that attention to the subject risks a return to repressive, Victorian taboos, while the other fears that allowing any sexual exploration by children is just the beginning of a slippery slope leading to incest and promiscuity (Ryan et al., 1987). Concern about the role of childhood sexual experiences in subsequent sexual abuse and dysfunction, however, has ultimately allowed a more dispassionate examination of the problem.

Any discussion of sexual development risks being clouded by cultural and even moral values. From earliest infancy, children receive messages from their parents about the appropriateness of touching their genitals or expressing interest in reproduction. Thus, behavior is, to some extent, modified by social norms. It is possible, however, to make some generalizations about psychosexual development in Western cultures (Rutter, 1971).

From the time they are physically capable of doing so, children manipulate their genitals as a source of stimulation and as a part of exploring their bodies. By the preschool years, children discover differences between the sexes and become intensely interested in their own genitals and how they may be different from those of other children or adults. Young children enjoy being naked, exhibiting themselves, and seeing what other children look like. When given a chance, they may want to touch the genitals of another child of either sex. Some of these actions may be misinterpreted by adults as having overtones of adult sexuality: competition for the attention of an opposite-sex parent may lead a preschooler to suggest that he would like to marry his mother or even have a baby. These discussions, although they may be part of the child's developing identity as a male or female, normally do not include references to adult sexual interaction.

By school age (age 6 through puberty), interest in sexual roles and activities increases, although most children have by now learned that these are subjects that are generally not discussed openly. Up to age 7 or 8, children play with friends of both sexes, but after that they tend to associate with same-sex friends, indicating that relationships with the opposite sex have taken on a new meaning. By age 10–12, many children have a sweetheart.

Pubertal changes in girls start about a 12–18 months earlier than in boys, with breast development beginning at around 8 years and pubertal growth at around 10. The time of onset of adult-type sexual activity is variable and shows cultural differences. In one survey of junior and senior high school students in a southern United States city, for example, at age 14 (range of 12–15 years in the survey) about 30% of white males and 11% of white females reported having had intercourse at least once (Smith and Udry, 1985). About 75% of black males of the same age and from the same school and about 40% of black females reported having had coitus.[1]

Little is known about the nature and impact of "normal" sexual contact among prepubertal children. In one survey of college students (Haugaard and Tilly, 1988) about 40% of respondents reported having had some sexual contact with another child (defined as someone under age 16) before they were 13. The average age was 9 at the time of the contact they remembered as "most meaningful." These contacts involved mostly hugging, kissing, fondling, and exhibiting genitalia, although 5–10% involved attempted intercourse. About 80% occurred with a friend, most of the remainder being with acquaintances or relatives; 70–80% involved heterosexual contact, with girls being slightly more likely to report contact with another girl. About 50% of males said that they were the person initiating the contact, while only 10% of the females reported being the initiator. Initiators were generally about 1.5 years older than the other child.

The students were also asked to remember both their reactions at the time and how they felt now about these encounters. Negative reactions were associated with encounters involving coercion, an individual the child did not know well, and contact with a child of the same sex. The type of sexual activity, fondling or touching versus attempted intercourse, did not seem to affect whether the reaction was positive or negative. Some of the students reported having had sexual contacts with both other children and adults; importantly, they rated coercive contacts with other children just as negatively as coercive contacts with adults.

In another survey of college students, Finkelhor (1980) found that about 15% of females and 10% of males reported having had a childhood sexual contact with one of their own siblings. As with the college survey discussed above, the peak age for these contacts was from 8 to 11, although 40% occurred when one of the children was under 8. As in the other survey, about three-quarters of the contacts were heterosexual. The type of sexual activity reported varied with age, although again, most involved fondling and exhibiting. These activities accounted for about 90% of the contacts of children under age 9 and about 80% of those of children ages 9–12. In the older group, however, attempted or completed intercourse started to take place; these encounters took place in nearly 20% of the contacts among those over 12. About a third of the sexual contacts with siblings happened only once, but about a quarter of the students reported contacts that recurred over a year or more. About a quarter of the contacts were said to involve some degree of force or coercion on the part of the initiator. In 70–80% of the cases in which the initiator used coercion or was 5 or more years older than the other sibling, the victim of the contact was female.

As in the previous survey, students in Finkelhor's study were asked if they remembered their sexual encounters with siblings in a negative light. Again, force and a larger age difference between the children made it more likely that an encounter would be perceived negatively. The most negative contacts, those which seemed most likely to have a long-term impact on the child's self-esteem, were those involving a child under 9 and a much older sibling.

From these and other results, Finkelhor proposed guidelines for evaluating sexual contacts between prepubertal or young adolescent children. Acceptable contacts may include those that involve children of the same age, are mu-

---

[1] It is important to note that this early coitus does not always involve activity between two young persons. If one looks at the age of the fathers of children born to teenage mothers, one finds that a sizable minority of the fathers are adults. In 1983, among children born to black mothers age 16 and younger in Baltimore, about 14% of the fathers were 21 or older. These figures are even higher for children of white mothers in the same age range: 28% of the fathers were 21 or older (Hardy and Duggan, 1988).

tually initiated, are limited in time, and involve only touching or exhibiting. Contacts that are likely to be traumatic or that begin to raise questions about exposure to adult sexual experiences include those that involve force or coercion, more than a small age difference between the children, attempts at intercourse, sodomy, or fellatio, and long-standing or compulsive activity. Intervention in these cases seems clearly warranted, for the evidence suggests that coercive contacts among children can be just as traumatic as sexual abuse by adults.

There is not a great deal of knowledge about prepubertal children who are abnormally sexually active. Johnson (1988) reported the characteristics of 47 boys ages 4–12 who had been referred to a treatment program. All of these children had engaged in sexually explicit behavior (predominantly fondling but also sodomy, oral-genital sex, and digital penetration of the vagina) that involved force or coercion and an age difference of 2 or more years between them and their victims. About half of the victims were immediate family members, but all were acquaintances of the assaulting children. The victims were both male and female.

It was not clear what had caused these children to become sexually abusive. None were said to have evidence of major psychopathology. About half said that they had themselves been sexually victimized by an adult. This proportion increased among the younger children. Ten of fourteen boys who were 4–6 years old reported being sexually abused by an adult. This finding parallels Finkelhor's findings, concerning sibling sexual encounters, that victimization experiences in early childhood may have the most traumatic impact. As discussed below, one way that boys may react to these experiences is to reenact the trauma with other children as victims.

Somewhat more is known about adolescent sex offenders, although data are clouded by both epidemiologic and social problems. Most studies come from treatment or correctional programs, and thus their findings are altered by the types of patient referred to such facilities. Offenders admitted to inpatient units are found to have a high prevalence of psychiatric disorders, while those seen in outpatient settings present a more mixed picture. Sexual abuse by and of adolescents is generally felt to be underreported, at least in part because many parents are unwilling to come forward and seek help for their children. Parents of victims and perpetrators are especially unlikely to disclose abuse when the children involved are both male. Given the fact that over half of all male sexual abuse victims are said to be victimized by other juveniles (Rogers and Terry, 1984), this is a substantial problem for understanding and treating juvenile offenders.

The characteristics of boys referred to a more general evaluation program appear to illustrate the range of generally less assaultive acts engaged in by adolescents (Deisher et al., 1982). Among 83 boys ages 12–17, about half had been involved in what were called "indecent liberties" with other children or with adults. These included all sorts of touching contacts, ranging from clothed fondling to unclothed touching short of penetration. About 10% had been referred for rape, with the remainder having been involved in peeping, exposing themselves, making obscene telephone calls, and stealing underwear. Over 80% of the victims were female.

As in Johnson's 1988 study of preadolescents, about half of the boys who were involved in sexual contact with younger children said that they had themselves been victimized by adults. These boys, however, seemed to have more psychologic problems than the preadolescents. They generally had a history of poor relationships with peers and, in common with older and more violent offenders, tended to have little empathy for their victims and to minimize the seriousness of what they had done.

The boys who had violently assaulted other adults or children were clearly different from the rest of the offenders. Their assaults had been more likely to involve strangers and to have happened multiple times. The boys approached discussion of their acts in a smooth and manipulative fashion, showing an extremely limited ability to identify with their victims. Lewis et al. (1979), in a study of 17 boys who had been convicted of sexual assault and placed on an inpatient unit, found similar characteristics. All had a long history of interpersonal violence dating back to early childhood. This included both physical assaults on other children and animals as well as witnessing or being victims of physical violence. These boys were even more violent than the few assaulters in the series studied by Deisher et al.; their sexual crimes had been unusually brutal and involved beatings, the use of deadly weapons, and an attempted hanging. Not unexpectedly, these boys had a high prevalence of serious psychiatric symptoms, including depression, hallucinations, paranoia, and other thought disorders.

Thus, adolescent sex offenses appear to encompass a range of problems. At one extreme, some children with poor peer relationships and inadequate adjustment to their developing sexuality may engage in peeping or develop paraphilias, perhaps as a substitute for normal sexual outlets. Some children, especially boys, may have been victims themselves. Although boys and girls have many similar reactions to sexual abuse, some others seem relatively unique to boys (Rogers and Terry, 1984). These include attempts to reassert masculine self-esteem by becoming aggressive and the tendency to recapitulate the victimization by in turn becoming an abuser. At the other extreme are children who appear to have had long histories of disordered and violent relationships. The sexual aspects of their crimes may in some ways be secondary to their needs to be aggressive. What is important, however, is that all of these children's offenses be taken seriously. None of them are likely to remit spontaneously, and many of the children display a level of denial and lack of empathy that is characteristic of adult offenders. Their victims are likewise worthy of attention. Although it is true that some sexual contacts with other children may not be perceived by the participants as traumatic, those that involve force, large age differences, or same-sex contact can clearly be as traumatic and have as long-lasting effects as those involving adult perpetrators.

IMPLICATIONS FOR CLINICIANS

The research discussed above suggests that it is important for primary care clinicians to be aware of the prevalence of violence among children in general and sexually abusive relationships in particular. Thomas (1982) suggests that parents who bring these problems to the attention of practitioners often do so in an oblique manner, asking about more general behavioral problems (such as poor peer relationships or a negative attitude) or inquiring vaguely about the child's poor understanding of sexual behavior. These concerns can be probed tactfully and, if necessary, explored in private with the adolescent.

Given the tendency of parents to deny this type of problem and the general fear that disclosure will result in punishment or legal action, it may be necessary to involve outside authorities as a way of pressuring the family to seek treatment. Many of these cases will not fall into the usual child abuse reporting framework because the perpetrator was not in a caretaking role vis à vis the victim. Alternative means of intervention include urging the victim's family to report the incident to juvenile authorities or, if the parents refuse to seek help for the child, reporting the family for medical neglect.

As with other types of child maltreatment, confidentiality issues are complex and not always clear. On the one hand, if an adolescent discloses the identity of his victims to a clinician, it might appear to be a breach of confidentiality for the clinician to contact the victims' families or to report the crime to juvenile authorities. On the other hand, the precedent set by the Tarasoff case (see Chapter 19), although it does not strictly apply outside of California, implies a duty to warn that would transcend the bounds of confidentiality.

One difficult situation that the clinician may confront is the medical examination, on referral from a juvenile agency, of a child who is alleged to be a sexual assaulter. This examination may very appropriately be aimed at determining whether the child has also been a victim, but the clinician must still be careful to not violate the child's rights by eliciting statements about what the child has done himself. Because the clinician cannot keep these statements in confidence, eliciting them violates the child's right to not incriminate himself (Holder, 1985). The child should be encouraged to talk about what has happened, but only under the proper circumstances. Prior to any adjudication, such disclosure should be solely in the presence of his attorney, and thereafter in the company of a competent therapist.

References

Deisher RW, Wenet GA, Paperny DM, Clark TF, Fehrenback PA. Adolescent sexual offense behavior: the role of the physician. J Adolesc Health Care 1982;2:279–286.

Finkelhor D. Sex among siblings: a survey of prevalence, variety, and effects. Arch Sex Behav 1980;9:171–194.

Hardy J, Duggan AK. Teenage fathers and the fathers of

infants of urban, teenage mothers. Am J Public Health 1988;78:919–922.

Haugaard JJ, Tilly C. Characteristics predicting children's responses to sexual encounters with other children. Child Abuse Negl 1988;12:208–219.

Hilson R Jr. Risky games with Roscoe. The Evening Sun [Baltimore] 1 July 1985:A1.

Holder AR. Legal issues in pediatrics and adolescent medicine. New Haven: Yale University Press, 1985:288.

Johnson TC. Child perpetrators—children who molest other children: preliminary findings. Child Abuse Negl 1988;12:219–229.

Kellerman AL, Reay DT. Protection or peril? An analysis of firearm-related deaths in the home. N Engl J Med 1986;314:1557–60.

Lewis DO, Shankok SS, Pincus JH. Juvenile male sexual assaulters. Am J Psychiatry 1979;136:1194–1196.

Rogers CM, Terry T. Clinical intervention with boy victims of sexual abuse. In: Stuart IR, Greer JG, eds. Victims of sexual aggression. New York: Van Nostrand Reinhold Co Inc, 1984:150–170.

Rutter M. Normal psychosexual development. J Child Psychol Psychiatry 1971;11:259–283.

Ryan G, Lans W, Davis J, Issac C. Juvenile sex offenders: development and correction. Child Abuse Negl 1987;11:385–395.

Smith EA, Udry JR. Coital and non-coital sexual behaviors of white and black adolescents. Am J Public Health 1985;75:1200–1203.

Straus MA, Gelles RJ, Steinmetz SK. Behind closed doors: violence in the American family. Garden City: Anchor Press, 1981:76–94.

Thomas JN. Juvenile sex offender: physician and parent communication. Pediatr Ann 1982;11:807–812.

Wintermute GJ. Firearms as a cause of death in the United States, 1920–82. J Trauma 1987;532–536.

19

Reporting Suspected Child Maltreatment

REPORTING REQUIREMENTS

The requirement that suspected child maltreatment be reported to civil authorities sets it aside from nearly every other medical diagnosis with the exception of certain communicable diseases. In the United States, state child abuse reporting laws were first passed in 1963; within 4 years they had been enacted across the country. Similar laws exist in Canada, Australia, and other countries. Individual laws have evolved over the years to include broader definitions of maltreatment, wider categories of individuals required to report, and, in some cases, specific exceptions such as allowances for corporal punishment or religion-based refusals of medical care. As a result, no two jurisdictions have exactly the same reporting requirements. The following paragraphs outline general provisions in force in most areas; clinicians need to be alert for specific variations that apply to the sites in which they practice.[1]

Who Must Report

Early reporting laws often divided individuals into groups of those who were required to report cases of suspected abuse ("mandated" reporters) and those who were authorized to violate confidentiality or other restraints but not legally obligated to report ("permissive" reporters). Because permissive reporters made few reports, most laws now list only individuals who must participate. In most jurisdictions, mandated reporters include all health professionals (nurses, physicians, emergency medical technicians, psychologists, social workers, etc.), teachers, daycare workers, police officers, and virtually anyone else who comes into contact with children in some professional capacity. Some states, such as Maryland, extend mandatory reporting to the entire population. Maryland's reporting law (Family Law Code Annotated Sec. 5-901—911) includes anyone "who has reasons to believe a child has been subjected to abuse." Other states include the general public in the permissive category of reporters. Some states, such as California, specifically mandate reports from persons who process film or are involved with other media that might be used to create or distribute child pornography.

Reporting obligations often become confused within large organizations such as academic medical centers or schools. There may be differences of opinion as to whether a report is warranted or as to who is ultimately responsible for seeing that one is made. When state laws recognize these difficulties, they usually specify that subordinates report to the head of the institution, the chief of the medical service involved, or someone designated by those individuals. Many institutions incorporate this practice into their own operating procedures. In large hospitals, for example, staff members who suspect abuse or neglect are asked to contact a social worker who, in turn, is responsible for notifying the appropriate authorities.

Individual legal responsibilities in large organizations vary from state to state. In some states, reporting to a supervisor, regardless of his or her subsequent action, is held to be legally sufficient. In other states, the subordinate retains responsibility for seeing that a report is made. California has what is perhaps the most explicit law on this point [Penal Code, Sect. 11166(f)]. It states that

> ... the reporting duties under this section are individual, and no supervisor or administrator may impede or inhibit the reporting duties and no person making such a report shall be subject to any sanction for making the report.

Even such a law, however, does not necessarily help in situations in which responsible professionals disagree on the need for a report.

---

[1] A general reference on United States reporting laws and the basis for much of the information in this chapter is: Myers JEB, Peters WD. Child abuse reporting legislation in the 1980s. Denver: The American Humane Association, 1987.

One function of hospital- or community-based child abuse teams is to help clarify the factual basis for suspecting abuse and to elicit the basis for feelings generated by a case. Frequently, the result can be a new consensus as to whether it is reasonable to suspect abuse and therefore whether a report is required. Regardless of local laws, however, institutions should have a policy supporting any staff member who has objective, responsible reasons for making a report, even if others see the situation differently.

When to Report

Reporting laws vary immensely in the detail with which they describe the acts of abuse or neglect that are to be reported. They also vary in descriptions of the amount of suspicion required to trigger a report and the time frame within which a report must be made.

The broad language used to define maltreatment stems both from a desire to cast the widest net possible and from the many difficulties involved in writing explicit definitions of the various forms of child abuse or neglect (see Chapter 1). Definitions have also been amended or expanded as mandated by federal legislation or pressure to strengthen the response to specific types of injury. Attempts to challenge reporting laws, premised on the potential unconstitutionality of their broad language, have, with a few exceptions, not been upheld (Smith and Meyer, 1984).

One precision that is sometimes important, depending on the details of local laws, is whether child protective service agencies will handle cases in which the alleged abuser is not a caretaker. Abuse and neglect are usually defined as actions taken by someone who is caring for the child in some way, even if only for a short time. Injuries by noncaretakers (adolescent peers, adult strangers who assault children on the street) may or may not be considered acceptable cases of child abuse by a local agency. In general, there is no legal obligation to report even violent crimes that do not fall within the definitions of child abuse.[2]

Clinicians often become confused about the level of certainty required before an abuse report becomes mandated. Laws use various language, including "reasonable cause to suspect or believe" or "knowledge" that a child is being neglected or abused. Regardless of the terminology, the intent of most laws is to trigger reporting of children who may be, but are not necessarily known for certain to be, abused or neglected. Reporters need not be able to prove that abuse or neglect has taken place. The only requirement is that there be some clinically sound reason for making the report. The observation or information that triggers the report should be verifiable and objective, and it should reflect reasonably established knowledge about the signs and symptoms of maltreatment.

This low threshold for reporting is a source of discomfort to many clinicians. Clinicians and parents frequently point out that it appears to reverse the usual direction of justice in that persons can be accused and actions taken that appear to presume guilt before anything can be proven. While in some cases this turns out to be true, in theory the process of reporting suspected abuse is not accusatory; it is intended to protect a child rather than punish an adult. In fact, many states do not require that reports name a suspected abuser, and reporters may always choose to omit this kind of information when they contact a social service agency. When police are involved in the response to a report, their decision to make an arrest is based on higher standards of proof or clearer evidence of an individual's dangerousness. Clinicians can serve an important role in helping police officers make these decisions by clearly stating when a report has been based on suspicions, which are unlikely to result in immediate police action, and when it has been motivated by more certain knowledge.

States also vary in requirements that individuals actually have had contact with a child for a report to be mandated. In some states, only those who "examine, attend, or treat" a child directly are required to report; those with secondhand knowledge may report but are not penalized for failing to do so. In other states, simply having knowledge (while working in one's professional capacity) of a child who may be abused or neglected mandates a professional's report. This distinction is important to persons who treat offenders, their spouses, or the siblings of abused children and who wish to avoid reporting. It is sometimes used as a justification for not reporting abuse disclosed by offenders

---

[2] Local laws usually do mandate reporting to police any injury thought to have been inflicted by a deadly weapon such as a gun or knife.

in the course of therapy or some unrelated treatment (see below).

Statutes are often silent on whether abuse that happened in the distant past can form a basis for a mandated report. The question may arise when an older child divulges facts about abuse that happened earlier or was perpetrated by a parent who has now left the family. This would appear to be an area in which clinicians can exercise some discretion. In many states, there is no statute of limitations (a legal limit on how long after a crime someone may be charged) for serious offenses such as child abuse. Certainly if the potential abuser is still in a position to harm the same child or other children, or if the abuse was particularly violent or cruel, a report may be indicated. Reporting may also be an important therapeutic step for both the abuser and the victim if one or the other has resisted seeking treatment and the issue of abuse continues to have a serious impact on their functioning.

Clinicians also frequently raise the question of how quickly reports of suspected abuse or neglect need to be made. Most reporting laws specify some time frame. In Maryland, for example, a written report is due to authorities within 48 hours of the "contact, examination, treatment, or other circumstance" that caused the reporter to believe that the child was abused or neglected. It is not unusual, however, for concerns to arise but for there to be controversy as to whether a report should be delayed in the hope that more information will soon come to light that will make the report more specific and credible. Again, this appears to be an area in which some clinical discretion may apply. There is often a great deal of stress immediately following a report, and children who were otherwise willing to talk about what happened may be reluctant to speak and may even recant. If a child is hospitalized and is being evaluated by a social worker, psychologist, or psychiatrist, it may be reasonable to delay reporting for a short period in the hope that a more detailed disclosure will be made. Delays may also be appropriate in cases that are likely to be viewed with skepticism by legal authorities. Cases of suspected Munchausen syndrome by proxy are often disbelieved by protective service workers or police. In such cases, it may be necessary to delay reporting until incontrovertible evidence can be accumulated, with strict surveillance (usually on an inpatient basis) to ensure a child's safety (see Chapter 15). The rationale for delaying is always the clinical judgment that a more therapeutic outcome for the family will result and will balance any additional risk to the child in the period before legal authorities are involved. Except in extreme cases such as Munchausen syndrome by proxy, prompt reporting, once a factual basis for concern is established, is the safest course.

Regardless of when a report is made, it is usually best to inform parents before authorities are contacted, preferably from the first point at which abuse or neglect is seriously entertained as a diagnosis (Racusin and Felsman, 1986). From an ethical viewpoint, the principle of autonomy suggests that patients have a right to be informed about the goals and risks of their medical treatment. In the case of abuse, it can be argued that the entire family is the patient. Not telling the family involves a deception which, once discovered, can have negative consequences for the clinician-patient relationship. It also may send the family a message that the clinician cannot talk about the issue directly and thus tacitly establish an agreement that neither party will speak openly.

Clinicians often counter that, in general, truth telling is not an absolute obligation. A "therapeutic privilege" is frequently invoked to withhold information that a clinician believes would be unnecessarily stressful or that could, in the short term, harm the course of therapy (Bok, 1983). In the case of suspected maltreatment, the specific concern is usually that telling the family will lead to an uncooperative stance in which the family will become angry, refuse further evaluation, or take the child from the premises. There is no doubt that this can happen, although there is the hope that it can be avoided by an empathetic presentation of the clinician's differential diagnosis, with ample opportunities for parents to reply. The risks of deceit have to be weighed against the expected benefits. Deceit may be justified when injury has been serious or the parents appear to be seriously disturbed or dangerous.

In some states, physicians are granted the authority to take children into protective custody without having first to obtain a court order or some other legal authority. In those settings, the parents' desire to remove the child can be directly countered. In most settings, however, clinicians cannot forcibly restrain parents from taking a child until a court order has been obtained or a parent is arrested. Sometimes allowing the child to leave the medical facility for even a brief time will be hazardous to the child's health, but in many if not most situations, the immediate hazard will be slight and the chances great that police or protective service workers will be able to find the family and ask them to return with the child. Clinicians also sometimes argue that deceit is necessary to avoid the risk that the family will refuse consent for a certain part of the maltreatment evaluation, such as a skeletal survey. Even if one could obtain the survey without the parents understanding why, in most jurisdictions the concern is unnecessary. In Maryland, for example, statutes define the medical evaluation of suspected abuse or neglect as "emergency medical treatment" for which no consent is required.

Who Receives Reports

Reporting laws vary regarding who is to receive reports of suspected abuse or neglect. As mentioned above, in schools or hospitals, reporting to a superior or a chief of service may be sufficient under the law. Individual reporters are often given a choice of whom to notify. Often both the police and the child protective service agency will receive reports, although in some jurisdictions protective service agencies must be notified first.

LIABILITY AND REPORTING

Most states have relatively mild criminal penalties for not reporting cases of child abuse or neglect when reporting would otherwise be indicated. In some states, failure to report can also be grounds for referral to a licensing board and thus possibly lead to professional disciplinary action. The legal risks of not reporting stem more from the general civil liability that may be incurred should a child be subsequently harmed and a claim made that reporting might have prevented the injury. In some states, reporting statutes specifically state that willful failure to report causes an individual to become civilly liable for damages that might be attributed to the failure. In most jurisdictions, however, civil liability must be derived from more general case law or from common law definitions of negligence (Myers and Peters, 1987).

One source of liability for not reporting comes from the duty a health care practitioner may have to warn potential victims of serious threats to their life or health. Some states, for example, have long had laws that require the notification of intimate contacts of persons with sexually transmissible diseases (Mills et al., 1986), although the epidemic of acquired immunodeficiency syndrome has caused these laws to be reexamined (Gostin and Curran, 1986). In the mental health field, the case of Tarasoff v. Regents of the University of California (17 Cal Rptr 3d 425, 1976; 529 P. 2d 533, 1975; 551 P. 2d 334, 1976) has been the key ruling defining a duty to warn of a possible assault. Although the Tarasoff decision was made by the California Supreme Court and thus strictly speaking does not establish a precedent elsewhere in the country, similar cases heard in other jurisdictions have tended to set out similar positions (Marcus, 1986).

The Tarasoff case involved a psychologist whose patient revealed that he was planning a murder. As described in court records, the patient said that he intended to kill a young woman, Tatiana Tarasoff, whom he would have liked to have had as his girlfriend. The psychologist reported this to the police, who detained the patient but later released him. The psychologist did not warn Tatiana or her family. The patient subsequently gained the confidence of Tatiana's family, even persuading her brother to share an apartment with him. He subsequently went to Tatiana's home and killed her. The majority opinion of the court ruled that

> ... the therapist owes a legal duty not only to his patient, but also to his patient's would-be victim, and is subject in both respects to scrutiny. ... Some of the alternatives open to the therapist, such as warning the victim, will not result in the drastic consequences of depriving the patient of his liberty. Weighing the uncertain and conjectural character of the alleged damage done the patient by such a warning against the peril to the victim's life, we conclude that professional inaccuracy in predicting violence cannot negate the therapist's duty to protect the threatened victim. ...

The implication of the Tarasoff case for child maltreatment cases rests largely on the belief that abuse is a phenomenon that tends to repeat and to increase in intensity. Thus, learning about abuse by encountering a child or hearing of it from a perpetrator creates a duty to help the child and the family seek protection from further harm. The Tarasoff case also suggests that reporting alone may not be enough. Clinicians may have a responsibility to follow up on their reports and assure themselves that a potential victim is being protected (Curran, 1977).

Physicians may also be found to be have been negligent if they encounter signs of abuse and subsequently fail to make a report. The landmark case in this area, Landeros v. Flood (551 P. 2d 389, 1976), was also heard by the California Supreme Court in 1976. An 11-month-old child was brought to an emergency room with a fractured leg. According to the court records, she had some scattered bruises and abrasions (of uncertain extent and meaning) but was treated and released. About 2 months later, she was brought to a second hospital with multiple injuries, including burns, puncture wounds, and bites. Her parents were ultimately convicted of child abuse. Her foster family brought a malpractice suit against the physician who had treated the fractured leg, claiming that he had negligently failed to diagnose and report the battered child syndrome and had thereby subjected the child to further risk. The California Supreme Court ultimately allowed a malpractice action against the physician and the hospital where the child was first seen. Although experts have debated the logic of the court's ruling (Curran, 1977), the case has come to imply that both failure to diagnose abuse and failure to report once abuse has been recognized are grounds for civil liability.

In contrast to the potential for liability for failure to report, all reporting statutes grant explicit immunity from civil liability for professionals who make "good faith" reports of suspected abuse. This protection is frequently extended to include anyone who participates in the investigation of a case, such as a clinician who is asked to examine a child who has already come to the attention of a department of social services. Some states go further and grant the presumption of good faith to the individual reporting. In other words, someone who challenges the appropriateness of the report has the burden of proving that it was made frivolously, as opposed to the reporter having to defend his or her action. This type of immunity does not mean that a suit cannot be initiated against a reporter (Roman v. Appleby, 558 F. Supp. 449, 1983), but it greatly reduces the chances that the action will be heard or that the truly good faith reporter will be found to be at fault. New challenges to the immunity of reporters will continue to arise, however. Each is likely to be based on strict interpretations of local reporting laws, but they may have a chilling effect that goes beyond the jurisdiction in which they are being heard. In one recent and well-publicized case, for example, the mother of a child who died after reportedly falling in a bathtub has sued the physicians who filed a report of suspected abuse regarding the child's injuries (Carlova, 1989). Her primary legal contention is that a "window of liability" opens after a report is made if clinicians appear to be advocating to authorities for a finding of abuse rather than simply reporting their suspicions.

CONFIDENTIALITY

General Legal Interpretations

The privacy of professional-client interaction is usually safeguarded in one or more ways. Professionals have an obligation to keep in confidence information that is revealed to them in the course of treatment. In addition, laws in most jurisdictions define specific "privileges" that apply to relationships between physicians, psychologists, social workers, clergy, or other individuals and their clients or congregants. In general, a privilege is the right of a patient or client to refuse to permit information from treatment to be disclosed in courtroom, legislative, or administrative testimony. The patient or client "owns" the privilege; it cannot be asserted by the professional independently. These laws vary among the professions and from state to state, so it is important to know their details on a local level. For example, some forms of information may be exempt from privilege when disclosed to social workers but not when disclosed to psychiatrists. Even more confusing are cases in which a single professional falls under two categories that have conflicting privilege statutes; psychiatrists, for example, may also be considered under a more general statute applying to physicians. Exacerbating the confusion about privilege, although the concept explicitly applies only to formal testimony, are some state rulings that have extended the principle to include disclosure in any setting, formal or informal (in Maryland, for example, Shaw v. Glickman 45 Md. App. 718, 726; 415 A. 2d 625, 1980). In the United States, other specific federal confidentiality laws apply to drug and alcohol treatment programs.

Most states specifically exclude concerns for child abuse and neglect from privilege statutes applying to professionals, with the exception of attorneys and their clients. Thus, for most professionals in most jurisdictions, the duty to report takes precedence over any client's right to confidentiality. Unfortunately, there may be important differences among states in how the relationship between reporting and privilege is interpreted. Controversies include whether privilege is waived only for a report containing minimal information, for informal cooperation with authorities during investigation, for full testimony in court, or for all three. State courts have also varied in opinions of whether the waiver applies only to civil or to both civil and criminal proceedings. Many of these issues may not be well defined, since often they are clarified only when a professional refuses to disclose or a client attempts to assert the privilege or to sue for inappropriate disclosure. Because parents involved in abuse cases often do not have an attorney who is knowledgeable in these areas, cases are not always made when they might be. Ambiguities also arise with information coming from drug and alcohol treatment programs, although it is generally accepted that federal laws requiring states to have abuse reporting mechanisms take precedence over other federal laws mandating confidentiality in programs that receive federal funds.

Offender Treatment

One of the major objections to mandatory reporting of abuse and neglect comes from clinicians who treat adults. These clinicians often claim that individuals who are seeking psychiatric help in general or treatment for child abuse in particular will be discouraged from seeking help by the knowledge that confidentiality cannot be guaranteed. Confidentiality, they assert, is an essential element of insight-oriented psychotherapy (Smith and Meyer, 1984). Proponents of this view have successfully advocated laws that exempt clinicians treating pedophiles from state reporting statutes (Maryland House Bills 377, 1319 [1988]). Some proponents favor barring the report of any abuse disclosed during treatment, whereas others would bar only reports concerning abuse that occurred before treatment was started.

Opponents of such exemptions base their position on two sets of facts. First, published data, with few exceptions, show that success rates for treatment of any type of abuse are relatively low. An evaluation of 11 federally sponsored abuse intervention demonstration projects found that 30% of enrolled parents committed severe, repeated abuse while under treatment; health care workers judged only 42% to be less likely to abuse once treatment had ended (Cohn, 1980). Although specific data regarding treatment of sexual offenders are difficult to interpret, most studies suggest that recidivism rates are also substantial (Finkelhor, 1986). These findings make it seem important that potential victims be warned and protected even though an offender is in treatment.

A second argument for mandatory reporting comes from therapists who treat sex offenders. The treatment of many pedophiles, they contend, does not fit the classic, insight-oriented psychotherapeutic model (Salter, 1988). Instead, sex offender treatment is based on a model more closely related to the treatment of addictions. Sex offenders have powerful abilities to deny and defend their offenses and to seduce their therapists into believing that they have been cured. Successful treatment is rarely carried through on an entirely voluntary basis. To these therapists, a full guarantee of confidentiality serves only the offender's interest in continuing undetected abuse. A clear stance that further abuse is wrong and will be punished, as well as a willingness to use information to verify and enforce compliance, is felt to be essential to this treatment approach.

Maine is one state that has attempted to seek a compromise on this issue (Maine Rev. Stat. Ann., Title 22, Sect. 4011). Legislation there allows professionals treating offenders to make a confidential report to a protective service agency and to negotiate the action to be taken. Outcomes of the negotiation could range from a full investigation to an agreement that no official action will be taken.

Sharing Information with Protective Service and Other Agencies

After a report of suspected abuse or neglect is made, law enforcement and social service agencies, or attorneys for parents, children, or alleged abusers, may request that a clinician provide them with medical records or other information. There is often a question about what information should be released and to which parties. In general, the fact that a report of suspected abuse has been made does not grant a clinician authority to release records or to discuss with authorities information that is not germane to the suspicion of abuse. Telephone calls frequently present a problem because it can be difficult to refuse a direct request for information. It is reasonable to discuss with police, prosecutors, or protective service workers details of a case that pertain directly to the suspicion and evaluation of maltreatment. These individuals are legally charged with investigating the situation, and clinicians in most jurisdictions are expressly protected from liability for cooperating with them. Calls from attorneys representing various parties to the case can be more troublesome. Attorneys for the child or for biologic or adoptive parents represent the clinician's "client" and are entitled to open discussions. This may be uncomfortable in cases where one of the parents is an alleged abuser, but cooperation is generally required unless the parent has temporarily or permanently lost custody of the child. A clinician might properly refuse to discuss a case with an attorney representing an abuser who is not a family member or a biologic or adoptive parent.

Requests for medical records should always be received in writing and include some legal authority for the request—either a consent for release of information from the patient or his proxies or a subpoena issued by a court. Police and social service workers often ask for a written copy of a medical report detailing a child's injuries or conditions without having either a release from the patient or a subpoena. In some states, special medical forms are used for this purpose. Patients provide signed consent for release of the information, and the form contains only information related to the investigation of abuse. Other states have enacted laws that automatically grant protective service workers access to a suspected victim's medical records (in Maryland, Family Law, Subtitle 7, Sect. 5–711). In other jurisdictions, clinicians may wish to write a letter or separate note elaborating on the abuse examination rather than providing the actual record. In large institutions, formal requests for records should be sent to the medical records department for processing. This procedure maintains equitable access to the records and protects the clinician from allegations that he or she provided different degrees of cooperation or different records to the various parties to a case.

One way in which information can be shared more freely is in the context of a multidisciplinary child protection team (Bross, 1981). Multidisciplinary teams may be based in the community or in a hospital and may have many functions, including diagnostic assessment of new cases and suggestion of plans for short- and long-term treatment. They consist of a variety of professionals, including social workers, attorneys, physicians, nurses, and representatives of community agencies. In many states, specific legislation provides for the existence of such teams and, within certain guidelines, for the free exchange of case information among professionals from different agencies and institutions. Even where specific legislation has not been enacted, members of a team sponsored by an organization such a hospital may also share information based on the premise that the team members, even those from outside the institution, can all be considered to be its "agents." This arrangement can be made more secure if the team has some written guidelines for operation and if written agreements are made with outside agencies for the participation of their representatives.

In any setting, however, clinicians must carefully choose the language used to describe a case of suspected abuse. Some cases evoke strong emotions about the child's injury or the guilt of the alleged perpetrator, tempting the clinician to move beyond objective presentation of the facts. At that point, the alleged abuser may well be able to convince a court that the report serves more to defame the adult than to protect the child.

One way that clinicians can avoid this situation is to scrupulously report objective findings rather than diagnoses. For example, unless a person's blood alcohol level has been measured, it is preferable to state that he or she smelled of alcohol, had an unsteady gait, or was intermittently somnolent rather than that the person was intoxicated. A second step is to avoid statements that imply an unwarranted absolute certainty. For example, serious head injury resulting from a fall out of bed is very unlikely but probably not impossible. Saying that a fall could never produce such injury may fuel a claim that the clinician prejudged the case or set out to victimize the parent (Carlova, 1989).

These cautionary notes do not mean that a clinician cannot work hard to ensure that a report of suspected abuse is properly considered by a law enforcement or social service agency. One might even claim, on the basis of the Tarasoff case, that clinicians have some degree of obligation to do so. The prudent child advocate, however, when personally involved in the evaluation of a case of suspected maltreatment, might well define advocacy as doing the most thorough and objective medical evaluation possible and then seeing that these findings are clearly and accurately represented in a report to the appropriate agency. These activities can reasonably be defined as part of good medical care for the suspected victim and the family. Investigation, developing proof that abuse has taken place, and identification of the perpetrator are the responsibilities of other professionals. Assuming these roles may entail taking on additional legal risk as well as jeopardizing one's ability to work with and on behalf of the family.

References

Bok S. Secrets. New York: Vintage Books, 1983.
Bross DC. Multi-disciplinary child protection teams and effective legal management of abuse and neglect. In: National Legal Resource Center for Child Advocacy and Protection, ed. Protecting children through the legal system. Washington, DC: American Bar Association, 1981:495–517.
Carlova J. Can a doctor go overboard in reporting child abuse? Med Econ 1989;Jan:58–62.
Cohn AH. The pediatrician's role in the treatment of child abuse: implications from a national evaluation study. Pediatrics 1980;65:358–360.
Curran WJ. Failure to diagnose battered-child syndrome. N Engl J Med 1977;296:795–796.
Finkelhor D. A sourcebook on child sexual abuse. Beverly Hills: Sage Publications, 1986.
Gostin L, Curran WJ. The limits of compulsion in controlling AIDS. Hastings Cent Rpt 1986;Dec:24–29.
Marcus FF. Case underlines psychiatric issue: to keep confidences or report threats. New York Times 23 May 1986:A10.
Mills M, Wofsy CB, Mills J. The acquired immunodeficiency syndrome: infection control and public health law. N Engl J Med 1986;314:931–936.
Myers JEB, Peters WD. Child abuse reporting legislation in the 1980s. Denver: The American Humane Association, 1987.
Racusin RJ, Felsman JK. Reporting child abuse: the ethical obligation to inform parents. J Am Acad Child Adolesc Psychiatry 1986;25:485–489.
Salter AC. Treating child sex offenders and victims: a practical guide. Beverly Hills: Sage Publications, 1988.
Smith SR, Meyer RG. Child abuse reporting laws and psychotherapy: a time for reconsideration. Int J Law Psychiatry 1984;7:351–366.

20 Physician Expert Testimony[1]
—Linda C. Anderson[2]

Testifying in a child abuse or neglect proceeding of any nature is often difficult. The legal standards for evidence of injury and the medical indicia of trauma do not always correspond, so the translation of data from one discipline to the other can be frustrating. Sometimes the legal inquiry will seem to focus more on minute details of the physician's curriculum vitae than on the injury itself. It may prove an unnerving experience for a clinician serving as an expert witness to have his or her qualifications parsed and attacked. To make matters worse, some lawyers incorporate into their examination styles either a subtle or an overt attempt to bully and ridicule the expert. Although this kind of hostility initially alienates a judge or jury, if the expert responds in kind, the lawyer's purpose is achieved. He or she can argue that the expert is emotionally invested in the diagnosis and thus biased.

The whole process of testifying, then, is much more sophisticated an interaction than the mere exchange of information. For physicians, this is often the most frustrating aspect of courtroom proceedings. Factors other than "the data" seem able to influence important judgments about whether a child has been abused or whether a defendant is innocent. This chapter is intended to give the medical expert guidance on the broad issues he or she can expect to encounter when called to testify as well as some insight as to how testimony can be most effectively given under a variety of circumstances.

---

[1] Portions of this chapter were adapted from: National Center on Child Abuse and Neglect. Discussion guide to film "The Medical Witness." In: National Center for Child Abuse and Neglect. We can help... A curriculum on the identification, reporting, referral and case management of child abuse and neglect. Washington, DC: US Government Printing Office, September, 1976:14-170–14-176.

[2] Attorney, U.S. Department of Justice. Formerly chair, Child Abuse Committee, State Bar of Texas. The views expressed are those of the writer and not necessarily those of the Department of Justice.

PREPARATION FOR COURT

Subpoenas

The physician's court involvement often begins with the arrival of a subpoena, a notification from the court that a hearing is taking place and that the physician is wanted as a witness. The subpoena will usually give the type of hearing (criminal or juvenile) and on whose behalf the physician is being called to testify: the state, the child, or the defense. The subpoena usually includes a telephone number for a court or witness assistance office. These offices can help the physician contact the lawyer who had the subpoena issued.

Occasionally, experts will not be subpoenaed if they have been assisting a lawyer with the case prior to trial and have agreed to testify, although being formally subpoenaed may offer some additional protection from a subsequent claim that the physician's participation in the case constituted an inappropriate breach of patient confidentiality. Physicians who are reluctant to participate as a witness may be tempted to evade court officials when they come to serve the subpoena. Evasion is rarely possible unless one plans to actually leave the country. Such tactics usually result only in postponing receipt of the subpoena until a more inconvenient time, such as the middle of the night. On the other hand, attorneys in hotly contested cases who are afraid that a physician will try to avoid being served have been known to arrange last-minute, surprise delivery of subpoenas, even though this tactic risks antagonizing a potentially friendly witness. The court itself, however, in the person of the judge, may be more respectful of the physician's need to schedule a court appearance and may help arrange a more convenient time for the testimony. Although subpoenas usually specify a date and time at which the witness must appear, the actual time of the expert's testimony may not be until hours or even days later. In some cases, hearings are canceled at the last minute because an agreement has been reached between the various parties or because one party has been granted a delay. In many juvenile or family court cases, attorneys may be able to "stipulate" as to what the expert would say if he or she was asked, and the expert, even though subpoenaed, would need to appear only if opposing parties in the case wanted to contest the expert's conclusions. Thus, it is usually reasonable for experts to ask if they can be placed on call for court, with the promise that they will be reachable and able to appear within a short time after being notified that their testimony is needed.

Records

The physician should thoroughly review his or her records and notes. Although it is not necessary to commit the contents of these records to memory, a court is particularly impressed by an expert's ability to discuss details of diagnosis and treatment without a great deal of reference to memory aids. The court will often wish to hear medical testimony in the chronology in which the case progressed, i.e., when the examination of the child began and what specifically occurred thereafter. It is therefore helpful to review the records in a chronological fashion. During the review process, the physician may wish to prepare visual aids to testimony, although doing so is not required. Charts and graphs help clarify the information for the court and jury and generally make the process of testifying easier on the physician.

Contact with the Lawyer

Once the physician has reviewed records and notes, he or she should talk with the lawyer for whom testimony will be given. This is the time for the physician to try to understand the legal case thoroughly. The legal case may differ from the medical case because of other information that has been gathered outside the medical setting and is not yet known to the physician or because the parties to the case have specific objectives (custody issues, for example) of which the physician is unaware. The physician needs to know where in the presentation of witnesses his or her testimony will occur and exactly what must be accomplished through that testimony. This will enable the physician to isolate and explain to the lawyer the medical facts that support what the lawyer seeks to prove. The physician may also wish to suggest additional witnesses or to clarify the role of witnesses that the lawyer has already retained. The physician may know of additional documents that could either refine or supplement the evidence already slated for presentation.

This is also the time to discuss the physician's qualifications. Some aspects of the physician's background may need to be detailed more thoroughly to the court or, alternatively, deemphasized. Emphasis on areas of expertise that are irrelevant to the case at hand tend to diminish rather than enhance the expert's credibility in the eyes of the judge or jury. Whatever qualifications are ultimately admitted into evidence, it is important to include experience in similar cases. Courts give particular credence to experts who specialize to some degree in the type of injury or syndrome in question.

Physicians can be specifically "qualified" before the court as experts in medicine, psychiatry, child abuse, or other specialties. To qualify as an expert, the witness will be asked to state facts about his or her education and experience. The opposing attorney or judge may ask further questions about the witness's expertise, and the judge will decide whether the witness qualifies as an expert. In each case, the judge has final discretion to decide whether a witness so qualifies.

Rehearsal

It is infrequently that a lawyer will review the specific questions to be asked of the expert at the trial, although this is the ideal. A rehearsal allows the lawyer to help the expert state his or her testimony in the most legally understandable and admissible form. The lawyer can also prepare the expert for cross-examination by role playing and by pointing out the kinds of questions that may be asked. At the very least, the expert and the lawyer should have a chance to review the case well before the trial date. The review will help both professionals participate more effectively.

Relationships with Opposing Parties

Sometimes a physician may be asked to function as an expert in a case in which he or she was also involved as a treating physician. The physician may be concerned about damaging the patient-doctor relationship, but there is little alternative to testifying if a subpoena has been issued. It is reasonable, however, for a physician who has made a report of suspected abuse to suggest that another expert be asked to offer an opinion as to whether abuse has actually occurred. An outside observer may be able to offer a more objective opinion, and the separation of roles may help the physician maintain a therapeutic relationship with the family.

Many physicians are uncertain, when subpoenaed by the state, as to whether they are allowed to talk with attorneys for the parents or the child before the hearing. There is no prohibition against such conversation. The physician should be aware, however, that on cross-examination these attorneys will be certain to raise any inconsistencies between what the physician told them informally and what is stated in court. This can be a particularly difficult area if the parents are separated or engaged in adversarial actions. To be safe from any accusation of bias, the physician can always insist on consent for release of information from both parents or issuance of a subpoena before discussion with counsel.

COURTROOM TESTIMONY

Physicians who have not testified in a trial may have expectations that are based on film depictions and descriptions in novels. Most of the time, the physician will be subpoenaed by lawyers for the local protective service agency to testify in a juvenile or family court adjudicatory hearing. The purpose of such a hearing is to determine whether there is sufficient evidence to believe that a child was abused or neglected and to determine a safe and therapeutic placement for the child. These proceedings may follow standard courtroom decorum or they may be quite informal, perhaps taking place in a judge's office with a court reporter present or in a courtroom but accompanied only by the other parties to the proceeding. Rules determining what sorts of evidence are permitted may also be relatively lax so that testimony can be more conversational and less elaborately orchestrated. In contrast, the physician may be called to testify in criminal prosecutions for child abuse or neglect. These proceedings follow strict procedural rules and have rigorous standards for the kind of testimony permitted.

The expert waits either inside or directly outside the courtroom until called to the witness stand. Expert witnesses are usually allowed to be in the courtroom during other testimony because they may be asked to comment on something that another witness has said. In contrast, witnesses who will be testifying only to facts (material witnesses) rather than giving opinions may be asked to remain outside so that they cannot be influenced by what they hear. Experts may also be asked to remain outside, especially in cases in which the various parties have recruited their own experts to support differing interpretations of the facts.

In some cases, the attorney may ask the expert not only to remain in the courtroom but to act as an advisor during the testimony of other witnesses. The expert's task usually will be to catch misinterpretations of medical facts by other witnesses or to formulate new arguments based on what other witnesses say. The expert can assess his or her role in the case and the nature of his or her relationship with the family involved and then determine whether this is an appropriate method of participation.

Testifying before a judge or jury can be intimidating for any witness. It is therefore helpful for the physician to remember that he or she will be perceived by the court as an authority in a given field and is likely to know more about that field than anyone else in the courtroom. For this expertise be fully utilized, however, the physician and attorney must work together on its presentation.

Testimony on Direct Examination

THE NATURE OF DIRECT EXAMINATION

The expert will testify in two phases of examination, direct and cross. In direct examination, it is usually the lawyer for whom the expert's testimony is sympathetic who will do the questioning. Direct examination is so named because the testimony presented is postured to prove directly the allegations made by the party that the examining lawyer represents.

Because the lawyer and expert witness are on the same "team" during direct examination, certain procedural limitations are placed on the lawyer's questions. For example, the lawyer cannot shortcut the question-and-answer process of testimony by asking questions that suggest answers to the physician. For example, the lawyer cannot ask, "Did your tests show that the child suffered a spiral fracture?" This is a leading question and may be objected to by the opposing attorney. If the opposing counsel objects, the court can require that the question be rephrased. The nonleading sequence of questions would be:

> Attorney: Did you perform tests to determine the nature of the child's injury?
> Physician: Yes.
> Attorney: What type of tests?
> Physician: An X ray of the child's arm.
> Attorney: What did the X ray show?
> Physician: The child suffered a spiral fracture.

The danger presented when a lawyer does not review the expert's testimony prior to trial is that the lawyer may not have the medical events clearly enough in mind to ask the proper sequence of questions. Under these circumstances, the attorney may have to ask questions such as "What happened next?" or "What did you do next?" Generally, these are legally permissible questions, but they put the burden of elaborating on the expert. There is also the risk, from the attorney's point of view, that such broad questions will elicit either an improper answer from the expert, to which opposing counsel can object, or an unexpected answer that could hurt the attorney's case. For example, a lengthy narrative answer that goes too far beyond the next step in the chronology of medical events is not allowed because, in theory, it wrests presentation of the evidence from the attorney and may lead to the introduction of objectionable material that it is the attorney's responsibility to exclude.[3] In general, a witness may answer only questions that have been asked; the witness cannot volunteer information on unrelated subjects, even if he or she thinks it is important to the case.

TECHNIQUES FOR RESPONSE TO QUESTIONS ON DIRECT EXAMINATION

Despite these cautions about narrative answers, the physician should not feel that the responses given during direct examination must be as brief as possible. A witness for one side of the case may purposely limit responses during cross-examination by the opposing side's lawyers, but during direct exam the attorney will wish to elicit a complete account in order to give the judge and jury the fullest possible understanding of the issues.[4]

During questioning, even a well-prepared attorney may slip into legal jargon or simply phrase a question awkwardly. Witnesses should not attempt to guess what a question means, but instead should ask that the question be clarified. Likewise, witnesses should not hesitate to say that they do not know the answer to a question. Credibility suffers when a physician vacillates after realizing the true meaning of a question that was initially misunderstood or when a reply is obviously vague or overqualified. To avoid giving the impression of vagueness, answers to questions should be as precise as possible. It is preferable to say "He had three fractures" instead of "He had several fractures." Phrases such as "I guess" or "I think" should be avoided unless one genuinely must be that conditional to be honest. To be precise, the physician will sometimes need to use medical jargon during testimony. Correct terminology should not be avoided, for it ensures that the facts are entered accurately into the trial record; when used properly, it bolsters the credibility of the expert's testimony. Proper use demands, however, that once medical terminology or jargon is introduced, it is then explained in lay terms.

Testimony on Cross-Examination

Cross-examination is the most difficult phase of testifying. The opposing attorney's job is either to discredit the physician's testimony or to turn it to his client's advantage. He or she will employ a variety of strategies to do so. The key to the physician's effective performance is adequate preparation, including close consul-

---

[3] The improper question counterpart to the narrative answer is the narrative question "Give the court the account of your involvement in this case."

[4] Many experts do not feel comfortable making a distinction between direct and cross-examination. In some cases, experts are willing to participate as advocates for one side or another. In most child abuse cases, however, the expert may wish to be as neutral as possible, striving simply for an objective presentation of facts for the court to consider. This position can often be established before the case goes to court, and frequently the attorneys involved will arrange joint access to the expert in preparation for the trial. The expert will still be subpoenaed by one side or the other and, if called to the witness stand, will still undergo direct and cross-examination.

tation with the lawyer who originally subpoenaed the physician about what questions are likely to be asked.

It is important to remain calm on cross-examination. Defensive, angry, or condescending responses diminish the expert's credibility and detract from his or her ability to respond competently to the questions asked. A strategy often used by the opposing lawyer is to closely question the expert's past involvement and experience with child abuse and neglect cases in an attempt to establish that he or she is not specifically experienced in those areas. Questions may include "How many cases like this have you seen previously, Doctor?" or "Have you ever had any training in the treatment of this type of injury?" This strategy is designed not only to expose weaknesses in qualifications but also to be upsetting. The physician should bear in mind that in the vast majority of cases, his or her overall professional background and experience will not be challenged by the court. These questions should be anticipated, however, so that they can be answered readily and confidently.

Another strategy opposing counsel uses to discredit the witness is a review of his or her notes, records, or charts to point out details to which the expert has testified but which are not in those documents. Physicians cannot be expected to precisely record every interaction and observation, although having records of key interactions obviously adds great credibility to the testimony. Opposing counsel may also attack the physician for failure to perform every medical test that might be needed to eliminate conclusively the possibility of some other cause for a child's injuries. If, in fact, the physician has not performed every possible test, he or she should be prepared to explain why the omitted tests were unnecessary.

It is important to remember several key principles of testifying during cross-examination. Only the questions asked should be answered, and no additional information should be volunteered. On the other hand, experts should resist pressure to make statements that are uninformative or only partially correct. There is no obligation to give yes or no replies to questions that require longer answers. It is proper to ask the judge to allow that a lengthier explanation be given. As a last resort, the witness can simply say that the question cannot be answered as posed. Likewise, as during direct examination, it is always acceptable to say that one does not know the answer to or does not understand a question. A particular ploy used by lawyers to confuse witnesses is to ask a complex question, one that actually contains a string of several queries. Complex questions are legitimate grounds for objection by the opposing attorney, but in an effort to save objections for more substantive issues, he or she may not come to the witness's rescue. If no objection is made, the witness may still ask that the questions be asked one at a time. This is always a good practice so that one question will not be forgotten while another is being answered.

Another trap the witness may fall into is reluctance to admit what is possible. If an attorney asks a hypothetical question that sets out an unlikely but possible scenario of what may have happened to a child, it is important to admit that it is, indeed, possible. One should, however, add a statement indicating that the scenario the attorney is proposing is "unlikely in this case" or "not likely from my experience."

The cross-examining attorney will often attempt to restate or redefine a witness's answer by using phrases such as "In other words, Doctor . . . " or "What you are saying is . . . " One should not agree with such a restatement unless it is exactly what was said or carries the intended meaning. Otherwise, testimony may be transformed into something favorable to the opposing party's position, and the opportunity for rebuttal may be lost.

"A Reasonable Degree of Medical Certainty"

Definitions of the words "possible" and "probable" constitute a crossover area of legal and medical jargon. Opposing counsel may carefully push the limits of the expert's ability to differentiate them in a legal context during cross-examination. The goal of cross-examination is often to show that what the expert claims is "possible" is not "probable" given the specific facts of the case at hand. One strategy is to try to demonstrate that the physician is not willing to state a totally unqualified opinion of how an injury occurred or totally rule out a diagnosis other than abuse. Experts should not hesitate to say that they cannot be 100% certain but that they have substantive reasons to believe that this is the most likely diagnosis.

The cross-examining lawyer will often use the phrase "reasonable medical certainty" in asking for an opinion about the likelihood that an injury represents abuse: "Can you say, Doctor, within a reasonable degree of medical certainty, that this fracture was caused by abuse?" It is important to realize that this phrase has no precise meaning in terms of numerical probabilities. If the physician's medical opinion is that the injury most likely resulted from abuse, the answer should be "Yes." "Reasonable medical certainty" is often a stumbling block because some jurisdictions require that the opinions be stated using that specific phrase (Little v. State 413 N.E. 2d 639, 646 [Ind., 1980]). Others take the position that the expert is not required to state those precise words if the testimony implies that there is "a reasonable medical probability" of a causal connection (Crocker v. State 573 S.W. 2d 190, 201, 203 [Tex. Ct. App., 1978]). The expert witness must know the phraseology that will be necessary in the jurisdiction where the case is being heard.

Another tactic aimed at parsing probabilities involves questioning the physician about each of a child's injuries separately, trying to demonstrate that any one injury, by itself, might have been accidental. The attorney then concludes by arguing that if each injury could have been accidental, all of the injuries could have been accidental and therefore there is no good evidence that any abuse has occurred. A physician should make it clear to the court and to opposing counsel that it is the existence of numerous injuries, often in different stages of healing, which indicates that the child has been abused.

THE PURPOSE OF EXPERT TESTIMONY

In general, there are two types of disputes in child abuse cases for which medical testimony is required. The first is whether an injury exists and, if so, its precise nature and extent; the second pertains to the cause of the injury. The physician need not be qualified as an expert to describe an injury or the way in which it was evaluated. Recognition as an expert by the court is required before the physician can offer an opinion about the cause of an injury or its possible future consequences for the child. These two areas of testimony can overlap, however. A physician may have to be recognized only as a properly trained medical professional to enable him or her to state diagnostic findings that are relevant to the case. The court may not insist on expert status, for example, for the physician to state that a child's injuries had the characteristics of bites or a gunshot wound so long as these are readily recognizable lesions and a great deal of subjectivity is not involved in making the identification. Likewise, a generalist clinician, not qualified as an expert in child abuse or forensics, could reasonably testify that these lesions were widely recognized as grounds for *suspecting* child abuse (and therefore the reason the clinician had made a report regarding the child), although he or she might not be allowed to offer an opinion as to whether the particular child in question had actually been abused.

Opinion testimony is procedurally more difficult to admit into evidence than testimony regarding facts. Except in rare cases, the physician witness has not actually observed the incident that caused a child's injuries, and therefore any testimony regarding causation must be based on speculation. Certain procedural safeguards are placed on speculation to ensure a high level of reliability. Beyond the requirement that the witness be qualified as an expert, testimony must follow certain rules of evidence that set limits on the kinds of opinions that may be rendered and the information that may be used in formulating these opinions. In the United States, federal courts have their own rules of evidence; state courts have either developed rules of their own or had them imposed by legislation. Although many newer court-developed or legislated rules are based on the procedures used in federal courts, there is still a great deal of local variation. The following paragraphs describe some of the evidentiary rules that apply most closely to cases involving abuse and neglect.

A basic concern of the court when hearing expert testimony is that the expert not usurp the court's role in evaluating the case at hand. This is the focus of two of the major rules of evidence that must be considered during a case of suspected abuse: a requirement that the expert not testify on matters of which the judge and/or jury are already knowledgeable, and a requirement that the expert not directly offer an opinion on the "ultimate issue" involved in the case.

In general, the purpose of expert testimony is to provide an evaluation of facts from a base of knowledge beyond that of the judge or jurors. Otherwise, in theory, there would be no need for an expert, only for someone to introduce the facts for the court's consideration. In some courts, and in particular those following Federal Rule of Evidence 702, this requirement may be relaxed: experts may testify about areas within the court's realm of knowledge so long as the court determines that doing so will be beneficial to its deliberations. In other jurisdictions, however, this point may be used as a way of limiting or excluding an expert's testimony. For example, a defense attorney may propose that many of the jurors are parents and therefore that an expert's testimony on the appropriateness of certain parenting skills is not required.

Similarly, experts are generally not allowed to testify on "ultimate issues of fact," those questions that the court itself has been called upon to determine. For example, in a juvenile or family court case involving physical abuse, the parents may claim that a child's injury was the result of an accident. The ultimate issue in the case thus becomes whether or not this claim is true, and therefore in some jurisdictions an expert may not be allowed to offer a direct opinion about the nature of the injury. Again, this rule may be liberalized in courts that follow the Federal Rules of Evidence (Rule 704).

SOURCES ON WHICH AN EXPERT OPINION IS BASED

The source of the information upon which the expert bases an opinion occasionally creates evidentiary difficulty. Sometimes the original examining physician will not have developed the expertise to testify about abuse causation. The lawyer will then call another child abuse expert to offer an opinion, but because this expert has not personally seen the injury, he or she must base that opinion on records made by the examining physician. The expert also will rely on his or her experience in other child abuse cases as well as a reading of the medical literature. These last two sources are not formally admitted into evidence, which technically makes it improper for them to serve as a basis for the opinion. The Federal Rules of Evidence, however, permit expert witnesses to rely on sources not admitted into evidence under certain circumstances. Rule 703 allows an expert to base an opinion regarding alleged causation on facts or other information known to him or her prior to trial so long as they are reasonably relied on by other experts in the field. Rule 705 permits the expert to give opinion testimony without disclosing underlying facts or data unless the court, or opposing counsel on cross-examination, requires otherwise.

Increasingly, however, courts are becoming more strict with expert testimony, especially if it involves the application of new diagnostic techniques or concepts that may not have gained widespread acceptance (Black, 1988). In the United States, testimony that involves scientific evidence, such as DNA analysis, to link an abuser with a victim or that touches on the relationship of a particular syndrome to child abuse must meet the so-called Frye test (Frye v. United States, 293 F. 1013 [D.C. Cir. 1923]). The Frye test requires that before an expert can offer testimony, "the thing from which the deduction is made must be sufficiently established to have gained general acceptance in the field in which it belongs" (Giannelli, 1980). For example, when the battered child syndrome was first described, its constellation of findings was not generally accepted as constituting evidence of inflicted injury. Today, however, most courts find it acceptable for a physician witness to say that a child has the physical findings of the syndrome and to use that as a basis for an opinion that the injuries were intentionally inflicted (Roberts, 1980; United States v. Bowers, 660 F. 2d 527, 529 [5th Cir. 1981]). This is not necessarily the case for other abuse-related syndromes such as Munchausen syndrome by proxy or the the rape-trauma syndrome and other posttraumatic disorders (Cohen, 1985–86). Before an expert attempts to testify about one of the lesser-known forms of child abuse, he or she should be able to state that this form of abuse is accepted by the general scientific community as a cause of certain types of injury and death. It may help to give attorneys copies of medical journal articles that describe important syndromes or findings. Sometimes these articles can be formally entered into evidence, and the expert can then describe their contents for the education of the court.

Rebuttal or Support of Exculpatory Statements

Opposing counsel will sometimes object to an expert's testimony regarding the cause of a child's injuries on the grounds that the expert did not personally observe the traumatic incident. Indeed, it appears that in the absence of an exculpatory statement of the trauma (an alternative, unintentional explanation offered by the defendant), the expert can introduce evidence of abuse causation but only through testimony about the battered child or some similar syndrome (People v. Kinder, 428 N.Y.S. 2d 375, 382 [A.D. 1980]). Testimony regarding the battered child syndrome can be introduced because it is not an opinion about whether any particular person has done something, which would be legally improper to offer. It simply indicates that a child who has sustained a certain type of injury has not suffered the injury by accidental means (People v. Henson 33 N.Y. 2d 63, 349 N.Y.S. 2d 657, 664, 304 N.E. 2d 358 [1973]; People v. Jackson, 18 Cal. App. 3d 504, 507, 95 Cal. Rptr. 919, 921 [1971]). However, if the caretaker has alleged an exculpatory theory of causation, courts allow the admission of expert testimony as a matter of course to show that the alternative explanation is probable or improbable. This testimony is allowed without the necessity of reference to the battered child syndrome (State v. Pennewell, 598 P. 2d 748 [Wash. App. 1979]), although evidence of the syndrome is also admissible to rebut the claim of accident (United States v. Bowers).

Battered Child Syndrome Testimony

The description of the battered child syndrome cited in many legal opinions is as follows: a child has received repeated, often serious injuries by nonaccidental means, characteristically inflicted by someone who is caring for the child (United States vs. Bowers at 529; People v. Jackson, 18 Cal. App. 3d 504, 506–507, 95 Cal. Rptr. 919, 921 [Cal. App. 1971]; People v. Ewing, 72 Cal. App. 3d 714, 717, 140 Cal. Rptr. 299, 301 [Cal. App. 1977]; Comm. v. Labbe, 373 N.E. 2d 227, 230–231 [Mass. App. 1978]; State v. Loss, 204 N.W. 2d 404, 407–408 [Minn. 1973]; State v. Wilkerson, 247 S.E. 2d 905, 911–912 [N.C. 1978]). Such testimony is not always labeled "battered child syndrome" testimony. Some lawyers consider "battered child" an inflammatory name and do not wish to encounter difficulty introducing it, so they label the syndrome differently. Terms used have included "traumatic periostitis," "parent-induced trauma," and "unsuspected trauma." The expert will want to agree on a name for the syndrome for the purposes of testimony.

Medical Records

Medical records are generally admissible as evidence. In cases involving medical institutions, it is best that the lawyer subpoena the records separately rather than have the expert collect them informally and bring them to court. This approach will allow the records to be more easily admitted into evidence because they will have always remained within the control of the official custodian. The expert should be aware that during cross-examination, opposing counsel has a right to see the reports and notes the expert uses while on the witness stand. The expert should be prepared to respond to questions about unsupported opinions, inaccurate information, or inconsistencies between the testimony given and those records and notes.

Photographs

Photographs can be introduced as evidence. This may be accomplished through the photographer's testimony about the camera, lens, film, time of day the photo was taken, and other details indicating the authenticity of a picture. Photographs also can be introduced by a physician, even if he or she did not take them, if they are illustrative of the witness's description of the scene depicted. For example, if a physician testified about the bruises and cuts observed on a child at the time of treatment and was then shown a picture of the child taken by the police at approximately the same time, the physician could testify that the photograph was a "true and accurate representation" of what he or she had seen. The photograph is then eligible for admission into evidence.

Hearsay

Generally, a witness can testify only about those facts that he or she knows personally, not about information from others (hearsay). Hearsay is usually inadmissible because its introduction violates a party's constitutional right to confront and cross-examine his or her accuser. There are an array of exceptions to the hearsay prohibition, such as statements made to the physician by the parents while they were experiencing the emotion of having the injury discovered ("excited utterances") or statements made by the child while in the course of medical treatment (see Chapter 6). These statements are considered to be more reliable because of the special circumstances that prompted their utterance. The physician should discuss with the lawyer all communications from parties in the case to discover whether it suggests any helpful testimony that may be admissible under one of the hearsay exceptions.

References

Besharov DJ. Proving child abuse: a guide for practice under the New York Family Court Act. Cornell University: Family Life Development Center, 1984.

Black B. Evolving legal standards for the admissibility of scientific evidence. Science 1988;239:1508–1512.

Cohen A. The unreliability of expert testimony in the typical characteristics of sexual abuse victims. 74 Georgetown Law J 429, 1985–6.

Giannelli PC. The admissibility of novel scientific evidence: Frye v. United States, a half century later. 80 Columbia Law Rev 1197, 1980.

Roberts M. Annotation: admissibility of expert medical testimony on battered child syndrome. 98 ALR 3d 306, 1980.

21 Treatment Decisions

Volumes have been written about the treatment of abused children, their families, and perpetrators (Sgroi, 1982; Jones and Alexander, 1987; Salter, 1988). As mentioned in Chapter 19, although the need to offer treatment is compelling, relatively little conclusive evidence is available to support its efficacy (Daro, 1988). This chapter does not attempt to provide a comprehensive guide to treatment options or a review of the literature on outcomes. Rather, it seeks to present an outline of immediate treatment considerations and long-term goals, as they are generally accepted, so that primary care clinicians can better participate in planning with their patients.

IMMEDIATE CONSIDERATIONS

Treatment of abused children and their families begins at the moment of disclosure. The sense of crisis and loss of control are similar regardless of whether a child has just been assaulted or whether long-term abuse has just been disclosed. The prototype reaction has been described by Burgess and Holmstrom (1974) and called the rape trauma syndrome. In the acute phase of the reaction, the victim is predominantly fearful and disorganized. He or she may be either openly distraught or seemingly in control. Both reactions represent coping mechanisms that overlay an attempt to process what has happened and come to terms with feelings of rage, helplessness, guilt, and shame (Martin et al., 1983).

At this acute stage, there are many ways in which clinicians can help victims. Victims especially need opportunities to feel in control. Particular care must be given to explain procedures, to seek consent, and to conduct the evaluation at a pace that is comfortable for the individual. On the other hand, both the victim and the family need to feel reassured about their safety, the medical condition, and the competency of the staff to handle the situation. Clinicians must be be able to show that they too are in control of their emotions and can approach the crisis in an objective and self-assured manner. Whenever possible, the victim and family should be continually accompanied by a supportive staff member for the duration of the initial visit. Opportunities should be made for expression of fear and shame; most importantly, this involves direct inquiry about how the victim and family are feeling, not just about the details of what has happened.

Both the victim and family can be helped by an open discussion of the feelings and reactions that often follow traumatic events. Family members can be prepared to accept regressive behaviors, rapid mood swings, sudden fears, and disruptions of sleep and appetite in the early period following the trauma. They can be cautioned to allow the victim to talk about what has happened and to not avoid the topic for fear of making things worse. The often protracted nature of recovery can also be mentioned, especially if a victim appears to be in control and thus may not be offered help. Families can also be told about the dynamics of recanting and the need to assure the victim that he or she is loved and not at fault.

Safe Placement for the Victim

A critical question when spouse or child abuse is seen in the acute care setting is whether it is safe for the victim to return home. If there are medical problems requiring hospitalization, an admission is indicated. Sometimes conditions that are otherwise treatable on an outpatient basis will require admission either for psychological support or because reliable care at home cannot be guaranteed. It is important that hospital staff be informed of the *medical* indications for such admissions. Patients classified as social admissions may not receive appropriate medical and emotional support.

The most difficult cases are those in which it is medically appropriate for the victim to go home but the safety of the home is uncertain. Several factors can be considered:

- Has the perpetrator been identified? If so, can he or she be kept from contact with the victim?
- Can the victim receive sufficient support and protection in the home? The home environ-

ment must be physically safe, but it must also be emotionally supportive. If other family members are sufficiently traumatized or angry about the disclosure, they may not be able to provide support for the victim. Particularly dangerous situations arise when an older child has disclosed abuse—especially incest—and the nonabusing parents seem not to believe the child's story. In these cases, not only will the victim fail to receive support, but the nonabusing parent cannot be counted on to protect the child should the abuser attempt to return to the home.

- How did the abusive crisis occur? Is it a general symptom of the family's level of stress or lack of resources? If abusing parents, for example, continue to show extreme anxiety and inability to cope, and if the stresses that contributed to abuse continue to exist, then the risk of further abuse may be high. Families that have a long history of dysfunction or that have no immediately available outside contacts may also be more likely to continue abusive behavior. These are points that a social worker must explore with a family in the emergency room or other acute care setting before the family can be released.

The tightening of public and private funding for all hospitalizations has led to a reluctance to admit children suspected of being abused unless they are seriously ill (Committee on Hospital Care, 1987). Hospitals may indeed be denied payment for some abuse or neglect-related admissions on the basis of standard utilization review criteria for medical necessity. This represents a situation in which clinicians must both advocate for children and find creative solutions to a genuine problem. The hospital remains a reasonable place to evaluate and protect these children: it offers a supportive environment and the intensive, comprehensive attention that can alter attitudes toward disclosure. As the caseloads of social service agencies become more overwhelming, hospitalization may help avoid overly hasty and incomplete evaluations of a child's immediate placement needs. Clinicians can ask these agencies to pay for stays that are lengthened while evaluations are pending and work more closely with adult- and family-oriented shelters that may be substitute safe environments.

Safety issues involving pedophiles and incest offenders may be especially difficult to evaluate. Dreiblatt (1983) points out that most sex offenders go through cycles of offense, remorse, and reoffense. In the remorseful state, they may convincingly seem to be under control and fully motivated to not reoffend. There will often be a "suppression effect" at the time of disclosure so that in the short term the offender appears to lose interest in children. Pedophile behavior, however, can be seen as a habituated behavior, like alcohol or drug abuse, over which the abuser initially has little control. For this reason, regardless of the abuser's initial appearance, many therapists consider separation of the sex offender and victim mandatory, at least until the victim is psychologically prepared and adequate safety can be guaranteed. Similar dynamics may occur in other forms of abuse. Remorse does not indicate that the abuser has learned how to handle the emotions or stresses that led to abuse.

Some other perpetrator behaviors that may be apparent to the clinician, even in the early evaluation of a case of suspected abuse, require immediate psychiatric consultation and raise the risk of serious danger to the child. Kempe and Kempe (1976) provide the following list of these less usual but very worrisome situations:

- When abuse has taken place for no apparent reason, without the family or personal stresses often found.
- When abuse was premeditated or characterized by torture or sadism, or the abuser shows evidence of sociopathic behavior (including violent outbursts and frequent previous involvement with legal difficulties).
- When the abuser seems to have been fixated on repeatedly injuring a specific part of the child's body.
- When the parent seems to have a particularly distorted view of reality or bizarre ideation.
- When the parent seems to be severely depressed or denies having any feelings at all.
- When the parent appears fanatical or extraordinarily rigid, especially if such thoughts are related to extreme religious or moral beliefs about child behavior or development.

Role of Child Protective Service Agencies

In the United States, child protective service (CPS) agencies are a branch of local or state government that have authority to carry out the state's mandate to protect children. Larger CPS agencies usually have several separate components, including personnel assigned to evaluation of new cases of suspected maltreatment, management of established cases, supervision of children in foster care, and sometimes supportive services for high-risk families in which maltreatment has not taken place. Communication among these components may not be rapid, and their actions may not be coordinated.

The precise criteria by which CPS agencies accept cases are rarely defined in law or regulation, and hence there may be great variability from jurisdiction to jurisdiction or even from shift to shift in the kinds of cases that are accepted for evaluation (Nelson et al., 1980). Recently, there has been a movement to reduce the range of cases accepted as a means of managing increased agency workloads. For example, in some agencies consideration has been given to not accepting cases solely on the basis of a concern for educational neglect or the use of illicit drugs during pregnancy. Clinicians who feel strongly that a case should be evaluated by a CPS agency must often work their way up a supervisory hierarchy until they can convince the agency of their concerns.

CPS agencies are usually mandated by law to evaluate a case within a certain period of time, shorter for physical and sexual abuse and longer for neglect. The initial response to the case may be carried out by the agency itself, or it may be delegated to the police if such an agreement has been made. These arrangements require clinicians to be prepared for contacts with investigators who may have little training in the area of family violence or who may consider it to be one of the more annoying or dangerous parts of the job. Investigation by a uniformed officer, often with weapons, ammunition, and a radio visible, may be stigmatizing to the family and frightening for the child. Clinicians can help by trying to arrange for these encounters at a neutral location such as a medical facility and by briefing the officer before he or she makes contact with the victim or family. Some facilities also prohibit visible weapons in the area in which abused children are being evaluated; many jurisdictions assign plain clothes officers to these duties.

CPS agencies may exert their authority in a variety of ways. The initial approach to a family is often to make a contract, sometimes written, in which voluntary arrangements are made for the child's safety and the abuser's conduct. The abuser may agree to stay out of the home, and the nonabusing parent may promise to call the police if the abuser returns. Alternatively, the parents may agree to have the child live with a close relative or family friend where his or her safety will be assured. If the family is unwilling to enter into any such agreement, the agency may go before a family or juvenile court and get an order, enforceable by the police, granting authority over the child's whereabouts to CPS. The child may still be placed at home, with relatives, or in a foster home, but now the action will have legal authority and the parents' consent is not required.[1]

Whenever possible, the offender and not the victim should be removed from the home. Sometimes, however, placement of the victim is unavoidable. In this case, some steps can be taken to ease the difficulty of separation (Broadhurst et al., 1980):

- To the extent possible, both parents and children should be involved in the decision to place the victim outside the home. Everyone should understand the rationale for placement, why other alternatives are not appropriate, and that the separation is temporary. Care must be taken that removal of children is not seen as a punitive step but rather as a move that will be therapeutic for both the victim and the abuser.
- From an emotional perspective, the best placements are with close family members or with a member of the extended family who can come and live with the child in the child's home. Whoever cares for the child must be

---

[1] Recently, attention has been focused on the practice of placing children with relatives rather than in designated foster homes (Daley S. Agency said to fail children placed in relatives' care. New York Times 23 Feb 1989:B1). Placement with relatives is appealing because it minimizes the emotional trauma of separation from parents, but in many cities children placed with relatives receive fewer services. In some cases, this is because children not formally placed in foster homes do not qualify for special assistance such as Medicaid or other financial benefits. This can place financial hardship on the relatives and diminish their desire to shelter the child. In other cases, the lack of services may stem from an agency's perceptions that children placed with relatives need less care.

prepared to help overcome guilt feelings that the child may have about causing the separation and must be careful not to vilify the offending parent.
- When possible, siblings should remain together and familiar objects and toys should accompany the children. At the least, preliminary plans for visitation should be discussed before the actual separation takes place.

TREATMENT RESOURCES

Physical Abuse

Treatment for families involved in physical abuse must address both acute and chronic problems as well as the needs of parents and children alike. Often, a variety of services are prescribed. They require close coordination from a single provider serving as a case manager. This is often a task performed by a protective service "continuing worker" or a primary health care provider.

TREATMENT FOR CHILDREN

Crisis intervention

In the short term, the child needs a chance to be relieved of any guilt or anxiety that he or she experiences for seemingly being at the center of the family's problems. The child may simultaneously be fearful of the parents' anger and frightened of losing their love. Which professional helps to meet these needs will depend on the child's condition. If the child is hospitalized, it may be a nurse, social worker, or child life therapist. If the child is at home or in foster care, these issues must be addressed in a follow-up visit to a medical or counseling facility. That visit should be scheduled within a few days of the initial disclosure of abuse.

SPECIFIC TREATMENT FOR CHRONIC MEDICAL PROBLEMS

At times, a child's chronic medical problems (asthma, a learning disability, a physical handicap) may put added stress on a family or serve as a trigger for abuse. Optimizing medical care of these conditions may help to reduce the risk of future injury.

PLAY THERAPY FOR PRESCHOOL CHILDREN

While preschool children are not usually able to verbally work through their reactions to abuse, they may benefit from individual play sessions that allow them to experience a "stable, reliable, and understanding relationship" (Kempe and Kempe, 1978). Through once- or twice-weekly individual play sessions, a child may learn to trust adults and begin to develop better social skills. Children who have become extremely withdrawn or overly aggressive may benefit most from this sort of therapy.

GROUP THERAPY

Group therapy can take place in therapeutic play or preschools specially dedicated to abused children or in mixed settings among other, nonabused children. These groups serve several purposes. First and foremost, they offer the child a place of total safety and acceptance, qualities often missing from the child's home environment. The child is helped to gain independence and self-confidence through separation from the parents and having a chance to try new skills without fear of being punished or ridiculed. The child can also learn better communication skills and more normal ways of interacting with other children and adults. Head Start programs in the United States are a successful model of therapeutic preschool that allow abused children to contact other children from the community. Extra help for abused children is also available in many regular nurseries and elementary schools. The child may receive special one-on-one attention in addition to the school's regular educational program. These special sessions may focus on both emotional and academic issues.

ROLE MODELS AND INDIVIDUAL SUPPORT IN THE HOME

Programs such as Big Brothers can help a child who has had little chance to build self-esteem and appropriate social skills. They also provide the parents a reprieve from child care responsibilities. It is important that volunteers commit themselves to work with a child for a fixed, extended period of time. Abused children are particularly vulnerable to feelings of loss and self-reproach when a meaningful relationship is unexpectedly ended.

FOSTER CARE

Foster care is often considered as treatment for many kinds of abuse. Ideally, it combines the assurance of safety with the provision of a nurturing and stable environment. Foster care may be provided by a relative or by families selected by public or private agencies. Unfortunately, foster care has many drawbacks. As Kempe and Kempe (1978) point out, whereas safety is often the primary concern of health care and social service workers, children entering foster care may be more concerned over losing the only love and consistency they have ever known, even if it came in the context of abuse or neglect. Thus, the child may see foster care more as punishment than as rescue. When foster care is used, it is important for the child to understand the necessity and to know that contact with the biologic parents will not be cut off.

Abuse has also been known to continue in foster care settings, and deaths of children in foster care have been reported. It is not known to what extent this is the fault of the foster families or CPS workers involved or to what extent the risk of abuse may have been increased by a child's own behavior. One of the most serious risks to children is that once placed in foster care they will be constantly shifted from one foster setting to another, never being returned to the family but never legally eligible for adoption or permanent placement. Children who remain in foster care for more than a short period of time are often never returned to their parents (Fanshel, 1981). Foster care is perhaps best seen as a treatment of last resort when no other alternatives are available and the risk to the child's safety is so great that it offsets the risks of placement.

TREATMENT FOR PARENTS

Treatment for abusing parents must be provided in a context of acceptance and approval; these individuals often have primary problems with low self-esteem and fear of rejection. They may not be sufficiently trusting or mature for insight-oriented therapy. Frequently, a combination of emotionally supportive services with practical parenting aids can provide a basis on which to later explore more deep-seated issues. The following resources may be appropriate for parents who express an interest in changing their behavior.

INDIVIDUAL THERAPY

Individual counseling or psychotherapy must ultimately involve both parents and later the entire family as a unit. Its goal is to aid the parents in developing new responses to dilemmas that they find overwhelming. Often the therapy will have specific behavioral objectives, and sessions will focus on replays of situations that cause the parents to become anxious or angry. Parents who are open to insight therapy may be helped to explore issues that underlie their propensity to abuse. Such treatment is usually planned to last from 6 months to 1 year.

GROUPS

Both supportive and explicitly psychotherapeutic groups can be effective means of helping parents confront their tendency to abuse and receive practical advice on the acquisition of new skills. The group is designed to be a major means of emotional support for the parents, in some instances substituting for a family when the abuser has none. In groups, parents are encouraged to express their feelings, deal with their poor self-esteem, and learn to accept some degree of social control (Holmes, 1978). Parents Anonymous is one example of a successful group that combines support and therapy in a community-based setting. Groups are conducted under the coleadership of lay therapists and professionals and are open to both acknowledged abusers and parents who feel that they have the capacity to abuse. Group work is usually an adjunct to individual counseling.

SUPPORTIVE SERVICES

A variety of concrete services are available to help parents with the kinds of life stresses that seem to precipitate abuse. Lay therapists and parent aides often have the advantage of coming from socioeconomic backgrounds similar to those of the parents. They may be able to model parenting and coping skills as well as provide a secure and uncritical friendship. They give parents a chance to build skills without exacerbating feelings of inadequacy.

Hot lines and crisis nurseries may serve two functions. First, their very presence can help a parent feel more confident in facing stress knowing that help is always available. Second, the parent can receive immediate support and concrete advice when required. Parents Anonymous members, for example, are urged to "pick up the phone" when they feel the impulse to harm a child. Crisis nurseries, which are facilities where parents can take children for short periods (usually less than 72 hours), can provide a useful alternative to foster care for parents who suffer intermittent periods of dysfunction.

A variety of concrete aids can help with day-to-day needs. Emergency funds for food or clothing (or for decreasing isolation by paying for telephone service or transportation) may be available from community relief organizations. Transportation may be provided on a regular basis for medical visits or simply to allow parents the opportunity to go shopping or visit family members. The parents' own medical problems also need attention, ideally from a primary care provider with whom the parents can establish an ongoing relationship.

Child Neglect

The treatment resources available for child neglect are very similar to those used in cases of physical abuse. Neglect, however, may prove much more difficult to treat. Neglectful parents may be more likely to have serious character disorders that lead to abuse. Those who are extremely apathetic or view life as futile may be especially hard to reach (Polansky et al., 1981). Marital counseling may be especially important to allow the parents to support and nurture each other. Groups may not be appropriate for many neglectful parents whose underlying problems make them extremely fearful of interactions with others. Home aides may be the best way to assure that the child's basic needs are being met and ultimately to provide a model for the parents of an organized, pleasurable approach to day-to-day tasks.

Treatment for Sexual Abuse

TREATMENT FOR CHILDREN

Crisis intervention

Victims of child sexual abuse are more likely to be totally rejected by both parents than are victims of other kinds of physical abuse. They need continued support and reassurance that they have taken the right step in disclosing abuse. Small children may have many of the symptoms of the rape trauma syndrome described above and in Chapter 2, coupled with regressive behaviors such as enuresis and sleep disturbances (Berliner and Ernst, 1984).

Individual and group therapy

Ongoing therapy for a sexually abused child has several goals. The first is to give the consistent message that the child is physically intact and will be able to have a normal life. Group treatment is especially important for older victims as a way of assuring them that abuse has not made them different from others. Abused children are often afraid to tell their peers about what has happened and may feel marked or damaged. Group treatment gives these children a safe place to share their experiences and the chance to see that abuse happens to other children, too. A second message given in groups is that the abuse is the responsibility of the abuser, not the child. The child is told that feelings of anger or ambivalence toward the abuser are understandable and that the purpose of therapy is to provide a protected place in which to state and cope with these feelings.

Treatment for sexual offenders

Treatment for sexual offenders may take several paths using group and individual counseling. Initially, offenders must take full responsibility for the abuse and make a commitment to change their ways and repair the damage they have done. In cases of intrafamilial abuse, abusers usually agree to leave the home for an extended period of time while still meeting their responsibilities to financially support the family (Salter, 1988).

Subsequent steps in therapy involve addressing the abusers' learned sexual arousal to children and their ability to overcome forces that would otherwise inhibit abuse. Treatment for alcoholism is often a part of this therapy. Offenders who are psychotic or sociopathic, or who have never been capable of arousal to adult sexual stimuli have a poor prognosis for treatment. One rarely speaks of cure, but rather of controlling offenders' behavior in the long term.

The final step in the treatment of intrafamilial abuse involves family sessions during which the offender reacknowledges responsibility for the abuse and family members agree on rules of conduct that will protect the children and foster a better relationship between the parents. Following such agreements, the abuser may be allowed to return to the home for a trial period.

References

Berliner L, Ernst E. Group work with preadolescent sexual assault victims. In: Stuart I, Greer JG, eds. Victims of sexual aggression: men, women and children. New York: Van Nostrand Reinhold Co, 1984:105–124.

Broadhurst DD, Estey RS, Hughes W, Jenkins JL, Martin JA. Child protection in military communities. DHEW Publ. (OHDS) 80–30260. Washington, DC: US Government Printing Office, 1980.

Burgess AW, Holmstrom LI. Rape trauma syndrome. Am J Psychiatry 1974;131:981–986.

Committee on Hospital Care. Medical necessity for the hospitalization of the abused and neglected child. Pediatrics 1987;79:300.

Daro D. Confronting child abuse: research for effective program design. New York: The Free Press, 1988.

Dreiblatt IS. Issues in the evaluation of the sex offender. In: Child Sexual Abuse Training Institute manual. Seattle: Harborview Medical Center, Social Work Department, 1983.

Fanshel D. Decision making under uncertainty: foster care for abused children. Am J Public Health 1981;71:685–686.

Holmes S. Parents Anonymous: a treatment method for child abuse. Social Work 1978;23:245–246.

Jones DPH, Alexander H. Treating the abusive family within the family care system. In: Helfer RE, Kempe RS, eds. The battered child. 4th ed. Chicago, University of Chicago Press, 1987:339–359.

Kempe R, Kempe CH. Assessing family pathology. In: Helfer RE, Kempe CH, eds. Child abuse and neglect: the family and the community. Cambridge: Ballinger, 1976:115–126.

Kempe RS, Kempe CH. Child abuse. Cambridge: Harvard University Press, 1978.

Martin CA, Warfield MC, Braen GR. Physician's management of the psychological aspects of rape. JAMA 1983;249:501–503.

Nelson GK, Dainauski J, Kilmer L. Child abuse reporting laws: action and uncertainty. Child Welfare 1980;59:203–212.

Polansky NA, Chalmers MA, Buttenwieser E, Williams DP. Damaged parents: an anatomy of child neglect. Chicago: University of Chicago Press, 1981.

Salter AC. Treating child sex offenders and victims: a practical guide. Beverly Hills: Sage Publications, 1988.

Sgroi SM. Handbook of clinical intervention in child sexual abuse. Lexington, Massachusetts: Lexington Books, 1982.

22
Causes and Prevention of Maltreatment

CAUSES OF ABUSE AND NEGLECT

The following paragraphs should be read with this caution in mind: the terms "child abuse" and "maltreatment" refer to a wide range of acts and omissions that are unlikely to be caused by any single set of factors. Theoretical models proposed to explain the phenomenon of maltreatment usually include influences of individual behavior (parent and child), family interactions, community characteristics, and cultural values (Belsky, 1980). Various, perhaps unique, combinations of these influences appear to cause specific types of maltreatment in specific families. Some themes, however, do seem to occur to some extent in all forms of maltreatment. This brief chapter addresses these common themes in the context of developing prevention efforts. More details about the etiology of specific forms of maltreatment are found in other chapters and in some of the many specific reviews available.

The Abuser's Childhood

Steele (1980) found that many abusive parents reported having suffered what could be labeled emotional abuse during their own childhood: a consistent lack of empathy from their parents, a lack of support for their development, and a chronic feeling of never having had their needs met. Altemeir et al. (1982) found further evidence of this in a prospective study of some 1400 parents, 2% of whom were later reported to have physically abused their children by the time they were of preschool age; 59% of the abusers, compared with 25% of the nonabusers, reported that they felt their parents had been displeased with them. Among the abusers, 57% said that they did not get along with their mothers, compared with 25% of the nonabusers.

Childhood physical and sexual abuse also appear to be more common among abusers than nonabusers. Evidence for this comes from the study of pedophiles. Gebhard and co-workers (1967), for example, found that 10–18% of adults incarcerated for having had sexual contact with young girls had themselves had sexual contact with an adult when they were children. One-third of adults jailed for having had sexual contact with boys reported victimization during childhood. Similar findings come from studies of other kinds of abuse, although comparison rates among nonabusing adults are not available. The American Humane Association (1979), in its compilation of United States national abuse reports, found that 20% of abusing parents said that they had themselves been abused as children.

Two points are important in considering the figures described above. The first is that while clinical observation has frequently remarked on the prevalence of childhood abuse among abusers, these essentially retrospective studies without control groups appear to overestimate the rate with which abuse is transmitted from generation to generation (Kaufman and Ziegler, 1987). When comparison groups or prospective studies are used, it appears that many if not most individuals who are abused as children do not go on to victimize a subsequent generation. For example, Finkelhor (1984) found that as many as 19% of college-age women and 9% of college-age men reported having had some episode of sexual victimization during childhood. The majority of these students had presumably not themselves become abusers.

A second point (Araji and Finkelhor, 1985) is that the observation of abuse during childhood still does not explain why adults abuse. In the case of sexual abuse, a number of theories have been advanced, including the need to "master" the traumatic experience by becoming an aggressor, the "damaged goods" syndrome which leads victims to believe they cannot have normal relationships, and the possibility that the early abuse conditions an "abnormal" pattern of sexual responses. Steele (1980) has proposed that one's experience as a child establishes what one then considers normal and acceptable for child rearing. Adults abused as children may consider that physical or sexual exploitation of children is implicitly accepted by society. They may also unconsciously attempt to rationalize their own experiences by perpetuating abusive behavior and thus establishing its "normality." These theories are as yet unproven, although they may be useful to clinicians evaluating individual cases.

Somewhat more information is available regarding factors that may decrease the likelihood that abused children will grow up to be abusers. These data come from longitudinal studies and not from trials of treatment programs, and they involve only physical abuse or neglect by mothers in the first few years of a child's life, but they suggest both interventions and means of identifying individuals who may be at higher risk of perpetuating abuse (Hunter and Kilstrom, 1979; Egeland et al., 1988). One apparently protective factor was the mother's ability to confront the issue of her own abuse. Women who were able to talk of it openly and who felt less ambiguity about parenting their own children were less likely to become abusers. Having had at least one supportive parent or a relatively secure relationship with an adult outside the family was also protective, as was the quality of the mother's support system as an adult. Having a satisfying and nonabusive relationship with a mate was associated with a decreased chance of becoming abusive. One of the main mechanisms by which men abuse their children may be this indirect pathway of neglect of the family as a whole and abuse of the wife in particular (Egeland, 1988).

Family Stresses and Supports

Another factor in the etiology of abuse appears to be excess stress on the parent or family, possibly causing a breakdown of inhibitions and a release of frustration upon a child. Stress may come from a variety of sources: financial difficulties, health, job, or marital problems, or the death of someone close. Stress was a factor in the intergenerational studies just described and was explored by Straus and colleagues (1980) in the 1976 National Family Violence Survey.

In that survey, physical violence against children increased as a function of the number of reported stresses in the family. Even in the highest-stress groups, however, the rate of violence remained under 35%. As Straus points out, the majority of highly stressed parents did not abuse their children. Several factors appeared to present an increased likelihood of abuse. Dissatisfaction with marriage, approval of physical violence between the spouses, and the expectation, when frustrated, that the husband should be the dominant family decision maker were associated with a twofold increase in the rate of abuse. Having many members of the extended family nearby was associated with more intrafamilial violence; the reasons for this were not clear. Participation in nonfamily social, business, or religious activity was associated with lower rates of abuse. These findings, it should be noted, were from a cross-sectional study in which it was not possible to determine whether abuse followed or preceded the factors examined.

Socioeconomic and Minority Status

In the National Family Violence Survey, job classification (blue versus white collar) and educational level had little to do with the occurrence of violence toward children. Low income, however, was associated with a marked increase in violence (14 versus 25% of children abused). This finding agrees with data from the National Incidence Study of Child Abuse and Neglect, a nationwide study of child abuse conducted in the United States states during 1979–80 (US Department of Health and Human Services, 1981). This study used different definitions of abuse than the National Family Violence Survey but obtained many parallel results. Although abuse (all types taken together) occurred in all income groups, detected cases (drawn from schools, hospitals, and protective service and other agencies) occurred 10 times more frequently among children in the lowest-income families than among those in the highest (27.3/1000 versus 2.7/1000). For all income groups, the rate of abuse among white children was equal to or higher than that among all other ethnic groups taken together. These differences were most striking in the lowest-income group, where the rate of abuse among whites was nearly twice that of others.

Abusers as Adults

Maternal age at the time of a child's birth appears to influence the likelihood of abuse. Leventhal (1981) compared abused and nonabused infants, controlling for a number of factors, including sex, race, and source of medical care. Mothers of abused children averaged 2 years younger (21 versus 23 years) at the time of the child's birth and were about 1 year younger at the birth of their first child (19 versus 20 years).

Abusers do not fall into any particular categories of psychiatric disorders, and only a minority are considered to fit strict definitions of mental illness (Steele, 1980). In some types of abuse, however, particular patterns have been observed at the time the abuse is discovered (it is not certain, though, that these problems preceded and therefore caused the abuse). Parents who poison or otherwise create factitious illness in children may suffer from a form of delusional thinking that allows them to harm a child and convincingly deny having done so (see Chapter 15). These parents may also have abnormally close "symbiotic" relationships with their children (Waller, 1983).

The symbiotic relationship may be a general characteristic of abusing families. All human relationships are based to some degree on symbiosis, the mutual provision of support that makes life possible. Symbiosis goes too far, however, when adults cannot supply for themselves a minimal amount of self-esteem and self-determination. When these needs must consistently be met by others, especially children, the scene is set for frustration, difficulties with separation, and, it is thought, ultimately abuse (Justice and Justice, 1976).

Pedophiles are another class of abusers who may have a specific psychological problem. As a group, pedophiles (although less so incest perpetrators) appear to develop physiologic sexual arousal to child stimuli (Araji and Finkelhor, 1985). How these arousal responses develop and how they can be modified are not known. Although there is little evidence that pedophiles have particularly immature or dependent personalities (which might cause them to prefer relationships with children rather than adults), some do display evidence of increased anxiety in relationships with other adults. It is not known whether this anxiety precedes the onset of abuse.

Social Forces and the Promotion of Maltreatment

Many workers feel that the root causes of child abuse rest in wider social values, especially those that condone violent behavior and that define the social position of children as parental property (Surgeon General's Workshop, 1985). These values may serve to "disinhibit" persons who otherwise would not abuse children. Two main observations support disinhibition as an antecedent of abuse.

Russell (1984) compared rates of incestuous sexual relations occurring to women with and without stepfathers. It was hypothesized that stepfathers, especially those who did not take on primary parenting relationships, might lack some of the bonds or attachments to their stepdaughters that prevent incest between biologic parents and their children. A total of 930 randomly selected women were asked about childhood sexual experiences with their parents. Of 749 biologic fathers, 18 (2.4%) were reported to have initiated some sort of sexual activity with a daughter before her 14th birthday; 10 of 29 stepfathers (34.5%) were reported to have done so. The risk of incest was 14 times higher in families in which a stepfather was present. The use of alcohol in conjunction with sexual offenses against children has also been considered evidence that disinhibition is involved in the causation of abuse. Several studies found that up to half of all pedophiles either were chronic alcoholics or drank at the time of their assaults on children (Araji and Finkelhor, 1985).

CHARACTERISTICS OF CHILDREN AT RISK FOR ABUSE

Many clinicians feel strongly that the child is not a passive, random target for the abuser but rather that certain children are more vulnerable or may act in ways that precipitate abuse. There is evidence for this viewpoint from studies of both physical abuse in early childhood and sexual abuse of older children, as well as from the observation that abusing parents often single out one child for abuse and report that that child's actions precipitate episodes of violence. This is a delicate subject in that it appears to risk blaming child victims for their fate or offering excuses to abusers seeking a defense. Once abuse has occurred, adults must take full responsibility for their actions, no matter what the purported provocation on the part of the child. Identifying vulnerable children, however, may be a step toward prevention.

Some child vulnerabilities may start early in life and exist totally in the mind of the parents. Parents may develop specific negative perceptions of a child to justify the fact that the child was unwanted and designated "bad" even before birth. A parent's experience with a particular pregnancy may cause that child to be selected for abuse while other children are spared. Lynch (1976) compared 25 abused children with 35 nonabused siblings. Abnormalities of pregnancy, labor, and early childhood experiences, including concealment of the pregnancy, refusal of prenatal care, and extended separation of the mother and child in the first 6 months of the infant's life, were three times more common among the abused children.

Infants perceived by their parents as being fussy or slow to develop mentally or gain weight appear to be at a higher risk of abuse, as do children considered by their parents to have undesirable characteristics reminiscent of disliked family members (Herrenkohl and Herrenkohl, 1979). Children who actually have difficult temperaments (low regularity, little flexibility, predominantly negative mood) are more likely to evoke feelings of irritability and hostility in their parents. Abuse and blame for family problems may result when a child's temperament makes it difficult for the parents to feel competent and in control (Rutter, 1987).

Boys and girls may be vulnerable to abuse at different ages and for different reasons (Martin, 1983; Rutter, 1987). Boys in general are expected to be rough, active, and physically and verbally aggressive; girls, on the other hand, are generally expected to be conforming and quiet. Children who step out of these sex-specific roles may evoke the ire of parents. Boys may be more vulnerable to physical abuse because of the ways in which they react to stress. Parents seem more willing to argue in front of boys and are more likely to be aggressively punitive toward their behavioral problems. This is unfortunate, because boys seem more likely than girls to respond to family stress and punishment with increasingly disruptive and oppositional behavior. Discord and abuse in the family thus appear to provoke child behaviors that in turn provoke more abuse. Emotional, intellectual, and conduct problems are extremely common among children at the time that abuse is discovered to be taking place. How much this reflects underlying vulnerability versus behaviors cultivated in the abusive home is not known.

Some studies have reported increased rates of physical abuse and neglect among handicapped children (Oates, 1985). It seems plausible that the risk to these children should increase, as it does for others, when parents cannot understand or feel competent to manage child behaviors. The families of handicapped children, however, may need more emotional and logistical support to achieve this competency. Particular points of stress may arise, for example, during school vacations, when there is a sudden increase in the family's need to provide care for a handicapped child. Work schedules may be disrupted, siblings may be conscripted against their will into supervisory roles, and the handicapped child's behavior may change outside the structured school environment.

Pedophiles sometimes suggest that the children they assaulted encouraged abuse or even initiated sexual contact. Usually this is a rationalization elaborated by the abuser as part of his denial, although some children who have already been traumatized may mimic adult sexual behaviors (see Chapter 2). Normal children, however, do not behave seductively or solicit sexual activity with adults, although they may sometimes engage in activities (masturbating while being given a bath, curiously touching a parent's genital area) that can be interpreted as seductive by vulnerable adults (Sgroi, 1982). When children mimic adult sexual behaviors, it is because they have learned them, either through activity with adults or through exposure to explicit sexual materials.

Children who are socially and emotionally isolated appear to be at a higher risk of sexual abuse. In his study of female college students, Finkelhor (1984) found that both geographic isolation (living on a farm) and social isolation (having few friends, having a distant relationship with the mother, experiencing little affection from either parent) increased the risk of abuse. Isolated children, Finkelhor postulates, may be more open to an abuser's advances, even if they perceive them to be wrong, as a substitute for other relationships. It also may be harder for these children to reveal the abuse to others; when they do so, they may be less likely to get a supportive response. Finkelhor also speculates that abusers may choose children who appear to be shy or less assertive in the belief that these children will be less likely to reveal abuse.

These observations suggest ways in which

vulnerable children might be protected from abuse (Rutter, 1987). Self-esteem may be bolstered and isolation lessened by providing an object for secure attachment, such as a teacher, "big brother," or relative capable of relating to the child on a regular basis. Children who already have emotional or behavioral problems can be helped by breaking the cycle of negative reactions they often engender when they venture outside the family. Contacts in school or medical care settings may unwittingly recreate the abusive intrafamilial environment by responding harshly to the child's maladaptive social skills. Accepting the child and helping him or her learn new ways of reacting to stress may decrease the chances of abuse in the home.

PREVENTION

Preventing Physical Abuse and Neglect in Early Childhood

Several studies have tested systematic interventions in the newborn period and in early childhood. Although the results have been mixed, it does seem that rates of subsequent injury and neglect can be reduced. Gray et al. (1977) reported that home visits (by a public health nurse) and a program of regular pediatric care resulted in a reduction in physical abuse. No incidents occurred in a group of 25 treatment families versus 5 in a group of 25 "high-risk" controls. O'Connor et al. (1980) found a lower rate of hospitalization for parent-child problems in a group of children randomly assigned to room in with their mothers in the immediate postpartum period (1 of 143 versus 8 of 156 for controls). Olds et al. (1986) found a reduction in abuse and neglect among "high-risk" (poor, unmarried) teenage mothers who participated in a nurse home visitor program (1 of 22 versus 6 of 32 controls). Table 22.1 lists some observations in the immediate postpartum period that may signify an increased risk of abuse or neglect.

Olds speculated that an important part of the nurse visitor's intervention was teaching parents to interpret and understand their children's behavior. In the mother-infant pairs studied, this emphasized an understanding of basic temperamental differences among infants and taught appropriate responses to normal infant behaviors. Although not all perinatal and infancy programs have had similar success (Sie-

Table 22.1. Postpartum Observations: Parenting Problems and Possible Interventions

Concerning observations[a]
  Parent avoids eye contact and *en face* positioning of child
  Negative verbalization to or about child
  Disappointment or negative association with child's sex, name, or appearance
  Parent hopeless, helpless, or annoyed by crying
  Mother not receiving support from other family members

Special well-child care for high-risk neonates
  Promote maternal attachment: point out positive attributes and model pleasurable interaction
  Focus parent education on understanding infant temperament and behavior
  Provide specific information about responses to challenging behaviors and basic nurturing needs
  Use compliments rather than criticism; attend to parents' needs as well as those of child
  Contact with increased frequency after discharge

[a] Adapted from Gray JD et al. Prediction and prevention of child abuse and neglect. Child Abuse Negl 1977;1:45-58.

gal et al., 1980; Lealman et al., 1983), the generally positive results are encouraging for those who practice routine well-child care and family education. Caring and consistent contact, combined with attentiveness to parental emotional needs, may be an effective and widely applicable tool for the prevention of physical abuse and neglect, at least in early childhood (Kempe, 1976).

Prevention of Sexual Abuse

Attempts to prevent sexual abuse have taken several directions. Public awareness campaigns have been designed to facilitate recognition and reporting of abuse and help parents cope with disclosures. Other public programs have used theater and music to teach parenting skills and coping strategies. Dozens of teaching packages and approaches, from school curricula to coloring books, have been developed for children. These programs have several messages (Wolfe et al., 1976):

- Sometimes it's OK to say no, even to those we love and trust.
- If you feel angry, scared, or embarrassed, there might be a good reason why.

- It's not right for people to ask you to keep secrets.
- You can and should tell someone about uncomfortable experiences.
- It's not your fault, and your telling will only help everyone involved.

Studies have not yet been published to demonstrate that these programs are capable of preventing sexual abuse. Children over 5 do seem capable of understanding and repeating the messages they contain (Conte, 1985; Ray-Keil, 1986), although is not certain whether this knowledge leads to modified behavior. What does seem clear is that such programs have an emotional impact. Teachers using prevention curricula must be well trained and generally avoid extemporaneous additions that may generate fear. Teachers must also be prepared for children who, prompted by the program, disclose that they or someone they know has been abused. Such disclosures are frequent, and eliciting them may be one of the most important functions the program serves.

Legal and regulatory steps to prevent sexual abuse have been proposed or enacted in many jurisdictions. Among the most controversial is the requirement for criminal background checks of applicants for jobs in fields involving contact with children. The law may prohibit employment or merely require disclosure if a job applicant has ever been convicted of a crime against a child or a sexual crime of any kind. Similar screening takes place in other situations in which professionals or businesses must be licensed. In states where such laws have been enacted for child care workers, only a small proportion of those screened have been found to have criminal records. It is not known whether this low yield indicates that the procedure successfully discourages sex offenders from applying or whether the fact that many abusers never get convicted means that the background check is not the way to find them. In the long term, the efficacy of such procedures remains to be proven. Other legal measures, including the requirement that parents be notified of their right to visit a daycare setting at any time and without announcement, have been proposed. It has also been suggested that daycare centers be legally required to disclose concerns for or occurrences of sexual abuse in the center to the parents of all children who attend, regardless of whether the children are directly involved.

Parents may also be counseled on the selection of daycare facilities. Facilities should be licensed and staffed by persons with documented experience in child care. The facility should have a written policy that any suspected abuse is to be reported immediately to the authorities and to the parents of the child involved. There should be no restrictions on parental visitation, and parents should make such a visit, unannounced, before enrolling a child. The physical layout of the center should be such that play areas are open and visible. The lesson plan should not include times during which individual work with a child takes place outside of the common areas.

Krugman (1985) argues that one solution to ensuring safety in daycare is for employers and schools to offer it on a more widespread basis. The availability of child care at places of employment would make it less likely that parents would place children with marginally supervised providers and would increase access to children during the work day.

Prevention of Injuries

Injuries resulting from falls, motor vehicle accidents, burns, poisonings, and other presumed accidents cause over half of all deaths among children ages 1–14. The rate at which such deaths occur has increased rapidly over the past two decades. Most of these deaths are preventable; some authors have termed them "culturally condoned child abuse" (Wilson, 1983–85). In some cases, the burden of prevention falls on manufacturers or builders who design inherently dangerous products or dwellings, but in many cases parents have control over hazards in the home that threaten children. Failure to control all but the most serious of these hazards is not currently considered neglectful, but it is clear that taking certain relatively easy steps could prevent many serious childhood injuries. Eliminating some hazards, such as scalding hot tapwater, may also help decrease the morbidity associated with intentional injury.

Health care workers can help parents to recognize hazards and take preventive steps. Educational efforts, however, have not always been the best way to bring about environmental change. Clinicians can use their influence in the community to find other mechanisms (compliance with building codes, voluntary home safety inspections, giveaways of safety equipment) to promote control of injuries. Some of the most commonly encountered hazards and steps that can be taken to mitigate them include:

- Falls—Installation of stair and window guards and elimination of surfaces (such as small rugs) on which children can slip.
- Motor vehicle accidents—Use of seatbelts, safety seats, and helmets.
- Poisoning—Disposal of unused medications; proper storage and labeling of toxins; access to syrup of ipecac; ability to contact poison control centers.
- Burns—Installation of smoke detectors; planning for emergency evacuation of the home; proper installation and use of heating devices; reduction of hot water temperatures to below 130°F, thus reducing the risk of accidental and intentional scalds.
- Firearm injuries—Safe storage where children do not have access. It is estimated that a half of all United States homes have one or more firearms. Nearly 10,000 children are "accidentally" killed or wounded by firearms every year (Rivara and Stapleton, 1982). Adults should be encouraged to seriously evaluate the need to keep firearms in the home.

SUMMARY

For many abusers, the propensity to abuse seems to be rooted in childhood and is manifested by a general lack of self-esteem, satisfaction with life, and ability assume adult roles. Abusers look to children to fulfill emotional needs that should be provided by other adults and that make developmentally inappropriate demands on children.

Many abusers seem unaware of or able to disregard social rules that prohibit violence against or neglect of children. Alcohol may play a major role in this disinhibition. Day-to-day stresses may precipitate episodes of abuse, but other, more chronic factors, including poverty, marital discord, and interpersonal violence in the home, may make an adult more likely to abuse under stress. Social and physical isolation (of both the abuser and the victim) may also increase the risk of abuse.

An essential factor in the perpetuation of abuse is the dependence and trust of children. Children are dependent on adults to define socially correct behavior. They are also emotionally dependent on trusted adults and thus easily coerced into participating in and concealing acts against their will.

Much more remains to be discovered about the prevention of abuse. The idea of screening populations to define high-risk groups does not seem workable, for present knowledge does not allow such groups to be selected with sufficient precision. Some interventions, however, show signs of being both workable and effective and can be considered for use in the clinician's daily activities. These interventions fall into three groups:

- Perinatal and early childhood intervention.
- Establishment of relationships with children that enhance the child's self-esteem, decrease isolation, and facilitate disclosure of abuse.
- Individual and community efforts to reduce environmental hazards that can lead to childhood injuries.

References

Altemeir WA, O'Connor S, Vietze PM, Sandler HM, Sherrod KB. Antecedents of child abuse. J Pediatr 1982:100:823–829.

American Humane Association. Annual statistical report: national analysis of official child abuse reporting. Denver: American Humane Association, 1979.

Araji S, Finkelhor D. Explanations of pedophilia: review of empirical research. Bull Am Acad Psychiatry Law 1985;13:17–37.

Belsky J. Child maltreatment: an ecological integration. Am Psychol 1980;35:320–335.

Conte JR. An evaluation of a program to prevent the sexual victimization of young children. Child Abuse Negl 1985;9:319–28.

Egeland B. Fathers and child abuse [Book review]. Contemp Psychol 1988;33:302–303.

Egeland B, Jacobovitz D, Sroufe LA. Breaking the cycle of abuse. Child Dev 1988;59:1080–1088.

Finkelhor D. Child sexual abuse. New York: The Free Press, 1984.

Gebhard PH, Gagnon JH, Pomeroy WB, et al. Sex offenders. New York: Bantam Books, 1967.

Gray JD, Cutler CA, Dean JG, Kempe CH. Prediction

and prevention of child abuse and neglect. Child Abuse Negl 1977;1:45–58.

Herrenkohl EC, Herrenkohl RC. A comparison of abused children and their non-abused siblings. J Am Acad Child Psychiatry 1979;18:260–269.

Hunter R, Kilstrom N. Breaking the cycle in abusive families. Am J Psychiatry 1979;136:1320–1322.

Justice B, Justice R. The abusing family. New York: Human Sciences Press, 1976.

Kaufman J, Ziegler E. Do abused children become abusive parents? Am J Orthopsychiatry 1987;57:186–192.

Kempe CH. Approaches to preventing child abuse: the health visitors concept. Am J Dis Child 1976;130:941–947.

Krugman RD. Preventing sexual abuse of children in day care: whose problem is it anyway? Pediatrics 1985;75:1150–1151.

Lealman GT, Haigh D, Phillips JM, Stone J, Ord-Smith C. Prediction and prevention of child abuse—an empty hope? Lancet 1983;i:1423–1424.

Leventhal JM. Risk factors for child abuse: methodologic standards in case-control studies. Pediatrics 1981;68:684–690.

Lynch M. Risk factors in the child: a study of abused children and their siblings. In: Martin HP, ed. The abused child: a multidisciplinary approach to developmental issues and treatment. Cambridge: Ballinger Publishing Co, 1976:43–56.

Martin J. Gender-related behaviors of children in abusive situations. Saratoga, California: R&E Publishers, 1983.

Oates K. Child abuse and neglect: what happens eventually? Sydney: Butterworths, 1985.

O'Connor S, Vietze PM, Sherrod KB, Sandler HM, Altemeir WA. Reduced incidence of parenting inadequacy following rooming- in. Pediatrics 1980;66:176–182.

Olds DL, Henderson CR, Chamberlin R, Tatelbaum R. Preventing child abuse and neglect: a randomized trial of nurse home visitation. Pediatrics 1986;78:65–78.

Ray-Kiel A. Summary of evaluations of Committee for Children materials and training. Seattle: Committee for Children, 1986.

Rivara FP, Stapleton FB. Handguns and children: a dangerous mix. J Dev Behav Pediatr 1982;3:35–38.

Russell DEH. The prevalence and seriousness of incestuous abuse: stepfathers vs. biological fathers. Child Abuse Negl 1984;8:15–22.

Rutter M. Psychological resilience and protective mechanisms. Am J Orthopsychiatry 1987;57:316–331.

Siegal E, Bauman KE, Schaefer ES, Saunders MM, Ingram DD. Hospital and home support during infancy: impact on maternal attachment, child abuse and neglect, and health care utilization. Pediatrics 1980;66:183–190.

Sgroi SM. Handbook of clinical intervention in child sexual abuse. Lexington, Massachusetts: Lexington Books, 1982.

Steele B. Psychodynamic factors in child abuse. In: Kempe CH, Helfer RE, eds. The battered child. 3rd ed. Chicago: University of Chicago Press, 1980:49–85.

Straus MA. Stress in child abuse. In: Kempe CH, Helfer RE, eds. The battered child. 3rd ed. Chicago: University of Chicago Press, 1980:86–103.

Surgeon General's Workshop on Violence and Public Health. Report. Leesburg, Virginia: Office of the Surgeon General, October 1985.

US Department of Health and Human Services. Executive summary: national study of the incidence and severity of child abuse and neglect. DHHS Publ. (OHDS) 81–30329. Washington, DC: US Government Printing Office, 1981.

Waller DA. Obstacles to the treatment of Munchausen by proxy syndrome. J Am Acad Child Adolesc Psychiatry 1983;22:80–85.

Wilson MH. Childhood injury control. Pediatrician 1983–85;12:20–27.

Wolfe DA, MacPherson T, Blount R, Wolfe VV. Evaluation of a brief intervention for educating school children in awareness of physical and sexual abuse. Child Abuse Negl 1986;10:85–92.

Index

Page numbers in *italics* denote figures; those followed by "t" denote tables.

Abandonment, 7
Abdominal injuries, 75–76
Abusers
  adolescent, 198–199
  as adults, 226–227
  childhood of, 225–226
  children as, 195–200
  treatment for
    physical abusers, 222–223
    sexual abusers, 223
Accommodation syndrome, 18–19
Acid phosphatase, in semen, 116–117
Acquired immunodeficiency syndrome, 112–113
  discrimination against children with, 127
Adjustment disorders, 18
Adolescent
  interview of, 36
  psychological impact of abuse on, 17
  sexual abuse by, 198–199
Aggressiveness, 7, 16
Alcohol abuse during pregnancy, 186, 188t
  medical indicators of, 189
  screening for, 189
American Humane Association, 3
Anal canal, 88
Anal sphincter, 89
Anal wink, 89
Anxiety, 15
Anxiety disorders, 18
Apathy-futility syndrome, 122
Arthritis, septic, 98
Assessment
  of cognitive abilities, 37
  of development, 143
  of diet, 144–145, 145t
  of family, 40
  of feeding, 145–146
  of nutrition, 143, 143t
  of temperament, 146, 146t
  vs. investigation, 23
Attachment, 13, 137–138
Attention-deficit hyperactivity disorder, 18
Autopsy, 178–179

Baby Doe regulations, 128–130
Bartholin's glands, 81
Battered child syndrome, 5
  testimony about, 216
Battle's sign, 68

Behavior. *See also* Temperament
  aggressive, 7, 16
  in children with failure to thrive, 146–147, 154
  in children with psychosocial dwarfism, 155
  in clinical setting, 29
  history taking about, 52
  maladaptive, 7
  parent questionnaires about, 52
Birth injuries, 98, 100
Bites, 54–57, *59–60*
  common locations of, 57
  forensic dentist's examination of, 57
  human vs. animal, 56
  photographing of, 57
  serial observations of, 57
  shape of, 55–56
  situations in which encountered, 56
  swabbing for saliva in, 57
Bonding, 137–138
Bone scans, 92–93
Bony injuries. *See* Fractures; Skeletal trauma
Bowel injury, 75
Brainwashing, 26–28
Breast-feeding assessment, 144–145
Bruises, 54–57, *56–58*
  color of, 55
  differential diagnosis of, 60–61
  patterns of, 54
  perirectal, 88
  photographs of, 55
  serial observations of, 55
  shape of, 55
"Bucket handles," 94
Burns, 61–65, *62, 64–65*
  characteristics suggesting abuse, 63, 65
  degree and extent of, 61–62
  hot solid objects causing, 63
  immersion patterns of, 63, *64–65*
  from microwave ovens, 65
  pain sensation and, 62
  prevention of, 230–231
  spill/splash patterns of, 63
  time and temperatures required for, 62, *62*

CAGE questionnaire, 189
Cardiopulmonary resuscitation
  retinal hemorrhage and, 70–71
  rib fractures and, 95

233

Caretakers, 2
Chain of evidence, 118
Chancres, 111
Child abuse. *See also* Emotional abuse;
    Neglect; Physical abuse; Sexual abuse
  adults who were victims of, 21–22
  causes of, 225–227
    abusers as adults, 226–227
    abuser's childhood, 225–226
    family stresses and supports, 226
    social forces, 227
    socioeconomic and minority status, 226
  children at risk for, 227–229
  cycle of, 22, 225–226
  definition of, 1
  duration of, 13–14
  evaluation of, 49–65
    interviewing child, 23–29
    medical history, 49–52
    physical examination, 52–65
  factors determining
    definition of caretaker, 2
    degree of harm, 2
    foreseeable vs. unfortunate harm, 2–3
    nature of act, 1–2
  fatal, 172–183. *See also* Fatal abuse
  by other children, 195–199
  physical effects of, 12
  prenatal/perinatal, 185–193
  prevalence of, 3–4
  prevention of, 229–231
  psychiatric diagnoses after, 17–19
    accommodation syndrome, 18–19
    post-traumatic disorders, 18
    separation problems, 19
  psychological impact of, 12–14
  reporting of, 3, 201–208
  responses to, 14–17
    aggressiveness, 15, 16
    anxiety, 15
    depression, 15
    developmental delays, 14
    empirical data on, 16–17
  responses to disclosure of, 19–20
    ambivalence and recanting, 19
    timing of disclosure and, 19–20
  responses to investigation of, 20–21
  terminology of, 1
  treatment of, 218–223. *See also* Treatment
  types of
    by age, 4–5, 5t
    by race, 5
    by sex, 5

Child Abuse Prevention and Treatment Act of 1974, 1–2
Child protective service agencies, 219–221
Chlamydia trachomatis, 102–105
  birth transmission of, 104
  cultures of, 104
  growth of, 102
  manifestations in adults, 102
  and sexual activity in children, 103–104
  tests for, 104–105
Christian Scientists, 130–132
Cigarette smoking during pregnancy, 186, 188t
Clavicular fractures, 98, 100
Coaching vs. truth, 26–28
Coagulation studies, 61
Cocaine abuse during pregnancy, 186–187, 188t
Condyloma acuminatum, 108–111. *See also* Human papillomavirus
Condyloma lata, 110
Confidentiality, 205–208
  general legal interpretations of, 205–206
  of offender treatment, 206
  sharing medical records and, 206–208
Conflict Tactics Scale, 6
Corporal punishment, 1–2, 6, 163–165
  acceptance of, 163–164
  alternatives to, 165
  basis of, 163
  consequences of, 164–165
  definition of, 163
  determining abusiveness of, 165
  rationale for, 164
  in schools, 164
  trends in, 164
Court testimony. *See* Physician expert testimony
"Crack" use during pregnancy, 186–187
Crisis
  characteristics of people in, 47
  intervention
    for physical abuse, 221
    for sexual abuse, 223
Critically injured child
  decision making for, 177–178
  physical examination of, 176–177
Custody, fake allegations of abuse in disputes over, 26–27

Deadly weapon injuries, 57–59
Death. *See* Fatal abuse
Depression, 15
  in adolescents, 17

infanticide and, 175
postpartum, 175
Deprivation, 7
Development
assessment of, 143
delay in, 14
emotional, 158–160
intellectual, 17, 154
stages of, 138–139
Diet
assessment of, 144–145, 145t
recommended daily intake, 145t
Differential diagnosis, 59–61
Disclosure
child's responses to, 19
timing of, 19–20
Drug abuse during pregnancy, 186, 188t
detection of, 189
medical indicators of, 189
Duodenal hematoma, 75

Education for All Handicapped Children Act, 126
Educational neglect, 7, 126–128
discrimination against ill children, 127
reasons for school nonattendance, 127–128
school phobia, 128
by schools, 126–127
types of, 126
underreporting of, 126
Emotional abuse, 10, 158–162
consequences of, 161–162
definitions of, 10, 160
diagnosis of, 160–161
incidence of, 10
proving in court, 162
reluctant recognition of, 158
treatment of, 162
Emotional development
forces affecting, 159–160
goals of, 158–159
Emotional neglect, 7–8
Endocrine disorders, 139–140
Epididymis, 87
Epidural hemorrhage, 74
Erythema multiforme, 60–61
Eye injuries, 68–72
from blunt trauma, 69
mechanism of, 69
retinal hemorrhage, 69, 70t, 71

Facial injuries, 68
Failure to thrive, 133–155

behaviors of child with, 146–147
child's temperament and, 134–135, 146, 146t
definition of, 133
diagnosis of
developmental assessment, 143
dietary assessment, 144–145, 145t
feeding assessment, 145–146
by growth parameters, 140–141
lab tests, 143–144
medical/social history taking, 141–142
nutritional assessment, 143, 143t
physical exam, 142–143
etiologies of, 133–140
early mother-child interactions, 137–138
endocrine disorders, 139–140
feeding interaction, 138–139
identifiable illnesses, 133–134, 134t
mechanical and developmental feeding problems, 135, 136t
parental factors, 135–137, 136t
temperament, 134–135
incidence of, 133
long-term effects of, 152–155, 153t
intellectual development, 154
personality and behavior, 154
physical abuse, 154–155
weight and height, 153–154
organic vs. nonorganic, 133
as reportable maltreatment, 152
response to refeeding in, 133
treatment of, 147–152
hospital discharge, 151–152
inpatient vs. outpatient, 147–148
nutritional, 148–150
ongoing therapy, 152
parental, 150–151
social/emotional, 150
Family
assessment of, 43–46
asking for problem statement, 43
asking questions, 44–45
clinicians' maladaptive responses during, 45–46
dysfunctional communication patterns, 43–44, 44t
observing communication process, 43
pros and cons of, 40
setting stage for, 43
behavioral influences of, 40
boundaries within, 41–42
characteristics of people in crisis, 47
children as bearers of symptoms of, 42

Family—*Continued*
    cycles of dysfunctional behavior in, 42–43
    data in medical history about, 51–52
    genogram for, 45
    stresses and supports in, 226
    structure of, 40–41
    subsystems of, 41
    talking to parents suspected of abuse, 46–47
    in which emotional abuse occurs, 161
    in which fatal abuse occurs, 174
    in which neglect occurs, 48
    in which physical abuse occurs, 47
    in which sexual abuse occurs, 47–48
Fantasy
    expression of, 29
    vs. reality, 24–25
Fatal abuse, 12, 172–183
    autopsy for, 178–179
    clinicians' reaction to, 172
    decision making for critically injured child, 177–178
    epidemiology of, 172–173, 172t–174t
    of infants, 173–175
        causes of, 174–175
        characteristics of, 173–174
    leading causes of death, 172t
    of older children, 175–176
    physical exam of critically injured child, 176–177
    postpartum mental illness and, 175
    prevention of, 182–183
    risk factors for, 182–183
    vs. sudden infant death syndrome, 179–182
Feeding
    assessment of, 145–146
    calculation of caloric needs, 145t, 148
    child behaviors and, 135, 136t
    developmental stages of, 138–139
    interactive process of, 138
    parental behaviors and, 135–137, 136t
    problems with, 135, 149
    starting of, 148
    what to feed, 148–149
Fetal abuse. *See* Pregnancy; Prenatal/perinatal abuse
Fetal alcohol syndrome, 186, 192
"Fisting," 87
Folk medicine practices
    intracranial bleeding due to, 73
    skin lesions due to, 56–57, 61
Foreign bodies, rectal, 87
Forensic procedures, 114–118
    chain of evidence, 118
    clothing, 115
    detection of semen, 115–117
        biochemical markers, 116–117
        skin examination, 115–116
        sperm, 116
    genetic fingerprinting techniques, 117–118
    photographic records
        camera, 118
        photographs, 118
    search for hair, 117
Foster care, 220–222
Fractures. *See also* Skeletal trauma
    at birth, 98, 100
    clavicular, 98, 100
    dating of, 93
    elbow, 97
    epiphyseal, 94
    metaphyseal, 94, *96–98*
    multiple, 96
    penile, 86
    rib, 94–95, *99*
    skull, 67, 72
        at birth, 100
        complex, 95–96, *99*
    spiral or oblique, 97
    tibial, 97
Frenulum, 80

Gardnerella vaginalis, 102
Genetic fingerprinting, 117–118
Genitalia
    female, 79–85, *86*
        anatomy of, 80–84, *81*, 83t
        congenital anomalies of, 80–81
        development of, 79–80
        examination of, 84–85
    male, 85–87
        anatomy of, 85–86
        examination of, 86–87
Genograms, 45
Gonorrhea, 103–107
    anal, 106
    diagnosis of, 106–107
    guarding against misidentification of, 107
    ophthalmologic disease due to, 105
    oropharyngeal, 106
    transmission of, 105–106
    urethritis due to, 106
    vaginal and cervical, 106
Group therapy
    for abused child, 221
    for abusive parents, 222

for sexual offenders, 223
for sexually abused child, 223
Growth
  emotional, 158–160
  failure of. *See* Failure to thrive; Psychosocial dwarfism
  measurement of, 140–141
  of premature or small-for-gestational-age infants, 141
Guilt, 23–24
Gunshot wounds, 57–59
  prevention of, 230–231

Hair loss, 67
Hazards, inattention to, 7, 230
Head injuries, 67–75
  eye injuries, 68–72
  facial injuries, 68
  inspection for, 67–68
  intracranial injuries, 72–74
  layers of head, 67t
  shaken baby syndrome, 74–75
  skull fractures, 67, 72
Health care
  history taking about, 52
  inattention to, 7
Hearsay rules, 50–51, 216–217
Hematoma
  duodenal, 75
  subdural, 72–74
Hemophilia, 61
Hemorrhage
  abdominal, 75–76
  epidural, 74
  ocular, 69–72, 70t, *71*
Hemorrhoids, 88
Henoch-Schönlein purpura, 60
Hepatic injury, 75
Hepatitis B, 113–114
Herpes simplex virus, 111–112
  diagnosis of, 112
  serotypes of, 111
  symptoms of, 111–112
  transmission of, 112
Homicide. *See* Fatal abuse
Human figure drawings, 29
Human immunodeficiency virus, 112–113
  adult seropositivity rates, 112–113
  perinatal exposure to, 113
  testing suspected abuse victims for, 112, 113
  transmission of, 113
Human papillomavirus, 108–111
  contact tracing for, 110

genital warts caused by, 110
genotypes of, 109
latent infection with, 109–110
nonsexual transmission of, 110
sexual transmission of, 109
Hymen, 82–84
  classification of, 82
  cleft or tear of, 84
  imperforate, 82
  inspection of, 82
  size of opening in, 82–84, 83t

Infant
  attachment patterns of, 13, 137–138
  failure to thrive of. *See* Failure to thrive
  fatal abuse of, 173–175
    causes of, 174–175
    characteristics of, 173–174
  fears of, 34
  interview of, 34
  premature or small-for-gestational-age, 141
  psychological impact of abuse on, 13
Infantile cortical hyperostosis, 98
Injury pattern studies, 95t
Injury prevention, 230–231
Intellectual development, 17
  in children with failure to thrive, 154
Interviewing children, 23–39
  approach to, 33–36
    adolescents, 36
    infants and toddlers, 34
    preschool children, 34–35
    school age children, 35–36
  behavior in clinical setting, 29
  characteristics of sexual abuse, 28–29
  child's memory and, 27–28
  dealing with anxious elaboration, 25–26
  dealing with guilt/shame, 23–24
  determining fantasy vs. reality/truth vs. lies, 24–25
  developmental considerations in, 34
  differentiating truth vs. coaching, 26–27
  documenting findings of, 39
  effects of bad technique in, 29
  initial interview, 31
  investigation vs. assessment, 23
  logistics of, 31–33
    accompanying persons, 32
    equipment, 32–33
    number of interviews, 31–32
    recording interview, 33
    setting, 32
    who conducts interview, 31–32

Interviewing children—*Continued*
  progressive confrontation method, 24
  steps in, 36–39
    asking questions, 38
    assessing child's abilities, 37
    establishing common vocabulary, 37–38
    first contact with child, 37
    greeting/introduction, 36–37
    questions about abuse, 38
    wrap-up, 38–39
  types of interviews, 31
  use of tests for, 29
Intracranial injuries, 72–74
Investigation process, 20–21
  vs. diagnostic assessment, 23

Jehovah's Witnesses, 130–131

Knife wounds, 57–59
Kwashiorkor, 142–143

Labia
  adhesions of, 80–81
  majora, 80
  minora, 80
Lead exposure, 144
Legal issues. *See also* Forensic procedures
  affecting critically injured child, 177–178
  Baby Doe regulations, 128–130
  documenting examination findings, 49
  hearsay rules, 50–51, 216–217
    admissibility of excited utterances, 50
    statements made to physician, 50
  investigation process, 20–21
  physician expert testimony, 209–217. *See also* Physician expert testimony
  proving emotional abuse, 162
  regarding suspected prenatal abuse, 190–193
  religious exemptions from medical neglect statutes, 130
  reporting suspected abuse, 201–208. *See also* Reporting of abuse
  school discrimination against ill children, 127
  state definitions of child abuse, 1
  treatment refusal
    on nonreligious grounds, 130
    on religious grounds, 130–132
Leukemia, 98

Maladaptive behavior, 7
Malnutrition. *See also* Failure to thrive
  assessment of, 143, 143t
  lab tests for, 143–144
Marasmus, 142
Medical history, 49–52
  in failure to thrive, 141–142
  goals of, 49
  hearsay rules, 50–51
  misleading, 49
  obtaining, 51
  review of systems, 52
  of sexual abuse, 77
  social history, 51–52, 141–142
Medical neglect
  Baby Doe regulations affecting, 128–130
  religious exemptions from statutes of, 130
  of sick and preventive care, 122–123
Medical records
  confidentiality issues and, 206–208
  of interview with child, 33
  legal admissibility of, 210, 216
  photographs, 55, 57, 118, 216
Memory, child's, 27–28
Meningococcal skin lesions, 60
Menkes's kinky hair syndrome, 98
Metaphyseal injuries, 94, *96–98*
Michigan Alcoholism Screening Test, 189
Minnesota Mother-Child Project, 16–17
Molluscum contagiosum, 114
Mongolian spots, 60
Mons pubis, 80
Munchausen syndrome by proxy, 167–170
  characteristics of, 167–169
  clinical presentations of, 167
  definition of, 167
  detection of, 169–170
    difficulty in, 169
    by hospital surveillance, 169–170
    warning signs for, 169
  father's role in, 168–169
  mother's role in, 167–168
  substances/maneuvers used in, 168t
  treatment of, 170
Murder. *See* Fatal abuse

National Committee for the Prevention of Child Abuse, 10
National Family Violence Survey, 6, 226
National Study of the Incidence and Severity of Child Abuse and Neglect
  determination of degree of harm constituting abuse, 2

prevalence data of, 3
by age, 4–5
  emotional maltreatment, 10
  neglect, 6–8
  physical abuse, 5–6
  by race, 5, 226
  sexual abuse, 8–9
  by socioeconomic status, 226
Neglect, 6–8, 121–132. *See also* Educational neglect; Emotional neglect; Medical neglect
  categories of, 7–8
  clinician's urge to rescue child from, 124
  diagnosis of, 124–125
  encouraging family caretaking, 125
  families in which it occurs, 48
  of ill/handicapped newborns, 128–130
  incidence of, 6–7
  legal interpretations of, 130–132
    religious exemptions from medical neglect statutes, 130
    treatment refusal on nonreligious grounds, 130
    treatment refusal on religious grounds, 130–132
  medical observations of, 122–124
    growth patterns, 122
    hazardous materials, 123
    injuries, 123
    lack of basic necessities, 123
    lack of preventive care, 123
    supervision, 123–124
    treatment delays, 122–123
  other maltreatment and, 8
  parental factors in, 121–122
    apathy-futility syndrome, 122
    economic forces, 121
    neuroses vs. character disorders, 121–122
    parents' personality, 121
    socioecological forces, 121
  prevention of, 229
  professional services for, 125
  social service involvement in cases of
    criteria for, 125–126
    threatening of, 124–125
  treatment resources for, 223
  underreporting of, 7
Neisseria gonorrhoeae, 105–107. *See also* Gonorrhea
Neuroblastoma, 98
New York Longitudinal Study, 134
"Nursemaid's elbow," 97
Nutrition. *See also* Feeding
  assessment of, 143, 143t

calculation of caloric needs, 145t, 148
therapy for
  feeding problems, 149
  observing weight gain, 149–150
  starting feeds, 148
  what to feed, 148–149

Oedipal dynamics, 34–35
Oppositional defiant disorder, 18
Osteogenesis imperfecta, 98
Osteomyelitis, 98
Osteoporosis, 97

Pediatric Symptom Checklist, 52
Penis, 85
  fracture of, 86
  tourniquet syndrome, 85
Peritonitis, 75
Photographs
  of bites, 57
  of bruises, 55
  legal admissibility of, 216
  obtaining of, 118
Physical abuse, 5–6
  corporal punishment, 163–165
  definition of, 5
  extent of injuries, 12
  families in which it occurs, 47
  following failure to thrive, 154–155
  historical recognition of, 5
  incidence of, 5–6, 6t
  other maltreatment and, 6
  prevention of, 229, 229t
  subtypes of, 6
  treatment resources for children, 221–222
    crisis intervention, 221
    foster care, 221–222
    group therapy, 221
    medical treatment, 221
    play therapy, 221
    role models/individual support, 221
  treatment resources for parents, 222–223
    group therapy, 222
    individual therapy, 222
    supportive services, 222–223
Physical examination, 52–65
  of bruises and bites, 54–57, *56–60*
  of burns, 61–65, *62, 64–65*
  child's general appearance, 53–54
  of critically injured child, 176–177
  differential diagnosis and, 59–61
  documenting findings of, 53
  extent of, 53

Physical examination—*Continued*
  of failure to thrive, 142–143
  of head, 67t, 67–68
  of injuries from deadly weapons, 57–59
  of sexual abuse, 77–79, 84–85
Physician expert testimony, 209–217
  in courtroom, 211–214
    concept of "reasonable degree of medical certainty," 213–214
    on cross-examination, 212–213
    on direct examination, 211–212
  preparation for court, 209–211
    contact with lawyer, 210
    records, 210
    rehearsal, 210
    relationships with opposing parties, 210–211
    subpoenas, 209–210
  purpose of, 214–215
  sources on which opinion is based, 215–217
    battered child syndrome testimony, 216
    Frye test, 215
    hearsay, 216–217
    medical records, 216
    photographs, 216
    rebuttal or support of exculpatory statements, 216
PL 93-247, 1–2
PL 94-142, 126–127
Placement, decisions immediately after abuse, 220–221
Play therapy, 221
Post-traumatic stress, 18
Posterior fourchette, 80
Postpartum mental illness, 175
Pregnancy
  determining feelings about, 187–189
  elective abortion of, 185
  spousal abuse during, 185
  substance abuse during, 186–187, 188t
    detoxifiction risks, 190
    medical indicators of, 189
    screening for, 189
    treatment goals for, 190
  treatment for high-risk mothers, 190
Prenatal/perinatal abuse, 185–193. *See also* Pregnancy
  interventions for, 187–189
  legal issues affecting, 190–193
  by men, 185
  treatment of, 192–193
Preschool child
  fears of, 35
  interview of, 34–35
  psychological impact of abuse on, 14

Proctitis, 88
Projective tests, 29
Prostitution, 9–10
Protein-energy malnutrition, 142, 143t
Psychiatric diagnoses, 17–19
  accommodation syndrome, 18–19
  post-traumatic disorders, 18
  separation problems, 19
Psychological impact of abuse, 12–14
  in adolescence, 17
  in elementary age children, 14
  factors affecting, 12
    duration of abuse, 12–13
    nature of abuse, 13
    psychological meaningfulness of perpetrator, 13
  in infancy, 13
  in preschool children, 14
  in toddlerhood, 13–14
Psychosocial dwarfism, 155–156
  behaviors of, 155
  definition of, 155
  diagnosis of, 156
  etiology of, 155
  treatment of, 156
Pubertal development
  in boys, 85, 87t
  in girls, 78t, 79–80
  precocious, 80
  sexual activity and, 197
Purtscher's retinopathy, 69–70

Radiological examination, 92–93
Rectal cultures, 114
Rectal injuries, 87–90
Reporting of abuse, 201–208
  confidentiality and, 205–208
    general legal interpretations, 205–206
    offender treatment, 206
    sharing medical records, 206–208
  immediate vs. delayed, 203
  informing parents before, 203
  liability and
    immunity for reporting, 205
    for not reporting, 204–205
  requirements for, 201–204
    when to report, 202–204
    who must report, 201–202
    who receives reports, 204
  underreporting, 3
Retinal hemorrhage, 69–72, 70t, *71*
  CPR and, 70–71
  mechanisms of, 71
  in newborn, 71
  ophthalmologic exam of, 71–72

Index

Retroperitoneal injuries, 75–76
Rib fractures, 94–95, *99*
Rickets, 97, 144
Roe vs. Wade, 190
Role reversals, 42
Rorschach test, 29
Runaway children, 9

Scapegoating, 42
School age child
  fears of, 35
  interview of, 35–36
  psychological impact of abuse on, 14
School phobia, 128
Schools
  corporal punishment in, 164
  discrimination against AIDS children by, 127
  educational neglect by, 126–127
  reasons for nonattendance at, 127–128
Scrotum, 85
Scurvy, 97
Semen detection, 115–117
  with biochemical markers, 116–117
  by recovery of sperm, 116
  by skin examination, 115–116
Separation problems, 19
Septic arthritis, 98
Sexual abuse, 8–10
  age of victims of, 8–9
  characteristics of history of, 28–29
  child prostitution, 9–10
  by children, 196–199
  children at risk for, 228
  crisis intervention for, 223
  definitions of, 8–9
  families in which it occurs, 47–48
  forensic procedures for, 114–118. *See also* Forensic procedures
  incidence of, 8
  individual/group therapy for, 223
  physical examination of, 77–79
    in boys, 86–87
    child/parent preparation for, 78
    child's reactions to, 78–79
    communication with child about, 79
    documentation of, 79
    in girls, 84–85
    interview before, 78
    perirectal exam, 90
    refusal of, 79
    timing of, 77–78
  prevention of, 229–230
  race and, 9

  rectal injuries, 87–90
  responses to, 15–16
  sex of victims of, 9
  socio-economic status and, 9
  treatment for offenders, 223
Sexually transmitted diseases, 101–115. *See also* specific disorders
  Chlamydia trachomatis, 102–105
  condyloma acuminatum, 108–111
  detection of, 114–115
    cultures, 114–115
    cytopathology, 115
    evaluation of skin or mucosal lesions, 115
    stained specimens, 115
    urinalysis, 115
    wet preps, 115
  genital organisms of prepubertal girls, 103t
  gonorrhea, 103–107
  hepatitis B, 113–114
  herpes, 111–112
  human immunodeficiency virus, 112–113
  molluscum contagiosum, 114
  syphilis, 111
  Trichomonas vaginalis, 107–108
  vulvitis and vaginitis, 101–102
Shaken baby syndrome, 74–75
  diagnosis of, 75
  mechanism of injury in, 74
  ophthalmologic exam in, 75
  symptoms of, 74–75
Shame, 23–24
Sibling abuse, 195–196
Skeletal trauma, 92–100. *See also* Fractures
  bone growth and injury in early childhood, 93–94
  differential diagnosis of, 97–100
  lesions seen in intentional and unintentional injuries, 96–97
  lesions suggestive of abuse, 94–96
    complex skull fractures, 95–96, *99*
    metaphyseal injuries, 94, *96–98*
    multiple fractures/multiple stages of healing, 96
    rib fractures, 94–95, *99*
  skeletal survey, 92–93
  stages of bone healing, 93–94
Skene's glands, 81
Skull fractures
  at birth, 100
  complex, 95–96, *99*
  detection of, 72
  palpation of, 67
Smegma, 85
Smoking during pregnancy, 186, 188t
Social history, 51–52, 141–142

Splenic injury, 75
Stomach injury, 75
Subdural hematoma, 72–74
Subpoenas, 209–210
Substance abuse during pregnancy, 186–187
　detection of, 189
　detoxification risks, 190
　maternal withdrawal syndrome, 193t
　medical indicators of, 189
　neonatal withdrawal syndrome, 192t
Sudden infant death syndrome, 179–182
　"apparent life-threatening events," 180–181
　definition of, 179
　diagnosis of, 179–180
　incidence of, 179–180
　risk factors for, 180
　in siblings, 180
　vs. accidental death, 181–182
Suicide potential, 17
Supervision, 7, 123–124
Syphilis, 111
　congenital, 98

Temperament, 134–135
　activity aspects of, 134
　assessment of, 146, 146t
　definition of, 134
　emotional aspects of, 134
　failure to thrive and, 135
　New York Longitudinal Study of, 134
　sociability aspects of, 135
Terson's syndrome, 69
Testes, 85
Testimony in court. *See* Physician expert testimony
Thematic Apperception Test, 29
Thrombocytopenia
　platelet count in, 61
　skin lesions of, 60

Toddler
　fears of, 34
　interview of, 34
　psychological impact of abuse on, 13–14
Treatment, 218–223
　for child neglect, 223
　immediate considerations in, 218–221
　　child protection agencies, 219–221
　　safe placement of victim, 218–219
　for physical abuse, 221–223
　　for child, 221–222
　　for parents, 222–223
　refusal of
　　on nonreligious grounds, 130
　　on religious grounds, 130–132
　for sexual abuse, 223
Triangle relationships, 42
Trichomonas vaginalis, 107–108
　diagnosis of, 108
　guidelines for detecting in children, 108
　transmission of, 108
Truth
　vs. coaching, 26–28
　vs. lies, 24–25

Urethral cultures, 114
Urinalysis, 115

Vagina, 81–82
Vaginal cultures, 114
Vaginitis, 101–102
Venereal warts, 108–111
Verbal abuse, 10
Vulnerable child syndrome, 176
Vulvitis, 101–102

Wet preps, 108, 115

X-rays, 92–93